Imaging of Thoracic Diseases

THORACIC
SURGERY CLINICS

www.thoracic.theclinics.com

Consulting Editor
MARK K. FERGUSON, MD

February 2010 • Volume 20 • Number 1

SAUNDERS an imprint of ELSEVIER, Inc.

W.B. SAUNDERS COMPANY
A Division of Elsevier Inc.

1600 John F. Kennedy Boulevard ● Suite 1800 ● Philadelphia, Pennsylvania 19103-2899

http://www.theclinics.com

THORACIC SURGERY CLINICS Volume 20, Number 1
February 2010 ISSN 1547-4127, ISBN-13: 978-1-4377-2268-0

Editor: Catherine Bewick

Thoracic Surgery Clinics (ISSN 1547-4127) is published quarterly by Elsevier Inc., 360 Park Avenue South, New York, NY 10010-1710. Months of publication are February, May, August, and November. Business and editorial offices: 1600 John F. Kennedy Boulevard, Suite 1800, Philadelphia, PA 19103-2899. Periodicals postage paid at New York, NY, and additional mailing offices. Subscription prices are $269.00 per year (US individuals), $367.00 per year (US institutions), $134.00 per year (US students), $343.00 per year (Canadian individuals), $464.00 per year (Canadian institutions), $183.00 per year (Canadian and foreign students), $365.00 per year (foreign individuals), and $464.00 per year (foreign institutions). Foreign air speed delivery is included in all *Clinics'* subscription prices. All prices are subject to change without notice. **POSTMASTER:** Send address changes to *Thoracic Surgery Clinics*, Elsevier Health Sciences Division, Subscription Customer Service, 3251 Riverport Lane, Maryland Heights, MO 63043. **Customer Service (orders, claims, online, change of address): Telephone: 1-800-654-2452 (U.S. and Canada); 314-447-8871 (outside U.S. and Canada). Fax: 314-447-8029. Email: journalscustomerservice-usa@elsevier.com (for print support); journalsonlinesupport-usa@elsevier.com (for online support).**

Reprints. For copies of 100 or more, of articles in this publication, please contact Commercial Rights Department, Elsevier Inc., 360 Park Avenue South, New York, NY 10010-1710. Tel: (212) 633-3812; Fax: (212) 462-1935; E-mail: reprints@elsevier.com.

Thoracic Surgery Clinics is covered in *MEDLINE/PubMed (Index Medicus)* and *EMBASE/Excerpta Medica.*

Printed and bound in the United Kingdom
Transferred to Digital Print 2011

Contributors

CONSULTING EDITOR

MARK K. FERGUSON, MD
Professor of Surgery, Section of Cardiac
and Thoracic Surgery, The University of
Chicago, Chicago, Illinois

AUTHORS

TSHERING AMDO, MD
Division of Pulmonary and Critical Care
Medicine, New York University-Langone
Medical Center, Tisch Hospital, New York,
New York

GERALD ANTOCH, MD
Department of Diagnostic and Interventional
Radiology, University of Duisburg, Essen,
Germany

F. ARBIB, MD
Consultant, Clinique de Pneumologie, CHU
Grenoble, France

YOUNG A BAE, MD
Clinical Assistant Professor of Radiology
and Attending Radiologist, Department
of Radiology, Center for Imaging Science,
Samsung Medical Center, Sungkyunkwan
University School of Medicine, Seoul;
and Department of Radiology, Hallym
University College of Medicine, Kyungki-do,
Republic of Korea

CATHERINE BEIGELMAN-AUBRY, MD
Professor, College of Medicine, Hôpital
Pitié-Salpêtrière, Assistance Publique-
Hôpitaux de Paris (APHP), Université
Pierre et Marie Curie Service de Radiologie
Polyvalente Diagnostique et Interventionnelle,
Paris, France

THOMAS BEYER, PhD
Department of Nuclear Medicine, University
of Duisburg, Essen, Germany

SANJEEV BHALLA, MD
Associate Professor of Radiology; Chief,
Cardiothoracic Imaging Section, Mallinckrodt
Institute of Radiology, Washington University
School of Medicine, Barnes-Jewish Hospital,
St Louis, Missouri

C. BITHIGOFFER, MD
Université J Fourier, Clinique Universitaire de
Radiologie et Imagerie Médicale, CHU
Grenoble, France

ANDREAS BOCKISCH, MD, PhD
Department of Nuclear Medicine, University
of Duisburg, Essen, Germany

PIERRE-YVES BRILLET, MD, PhD
Assistant Professor, Hôpital Avicenne,
Assistance Publique-Hôpitaux de Paris
(APHP), Service de Radiologie,
Université Paris XII, Bobigny, France

G.R. FERRETTI, MD, PhD
Professor of Radiology, Clinique Universitaire
de Radiologie et Imagerie Médicale, CHU
Grenoble, France; Université J Fourier,
Grenoble, France; and INSERM U 823, Institut
A Bonniot, la Tronche, France

LUTZ S. FREUDENBERG, MD, MA, MBA
Department of Nuclear Medicine, University
of Duisburg, Essen, Germany

MYRNA C.B. GODOY, MD
Department of Radiology, New York
University-Langone Medical Center, Tisch
Hospital, New York, New York

LAWRENCE R. GOODMAN, MD
Professor, Diagnostic Radiology & Pulmonary Medicine, Department of Radiology, Medical College of Wisconsin; Director, Section of Thoracic Imaging, Department of Radiology, Froedtert Memorial Lutheran Hospital, Milwaukee, Wisconsin

PHILIPPE A. GRENIER, MD
Professor of Radiology, Hôpital Pitié-Salpêtrière, Assistance Publique-Hôpitaux de Paris (APHP), Université Pierre et Marie Curie Service de Radiologie Polyvalente Diagnostique et Interventionnelle, Paris, France

HIROTO HATABU, MD, PhD
Clinical Director, MRI Program, Medical Director, Center for Pulmonary Functional Imaging, Department of Radiology, Brigham and Women's Hospital; Associate Professor of Radiology, Harvard Medical School, Boston, Massachusetts

TRAVIS J. HILLEN, MD, MS
Clinical Fellow, Division of Diagnostic Radiology, Section of Musculoskeletal Radiology, Mallinckrodt Institute of Radiology, Washington University School of Medicine, St Louis, Missouri

A. JANKOWSKI, MD
Université J Fourier, Clinique Universitaire de Radiologie et Imagerie Médicale, CHU Grenoble, France

CYLEN JAVIDAN-NEJAD, MD
Assistant Professor, Section of Cardiothoracic Imaging, Mallinckrodt Institute of Radiology, Washington University School of Medicine, St Louis, Missouri

JANE P. KO, MD
Department of Radiology, New York University-Langone Medical Center, New York, New York

JEAN KURIAKOSE, MBBS, MRCP, FRCR
Division of Cardiothoracic Radiology, Department of Radiology, University of Michigan Health System, Ann Arbor, Michigan

S. LANTUEJOUL, MD, PhD
Professor of Pathology, Département d'Anatomie et Cytologie Pathologiques, CHU Grenoble, France; Université J Fourier, Grenoble, France; and INSERM U 823, Institut A Bonniot, la Tronche, France

HWA YEON LEE, MD, PhD
Associate Professor, Department of Diagnostic Radiology, Chung-Ang University College of Medicine, Seoul, Korea

KYUNG SOO LEE, MD
Professor of Radiology and Section Director of Thoracic Radiology, Department of Radiology, Center for Imaging Science, Samsung Medical Center, Sungkyunkwan University School of Medicine, Seoul, Republic of Korea

DAVID P. NAIDICH, MD, FACCP
Department of Radiology, New York University-Langone Medical Center, Tisch Hospital, New York, New York

MIZUKI NISHINO, MD
Staff Radiologist, Department of Radiology, Dana-Farber Cancer Institute, Assistant Professor of Radiology, Harvard Medical School, Boston, Massachusetts

DAVID OST, MD, MPH
Division of Pulmonary and Critical Care Medicine, New York University-Langone Medical Center, Tisch Hospital, New York, New York; and Division of Pulmonary Medicine, MD Anderson Cancer Center, Houston, Texas

SMITA PATEL, MBBS, MRCP, FRCR
Department of Radiology, University of Michigan Health System, Cardiovascular Center, Ann Arbor, Michigan

C.A. RIGHINI, MD, PhD
Assistant Professor of ENT, Université J Fourier, Clinique Universitaire de'ORL, CHU Grenoble, France; and INSERM U 823, Institut A Bonniot, la Tronche, France

SANDRA J. ROSENBAUM, MD
Department of Nuclear Medicine, University of Duisburg, Essen, Germany

BRADLEY S. SABLOFF, MD
Department of Radiology, University
of Texas MD Anderson Cancer Center,
Houston, Texas

MYLENE T. TRUONG, MD
Department of Radiology, University
of Texas MD Anderson Cancer Center,
Houston, Texas

GEORGE R. WASHKO, MD
Division of Pulmonary and Critical Care
Medicine, Brigham and Women's Hospital;
Instructor in Medicine, Harvard Medical
School, Boston, Massachusetts

DANIEL E. WESSELL, MD, PhD
Assistant Professor, Division of Diagnostic
Radiology, Section of Musculoskeletal
Radiology, Mallinckrodt Institute of Radiology,
Washington University School of Medicine,
St Louis, Missouri

CHARLES S. WHITE, MD
Professor, Department of Diagnostic
Radiology, University of Maryland, Baltimore,
Maryland

SEUNG MIN YOO, MD, PhD
Assistant Professor, Department of Diagnostic
Radiology, CHA Medical University Hospital,
Bundang, Korea

Contents

a clinical HRCT scan protocol was developed. It has since been used for evaluation of diffuse lung disease with suspected airway abnormalities. It provides volumetric assessment of the entire thorax at end-inspiration and at end-expiration, and allows for detailed analysis of the airway and parenchyma. It offers a powerful adjunct to inspiratory HRCT in the detection of lung diseases involving the small airways. This article explores its clinical applications for chronic obstructive pulmonary disease, bronchiectasis, and sarcoidosis. It concludes that standardization of image acquisition and post-processing in CT examinations will be necessary for the real application of quantitative data derived from volumetric expiratory HRCT to daily clinical medical practice.

Evolving MDCT technology and high accuracy for pulmonary embolism detection has led to CT pulmonary angiography (CTPA) becoming a first-line imaging test. Rapid and accurate assessment for DVT and PE can be performed with a single test. Concerns remain regarding the radiation exposure incurred with CTPA and CT venography, especially in young patients. There are concerns also regarding radiation exposure in pregnancy and search for the best diagnostic test for PE in pregnancy. The increased detection of subsegmental emboli raises the question as to which emboli are significant and should be treated and which should be left alone. We review the current role of CT in the diagnosis of pulmonary embolism.

This article provides a summary of acute aortic syndrome (AAS), focusing especially on the multidetector CT technique and findings of AAS, as well as recent concepts regarding the subtypes of AAS, consisting of aortic dissection, intramural hematoma, penetrating atherosclerotic ulcer, and unstable aortic aneurysm.

Acute nontraumatic chest pain is a common presenting symptom to the emergency department. Often, it is evaluated by thin-collimation multidetector computed tomography scan (MDCT) using pulmonary embolism, aortic dissection, or coronary artery protocols. The parameters used for these protocols are very similar to those used in protocols for dedicated imaging of the musculoskeletal system. In essence, every MDCT of the chest is also a musculoskeletal examination of the chest. Familiarity with the MDCT-imaging appearance of common musculoskeletal causes of acute nontraumatic chest pain aids in interpretation of the images. This article discusses the MDCT appearance of a number of musculoskeletal causes of chest pain, including those of infectious, rheumatologic, and systemic causes.

In patients who have lymphoma, the presence and distribution of thoracic involvement is important in both tumor staging and treatment. Thoracic involvement in Hodgkin lymphoma (HL) is more common than in non-Hodgkin lymphoma (NHL). In HL, mediastinal lymphadenopathy with contiguous spread is a hallmark, and lung parenchymal involvement at the initial presentation is almost always associated with mediastinal lymphadenopathy. NHL is more heterogeneous and generally presents at a more advanced stage than HL. Most often, mediastinal involvement occurs as a disseminated or recurrent form of extrathoracic lymphoma. Bulky mediastinal disease with compression of adjacent structures can occur, particularly with high-grade subtypes of NHL and isolated lung disease without mediastinal lymphadenopathy can occur in contrast to HL.

Thoracic Surgery Clinics

THE CLINICS ARE NOW AVAILABLE ONLINE!

Access your subscription at:
www.theclinics.com

Foreword

Advanced imaging technology has greatly improved the practice of thoracic surgery in the past 35 years. Those among us who began training before the advent of computed tomography (CT) remember the startling improvements in identification and staging of lung cancer that this modality offered. Among many other benefits, the advances decreased the rate of futile thoracotomy for this disease from more than 20% in the 1970s to the current incidence of only a few percent. This issue of *Thoracic Surgery Clinics*, which provides updates about recent advances in imaging of thoracic diseases, celebrates the 30th anniversary of the awarding of the Nobel Prize for Medicine to Allan M. Cormack and Godfrey N. Hounsfield for the development of CT technology.

Most thoracic surgeons are becoming familiar with the new technologies that have developed in the field of thoracic radiology in the past decade. Positron emission tomography (PET) and PET/CT, which are compared in this issue, are well known for their utility in evaluating lung nodules and in staging thoracic malignancies. Multidetector CT technology, which is not yet universally available, offers advantages over standard CT that are only beginning to be appreciated. Multidetector scanners currently available commercially offer 64-slice systems with gantry rotation times of 0.33 seconds and a spatial resolution of 0.4 mm, far better than the previous standard 16-slice scanners. These advanced features lend themselves well to three-dimensional visualization and promise to provide functional information in the future as well.

The technological advances, as evidenced by the contributions in this issue, have been applied to a wide variety of thoracic conditions. Among the intuitive applications are three-dimensional imaging of the aorta, major airways, and chest wall. Less obvious, but equally interesting, are developments that improve visualization of pulmonary parenchyma. These applications are designed to assist in the evaluation of such conditions as bronchiectasis and pulmonary embolism, and of such parenchymal abnormalities as emphysema.

The advancing technologies and new clinical applications present a host of challenges for the radiologist and clinician. Ordering the specific technique needed to evaluate a given condition requires much better communication between clinician and radiologist than has historically been the case. I hope this issue of *Thoracic Surgery Clinics* will help practicing thoracic surgeons understand how to best frame requests so that the most useful information emerges from an examination. From the radiologist's perspective, the speed with which scans are now completed requires the development of new algorithms for when and how quickly to administer intravenous contrast. The growing interface between three-dimensional imaging and endoscopic techniques creates an opportunity for clinicians and radiologists to collaborate on optimal use of technology for diagnosis and staging of central thoracic conditions.

This issue of *Thoracic Surgery Clinics* is the first of its kind for this publication and represents a nascent opportunity to make use of the considerable talents of individuals outside of the specialty of thoracic surgery. The demands of our specialty mandate that we improve diagnosis, management, and outcomes for our patients, and this can occur most effectively by interfacing with our colleagues in the radiologic sciences. Thus, the majority of the papers in this issue were published almost simultaneously in other *Clinics* series, permitting specialists from many different fields to benefit from the outstanding expertise of the contributing authors.

It is my hope that readers of this issue will develop a new understanding of the science behind advances in thoracic radiology, and perhaps will encourage their colleagues in radiology to develop even better tools for improving the care of thoracic surgery patients. I thank the authors of these articles, who kindly consented to have their work republished. I also thank Catherine Bewick, executive publisher of *Clinics*, for her innovative thinking and steadfast support.

Mark K. Ferguson, MD
Department of Surgery
The University of Chicago Medical Center
5841 S. Maryland Avenue
MC 5035, Chicago, IL 60637, USA

E-mail address:
mferguso@surgery.bsd.uchicago.edu

Thorac Surg Clin 20 (2010) xiii
doi:10.1016/j.thorsurg.2010.01.001
1547-4127/10/$ – see front matter © 2010 Elsevier Inc. All rights reserved.

The Beatles, the Nobel Prize, and CT Scanning of the Chest

Lawrence R. Goodman, MD[a,b],*

KEYWORDS

- Tomography • Radiograph computed • Radiography
- Thorax • Diagnostic imaging • Imaging history

On June 6, 1962, the Beatles (**Fig. 1**A) had their first recording session with Electrical Musical Industries, Ltd (EMI). Their meteoric success changed the history of modern radiology and medicine forever. The money generated by record sales enabled the EMI basic science researchers to thrive in a cash-rich environment,[1–3] including the research of Dr Godfrey Hounsfield, an electrical and computer engineer. He had spent years exploring whether back projection methods of producing an image could use differential X-ray attenuation values.

"YESTERDAY ... SEEMED SO FAR AWAY"

In 1967, the first experimental computer axial tomography (CAT) scan was constructed on an old lathe, using americium as a gamma ray source.[2] The scan of a mouse took 9 days to complete. It required 2.5 hours of main frame computer time to reconstruct, but produced a recognizable image.[4] Four years later, in October of 1971, the first head scan of a living patient was performed using an EMI "Mark I" scanner.[2,4–6] The equipment used a translate-rotate gantry (step and shoot), an 80 × 80 matrix yielding a spatial resolution of 0.5 cm, and required a water bag for stabilization and normalization of the head. Reconstruction took all night but produced a recognizable image of a brain tumor. "My God, it does work!" exclaimed Hounsfield. The first EMI production model required 4 minutes per slice and 7 minutes per reconstruction. The first description of a CAT scan in the radiology literature by Hounsfield and colleagues[4–7] was in the British Journal of Medicine in 1973.

Hounsfield apparently was unaware of prior work. In the 1960s, Dr Allan Cormack of South Africa, and later Tufts' University, a particle physicist, and Dr William Oldendorf, a Colorado neurologist, independently showed that multiple measures of radiograph attenuation around a target enabled one to compute an image of that target.[8,9] Unfortunately, without more powerful computers, there was little practical application of this concept.

Although Cormack (PhD) and Hounsfield (no formal degree) never met, and neither had a medical background or interest in medicine, both received the Nobel Prize in Physics and Medicine, in 1979, for the CAT scan, the "greatest advance in radiologic medicine since the discovery of the X-ray."[2] Cormack was cited for his math analysis that led to the CAT scan and Hounsfield for its practical development (**Figs. 1**B and **2**).[10] As CAT scans became more sophisticated, new areas of investigation opened up in radiology. Many opened up new approaches to surgery, and new understandings of medical conditions emerged.

"WITH A LITTLE HELP FROM (OUR) FRIENDS"

EMI estimated it needed to sell 25 CAT scanners worldwide to make it a commercially viable

This article originally appeared in *Radiologic Clinics of North America*, Volume 48, Issue 1, January 2010.
a Department of Radiology, Medical College of Wisconsin, 9200 West Wisconsin Avenue, Milwaukee, WI 53226-3596, USA
b Section of Thoracic Imaging, Department of Radiology, Froedtert Memorial Lutheran Hospital, 9200 West Wisconsin Avenue, Milwaukee, WI 53226-3596, USA
* Department of Radiology, Medical College of Wisconsin, 9200 West Wisconsin Avenue, Milwaukee, WI 53226-3596.
E-mail address: lgoodman@mcw.edu

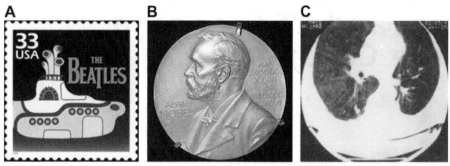

Fig. 1. (*A*) The Beatles. (*B*) The Nobel Prize Medallier. (*C*) Early chest CT scan from 1973. (**Fig. 1**C. *From* Sheedy PF 2nd, Stephens DH, Hattery RR, et al. Computed tomography of the body: initial clinical trial with the EMI prototype. AJR Am J Roentgenol 1976;127:23–51; with permission.)

product. Others were more optimistic. Over the next few years, 18 companies, large and small, competed for the growing scanner market. Over the first decade, many companies disappeared, leaving several major manufacturers as survivors.[9]

Gradually, computed axial tomography (CAT scanning) morphed into computed tomography (CT scanning). The first body CT scanner, which required no water bag, was developed at George-town Hospital by Dr Robert Ledley, a dentist (**Fig. 3**).[11] The automatic computerized transverse axial (ACTA) scanner was commercialized by Pfizer, with 30 photomultiplier tubes and a 256 × 256 matrix. The race to perform faster and better CT scans was on! Improvements in the translate-rotate scans by several manufacturers brought scan time down to 2 minutes per image (**Fig. 4**). By 1974, second-generation scanners from EMI, Ohio Nuclear, and Siemens brought scan time down to 1 minute, and then to18 seconds (**Figs. 5 and 6**).[9,12] A 320 × 320 matrix replaced an 80 × 80 matrix.

In 1974, General Electric (GE) abandoned the translate-rotate approach and proposed a fan

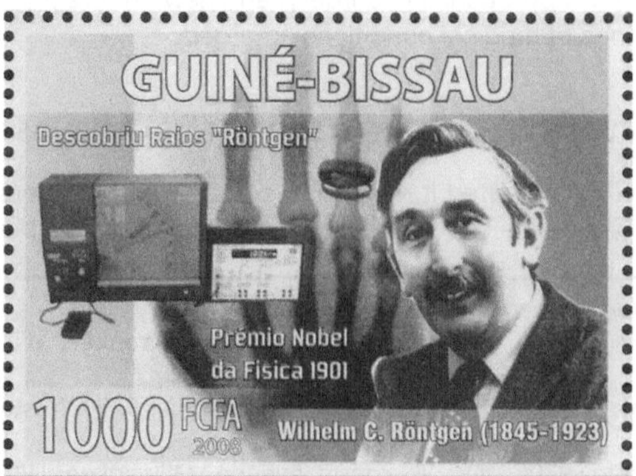

beam, which rotated around the patient (rotate-rotate) in synchronicity with a small curvilinear detector (300–700 elements) (see **Fig. 4**). This was a small scanner prototype large enough to image the breast and, eventually, the head. By 1976, they produced a third-generation body scanner capable of producing 10 mm axial images with 9.5-second gantry rotation per image. Within a few years, GE and Siemens were the dominant producers of third-generation scanners.

Fourth generation scanners, produced by Tech-nicare (Johnson & Johnson), mounted a thousand stationary detectors around the gantry with a rotating radiograph tube. Technical problems eventually defeated this technique.[9,12] Imaging changed dramatically in 1989, when the first helical or spiral scanners were produced by Siemens. The tube rotated continuously as the patient moved through the gantry. Elscint produced a two-detector scanner and the multide-tector race was on.

"YOU REALLY GOT A HOLD OF ME"

The life of the radiologist, and every physician, hospital, and patient, was never the same again. Although the original images were quite crude, the machinery was expensive, and validating studies were lacking, the CT scans were an instan-taneous success.[1] It required only a brief look to realize that the CT scans were special and would replace many conventional techniques. By 1979, 6 years after its clinical introduction, 1,300 CT scanners were in use in the United States. By 1980, 3 million CT scans were performed and, by the year 2000, 62 million CT scans were performed annually.[1,13] With each generation of scanner, new applications arose, much of it made possible by the rapid increase in computer power and the markedly decreasing cost of memory.

The first published images of chest CT scans were in February of 1975, using the ACTA

Fig. 2. Confusion on stamp from Guine-Bissau. It describes Roentgen's 1901 Nobel Prize but has a picture of Hounsfield, the 1979 Nobel Laureate.

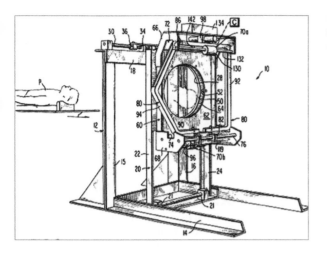

Fig. 3. Patent diagram of Ledley's 1974 ACTA scanner provided for "do it yourselfers." (U.S. patent #3,922,552; Nov 25, 1975.)

scanner.[14] Images were 7.5 mm thick and used a raster of 160 × 160. Images were displayed on a 19-in color monitor, photographed directly with a Polaroid camera, and the snapshots were archived. Later, in 1976, others showed similar images obtained with EMI equipment (**Figs. 1C, 5** and **6**).[15,16] Predictions about the value of chest CT scans were mixed, "Considering that the scanning cycle takes about five minutes, one would expect that scanning of body parts containing moving organs, such as the chest and abdomen, would present a problem. However, we have been favorably impressed in particular by the quality of chest films obtained. Clear visualization

of the lungs, heart, and mediastinal formations was possible."[16] Others expressed some doubt, "In the thorax, CT scans rarely surpass the diagnostic accuracy of conventional radiologic studies."[15]

"NOW MY LIFE HAS CHANGED IN OH SO MANY WAYS"

As this new expensive equipment spread, governments and insurers attempted to limit purchases. Certificates of Need were required in many states before a CT scanner could be purchased. However, the undeniable value of CT scanning—for both

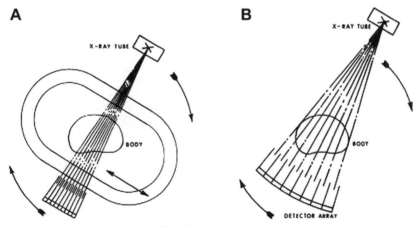

Fig. 4. (*A, B*) Translate-rotate detector versus fan beam detector. Original legends: "(*A*) Moving fan beam with rotation system. Fan beam produced from X-ray tube falls on X-ray detector and scans backward and forward, linearly, across the patient. At each scanning stroke, angle of scanning traverse changed by an amount equal to the angle of the fan beam. In this rotational method, all possible angles of scan across entire body will have been recorded after a 180 degree rotation. (*B*) Rotating fan beam system. X-ray tube produces fan beam as wide as large patient to be scanned. This was on wide array of 300 detectors. To obtain picture, assembly rotated around patient 360 degrees." (*From* Hounsfield GN. Picture quality of computed tomography. AJR Am J Roentgenol 1976;127:3–6; with permission.)[28]

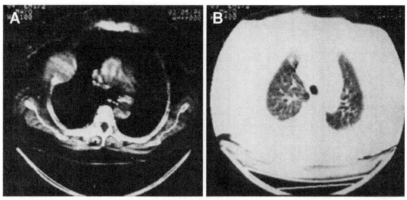

Fig. 5. Original legend: "CT scan of a 79-year-old woman who had subtotal thyroidectomy, three years earlier, for papillary adenocarcinoma. Destructive lesion had recently developed in the right third rib and in the right side of the pelvis. (*A*) Tomographic section through the chest revealing large destructive lesion in rib on right. Large potion of the mass projects into the chest, and tumor extends considerably into chest wall. (*B*) Lung parenchyma revealed after adjusting window height and width. Note tiny nodule in apex of right lung anteriorly, which was not appreciated on chest film." (EMI Body Scanner) (*From* Sheedy PF 2nd, Stephens DH, Hattery RR, et al. Computed tomography of the body: initial clinical trial with the EMI prototype. AJR Am J Roentgenol 1976; 127:23–51; with permission.)

diagnosis and patient management—eventually overwhelmed attempts to control dissemination.[1] In the United States, in 2000, it is estimated that over 62 million CT scans were performed annually.[13] Today, approximately 30% of CT scans are of the thorax. Initially, most scanning was done for lung and mediastinal disease. With the advent of helical scanning, vascular and cardiac imaging

has become a major focus. With each technical advance, new CT scan applications arose.

Lung

Initial scanning concentrated on parenchymal consolidation and tumor, as the peripheral anatomy of the lung was not well demonstrated

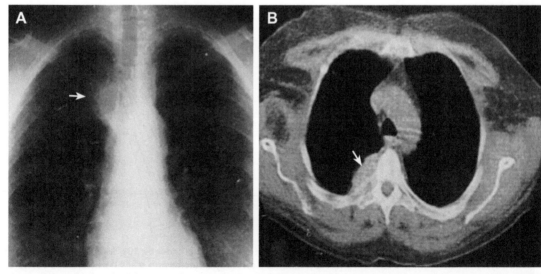

Fig. 6. Original legend. "(*A*) Currently asymptomatic 57-year-old with known multiple myeloma. A chest radiograph demonstrating 4 cm mass (*arrow*) in right posterior mediastinum. (*B*) CT scan showing the posterior mediastinal mass arises from contiguously destroyed posterior aspect of the right fourth rib (*arrow*), a manifestation of her known multiple myeloma." (EMI Body Scanner) (*From* Stanley RJ, Sagel SS, Levitt RG, et al. Computed tomography of the body: early trends in application and accuracy of the method. AJR Am J Roentgenol 1976; 127:53–67; with permission.)

on 10 mm slices with long breath holds (**Figs. 1C, 5 and 7**). With improved equipment, thinner and thinner scans became available. The first English language report of high-resolution CT (HRCT) scanning (1 mm slice every 10 mm, high-resolution algorithm) was in 1985.[17] HRCT became the hot new area in the late 1980s and 1990s. Multislice CT scanning now permits one to obtain sub-millimeter images using isotropic voxels and to perform high-quality multiplanar reconstructions. Now, lung detail and distribution of disease can be assessed at the sub-millimeter level in any plane. HRCT scanning has led to new understanding, classification, and reclassification of various forms of interstitial lung diseases and bronchial diseases. HRCT scanning has dramatically changed the way radiologists, pathologists, and clinicians diagnose and understand interstitial lung disease. As with most advances, as some areas become better elucidated, new questions arise.

Mediastinum

CT scanning was immediately embraced as the method for evaluating the mediastinum. Conventional radiographs and conventional tomography often failed to detect or adequately characterize mediastinal pathology because of lack of contrast between the normal structures and the pathologic structures (**Figs. 5 and 6**).[18] Because the mediastinum is less prone to respiratory motion, and intravenous contrast (administered by drip) provided sharp contrast boundaries, CT scanning rapidly became the modality of choice. It was soon touted as both sensitive and specific for staging lung cancer metastasis. With time, it was realized that CT scanning was an improvement, but fallible, for cancer staging. The recent fusion of CT and

positron emission tomography scanning has overcome many of those problems.

Fast-drip intravenous contrast infusion was a valuable asset in distinguishing the major vessels from other structures, but little thought was given to using CT scans for evaluating the vessels beyond the superior vena cava and aorta. As axial imaging became faster, more detailed vascular evaluation became possible.[19–21] Early studies of the aorta for trauma, dissection, or aneurysm were limited by motion and had limited acceptance in the radiologic and the surgical community. Aided by power injection of contrast, single-detector helical and then multidetector helical scanning, CT scanning is now the procedure of choice in the majority of patients with suspected aortic disease.

The first CT scan report on pulmonary embolism, in 1977, looked at parenchymal changes but did not even mention the visualization of intravascular clot.[22] The first mention of prospective evaluation for pulmonary embolus involved three cases using "rapid sequence of up to twelve 2.4-second scans, with a one-second delay between scans" (**Fig. 8**).[23] Although large pulmonary emboli could be visualized with axial CT scanning it was not until the advent of helical CT scan that large and midsized pulmonary vessels could be imaged routinely.[24] Single-detector helical scanning allowed one to scan only 12 cm of the chest in a 24-second breath hold at 5 mm intervals. Multidetector scanners shortened the breath hold to

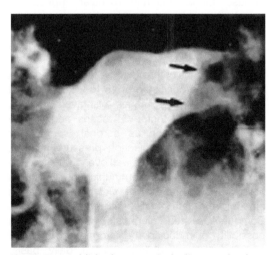

Fig. 8. First published prospectively diagnosed pulmonary embolism. 1977 Axial image using a fan beam/rotating detector with 9.5 second gantry rotation. (*From* Godwin JD, Webb WR, Gamsu G, et al. Computed tomography of pulmonary embolism. AJR Am J Roentgenol 1980;135:691–5; with permission.)

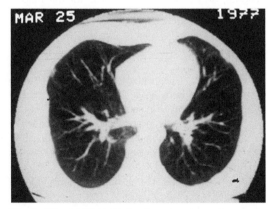

Fig. 7. CT scan on early fan beam scanner. Scan rotation time was 9.5 seconds and the slice thickness was 10 mm. (GE 5000 Scanner.)

a few seconds, provided subsecond rotation time and submillimeter resolution. Helical CT scanning rapidly replaced perfusion scanning and angiography as the clinical procedure of choice and is now the gold standard.[25]

The same improvements, with 16-detector scanning and above, have made cardiac imaging and coronary artery imaging possible. Elegant 2- and 3-dimensional (D) reconstructions add a new dimension. CT scanning's role is yet to be defined, as there are many competing modalities.

Lung Cancer Screening

CT scan screening for lung cancer is another recent addition to the diagnostic armamentarium. High-end scanners provide relatively low-dose images, capable of detecting even the smallest cancers.[26] Unfortunately, other clinically irrelevant nodules are seen with great frequency. The eventual role of lung cancer screening is still being debated.[27]

Other Developments

Many of the high-end applications discussed above are possible because of high quality 2D and 3D reconstruction. The development of the isotropic voxel has provided high-quality volumetric scanning and reconstruction in any two-dimensional plane or as three-dimensional images. Lung applications are numerous, including bronchiectasis and interstitial lung disease. Mediastinal and vascular applications include the trachea, the aorta, the great vessels, the pulmonary vessels, and cardiac applications—especially when gating is applied—include cardiac and coronary evaluation.

Early CT scans of the chest were 10 mm each. A chest CT scan consisted of 15 to 20 mediastinal and 15 to 20 lung images displayed on film. Now, with multidetector CT scans and routine reconstructions, such as coronal, sagittal, or maximum intensity projection pressure images, the chest CT scan is often well over 1,000 images. Picture archiving and communications systems have made it practical to view the staggering amount of data that each case presents. Computer-assisted diagnosis (CAD) offers a possibility of reducing the information overload confronting the radiologist on a daily basis. Sophisticated nodule detention and nodule quantization software promises to make these two tasks less burdensome. In addition, CAD programs, now in testing, can also detect pulmonary emboli to the subsegmental level and quantify emphysema.

"WILL YOU STILL NEED ME . . . WHEN I'M 64?"

As this article is written, the 64-slice multidetector scanner is the dominant CT scanner. Although it is a current workhorse, the industry is rapidly moving forward.

Phillips now has a functional 256-slice multidetector scanner that can provide images of the entire thorax within seconds and of the heart, in less than 2 beats. Toshiba (320 slice) can image the entire heart in one rotation. These newer scanners show the most promise for cardiac and coronary imaging and other small organ imaging. Technical limitations currently limit more general use.

Dual-energy scanning also has multiple potential applications in the lung. With dual energy, calcification can be more easily assessed and perfusion scanning of the lung is possible. This has potential applications for evaluation of pulmonary emboli and other clinical scenarios where perfusion information is helpful. Unlike nuclear studies, it provides both anatomic and functional information in the same scan. Myocardial infarct imaging, and perhaps coronary calcium removal, may be in the future. Dynamic respiratory imaging for airflow obstruction, tracheobronchial mechanics, and diaphragm motion are also possible with faster scanners.

SUMMARY

Chest CT scanning has come a long way since 1975. Anatomic images are now superb and functional imaging is in its early stages.

ACKNOWLEDGMENTS

Thanks to Dr Stanley Fox, PhD, for his historical insights, and to Mrs Sylvia Bartz, for her help in preparing this manuscript.

REFERENCES

1. Berland LL. Commentary on "Computed tomography of the body: initial Clinical Trial with the EMI Prototype" and "Computed tomography of the body: early trends in application and accuracy of the method". AJR Am J Roentgenol 2008;191:16–8.
2. Ambrose J. CT scanning: a backward look. Semin Roentgenol 1977;12:7–11.
3. The beatles. Available at: http://Wikipedia/org/wiki/beatles. Accessed August 1, 2009.
4. Ambrose J. Computerized transverse axial scanning (tomography): part 2. Clinical application. Br J Radiol 1973;46:1023–47.

5. Hounsfield GN. Computerized transverse axial scanning (tomography): part 1. Description of system. Br J Radiol 1973;46:1016–22.

6. Richmond C. Obituary. Geoffrey Newbold Hounsfield, engineer (b 1919, CBE, FRS), d 12 August 2004. BMJ 2004;329:687.

7. Perry BJ, Bridges C. Computerized transverse axial scanning (tomography): part 3. Radiation dose considerations. Br J Radiol 1973;46:1048–51.

8. Bui-Mansfield LT, Sutcliffe JB. Nobel prize laureates who have made significant contributions to radiology. J Comput Assist Tomogr 2009;33:483–8.

9. Robb WL. Perspective on the first 10 years of the CT scanner industry. Acad Radiol 2003;10:756–60.

10. Montgomery BJ. CT scanning recognized with Nobel Prize. Medical news. JAMA 1979;242:2380–1.

11. U.S. Patent #3,922,552 applied for Nov 25, 1975. Information for patent. Available at: http://patft.uspto.gov.

12. Eisenberg RL. Computed tomography. In: Eisenberg RL, editor. Radiology, an illustrated history. St. Louis (MO): Mosby-Year Book; 1992. p. 467–77.

13. Brenner DJ, Hall EJ. Computed tomography – an increasing source of radiation exposure. N Engl J Med 2007;357:2277–84.

14. Schellinger D, Di Chiro G, Axelbaumn SP, et al. Early clinical experience with the ACTA scanner. Radiology 1975;114:257–61.

15. Stanley RJ, Sagel SS, Levitt RG, et al. Computed tomography of the body: early trends in application and accuracy of the method. AJR Am J Roentgenol 1976;127:53–67.

16. Sheedy PF 2nd, Stephens DH, Hattery RR, et al. Computed tomography of the body: initial clinical trial with the EMI prototype. AJR Am J Roentgenol 1976;127:23–51.

17. Nakata H, Kimoto T, Nakayama T, et al. Diffuse peripheral lung disease: evaluation by high-resolution computed tomography. Radiology 1985;157:181–5.

18. Mink JH, Bein ME, Sukov R, et al. Computer tomography of the anterior mediastinum in patients with myasthenia gravis and suspected thymoma. AJR Am J Roentgenol 1978;130:239–46.

19. Heiberg E, Wolverson M, Sundaram M, et al. CT findings in thoracic aortic dissection. AJR Am J Roentgenol 1981;136:13–7.

20. Heiberg E, Wolverson MK, Sundaram M, et al. CT in aortic trauma. AJR Am J Roentgenol 1983;140:1119–24.

21. Moncada R, Salinas M, Churchill R, et al. Diagnosis of dissecting aortic aneurysm by computed tomography. Lancet 1981;1:238–41.

22. Sinner WN. U.S. Patent #3, 922,552; 11/25/75. J Comput Assist Tomogr 1978;2(4):395–9.

23. Godwin JD, Webb WR, Gamsu G, et al. Computed tomography of pulmonary embolism. AJR Am J Roentgenol 1980;135:691–5.

24. Remy-Jardin M, Remy J, Wattinne L, et al. Central pulmonary thromboembolism: diagnosis with spiral volumetric CT with the single-breath-hold technique–comparison with pulmonary angiography. Radiology 1992;185:381–7.

25. Stein PD, Fowler SE, Goodman LR, et al. Multidetector computed tomography for acute pulmonary embolism. [PIOPED II]. N Engl J Med 2006;354(22):2317–27.

26. Henschke CI, McCauley DI, Yankelevitz DF, et al. Early lung cancer action project: overall design and findings from baseline screening. Lancet 1999;354:99–105.

27. Unger M. A pause, progress, and reassessment in lung cancer screening [comment]. N Engl J Med 2006;355:1822–4.

28. Hounsfield GN. Picture quality of computed tomography. AJR Am J Roentgenol 1976;127:3–6.

Multidetector CT of Solitary Pulmonary Nodules

Mylene T. Truong, MD[a],*, Bradley S. Sabloff, MD[a],
Jane P. Ko, MD[b]

KEYWORDS

- Chest imaging • CT • Lung • PET/CT
- Pulmonary nodules

A solitary pulmonary nodule is defined as "a round opacity, at least moderately well-marginated and no greater than 3 cm in maximum diameter."[1] The adjective *small* is occasionally used to characterize a nodule with a maximum diameter of less than 1 cm.[1] With the increasing use of multidetector CT (MDCT), small nodules are being detected with increasing frequency. In one screening study, the majority of patients who were screened had at least one nodule.[2] Although most incidentally discovered nodules are benign (usually the sequelae of pulmonary infection), malignancy remains an important consideration in the differential diagnosis of solitary pulmonary nodules (**Table 1**). According to the American Cancer Society,[3–5] 1 in 13 men and 1 in 16 women will be diagnosed with lung cancer and it is estimated that 20% to 30% of these patients will present with a solitary pulmonary nodule. Because many patients with early-stage lung cancer can present with a solitary pulmonary nodule, one of the main goals of imaging is to accurately differentiate malignant from benign lesions. Techniques for noninvasive image-based assessment and management of these nodules have rapidly evolved recently in large part because of data from ongoing screening studies and from thin-slice helical MDCT studies examining nodule morphology.

MDCT has improved nodule detection and characterization by increasing spatial and temporal resolution and decreasing misregistration artifacts. Typical reconstructions comprise 3- to 5-mm slice collimation for a nontargeted field of view. Obtaining images through the region of interest using a slice collimation of 1 to 1.5 mm improves spatial resolution and is useful in reducing partial volume averaging. If a 1.25-mm slice collimation has been used, as is common in CT angiography protocols to evaluate for pulmonary emboli, differentiating a vessel from a small central nodule is difficult and can be addressed with postprocessing techniques, such as maximum intensity projection, volume rendering, and cine viewing.[6–8] This article reviews the role of imaging in the detection and characterization of solitary pulmonary nodules. Strategies for evaluating and managing solitary pulmonary nodules are also discussed.

CLINICAL ASSESSMENT

How a nodule is managed depends on the probability of malignancy. Clinical factors associated with an increased risk of developing lung cancer include older age, presenting symptoms, smoking, and exposure to asbestos, uranium, or radon. In terms of clinical presentation, patients with hemoptysis are at increased risk for malignancy.[9] Past medical history is important as there is an increased risk of lung cancer in patients with

This article originally appeared in *Radiologic Clinics of North America*, Volume 48, Issue 1, January 2010.
[a] Department of Radiology, University of Texas MD Anderson Cancer Center, 1515 Holcombe Boulevard, Unit 371, Houston, TX 77030, USA
[b] Department of Radiology, New York University Langone Medical Center, 560 First Avenue, IRM 236, New York, NY 10016, USA
* Corresponding author.
E-mail address: mtruong@mdanderson.org (M.T. Truong).

Thorac Surg Clin 20 (2010) 9–23
doi:10.1016/j.thorsurg.2009.12.002
1547-4127/10/$ – see front matter © 2010 Elsevier Inc. All rights reserved.

Table 1
Differential diagnosis of solitary pulmonary nodules

Type of Cause	Disease
Neoplastic malignant	Primary lung malignancies (non–small cell, small cell, carcinoid, lymphoma); solitary metastasis
Benign	Hamartoma; arteriovenous malformation
Infectious	Granuloma; round pneumonia; abscess; septic embolus
Noninfectious	Amyloidoma; subpleural lymph nodule; rheumatoid nodule; Wegener granulomatosis; focal scarring; infarct
Congenital	Sequestration; bronchogenic cyst; bronchial atresia with mucoid impaction

a history of a prior neoplasm and in patients with pulmonary fibrosis.[9,10] Family history also plays a role in determining the likelihood of malignancy. In this regard, a susceptibility gene to lung cancer has been reported and the risk of developing lung cancer increases in patients who have a first-degree relative with lung cancer.[11] The overall assessment of a patient's risk for malignancy is important in the decision analysis concerning management. For example, in a patient presenting with fever, cough, and a new focal pulmonary opacity, radiographic follow-up to resolution may be all that is necessary to exclude malignancy and confirm a diagnosis of round pneumonia. However, if a new nodule is detected in a patient with a prior history of pulmonary sarcoma, the probability that this is a metastasis is high and tissue should be obtained for diagnosis (**Fig. 1**). For patients with a prior history of cancer, Ginsberg and colleagues[12] showed that nodules 5 mm or smaller were malignant in 115 of 275 (42%) patients undergoing video-assisted thoracoscopic resection of nodules. To identify independent predictors of malignancy, quantitative models have been developed using multiple logistic regression analysis. Independent predictors of malignancy include older age, current or past smoking history, and history of extrathoracic cancer more than 5 years before nodule detection.[13]

RADIOLOGICAL EVALUATION

Although CT detects an increasing number of solitary pulmonary nodules either incidentally or as part of a lung cancer screening study, many nodules are still initially detected on chest radiographs. If the nodule is diffusely calcified or if a comparison with older radiographs shows stability in size for more than 2 years, the nodule

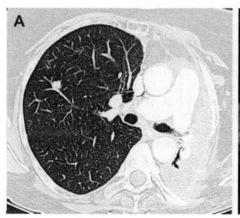 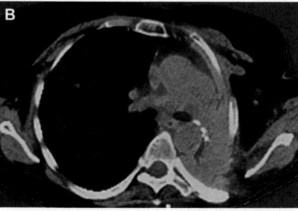

Fig. 1. Sixty-eight-year-old woman with a prior left pneumonectomy for a sarcoma. (*A*) Contrast-enhanced CT and (*B*) positron emission tomography/CT show a hypometabolic irregular right upper lobe nodule with standardized uptake value of 1.4. With advances in positron emission tomography technology, evaluation of nodules as small as 7 mm is possible. However, a negative positron emission tomography does not preclude malignancy. Because of the high clinical suspicion of malignancy with regards to the age of the patient and history of prior lung malignancy, transthoracic needle aspiration biopsy was performed and revealed an adenocarcinoma.

is presumed to be benign and no further evaluation is recommended. However, many nodules require further imaging evaluation. MDCT optimally evaluates morphologic characteristics of the nodule and is useful in assessing for growth on serial studies. Nodules may be missed on MDCT because of a variety of factors, including central location, small size, low attenuation, and location in the lower lobes or adjacent to another abnormal pulmonary opacity, such as inflammatory change.[8] Difficulty with interpretation also occurs with CT as it may not be possible to determine whether a small opacity is a nodule, a vessel, or- due to partial volume averaging of adjacent intrathoracic structures. However, the use of thin-section CT together with postprocessing techniques, such as maximum intensity projection, volume rendering, and cine viewing of images at a picture archiving and communication system workstation, has improved the ability to correctly determine whether a pulmonary opacity is a nodule.[8,14]

Nodule Morphology

Although there is considerable overlap in the morphology and appearance of benign and malignant solitary pulmonary nodules, several morphologic features are useful in assessing a nodule's malignant potential. These features include the size, margins, contour, internal morphology (attenuation, wall thickness in cavitary nodules, air bronchograms), presence of satellite nodules, halo sign, reverse halo sign, and growth rate.

The risk of malignancy correlates with nodule size. However, small nodule size does not exclude malignancy. In this regard, the widespread use of MDCT, coupled with the recent interest in CT screening for lung cancer, has resulted in the frequent and incidental detection of small nodules (1–5 mm).[15–17] While the majority of these nodules are benign, studies of resected small nodules have shown that a considerable number are malignant—as high as 42% for patients with a known malignancy undergoing video-assisted thoracoscopic resection of nodules 5 mm or less.[12]

Typically, benign nodules have well-defined margins and a smooth contour while malignant nodules have ill-defined or spiculated margins and a lobular or irregular contour.[9,18,19] Lobulation is attributed to differential growth rates within nodules, while the irregular or spiculated margins are usually due to growth of malignant cells along the pulmonary interstitium.[20] However, there is considerable overlap between benign and malignant nodules regarding margins and contour. For example, although a spiculated margin with distortion of adjacent bronchovascular bundles (often described as a sunburst or corona radiata) is highly suggestive with a 90% predictive value of malignancy,[21] benign nodules due to infection/ inflammation can also have this appearance (**Fig. 2**). Additionally, a smooth nodule margin does not exclude malignancy. Up to 20% of primary lung malignancies have smooth contours and well-defined margins and most metastatic nodules typically manifest as smooth margins.[9,19]

The halo sign is a poorly defined rim of ground-glass attenuation around the nodule (**Fig. 3**). This halo may represent hemorrhage, tumor infiltration, or perinodular inflammation. Originally described as a sign of invasive aspergillus infection, the CT halo sign may also be seen with bronchioloalveolar carcinoma.[22] Conversely, the reverse halo sign is a focal round area of ground-glass attenuation surrounded by a ring of consolidation (**Fig. 4**).

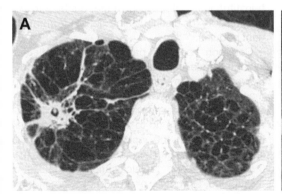 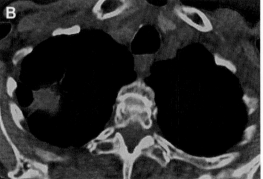

Fig. 2. Seventy-eight-year-old woman presenting with a chronic cough. (*A*) Contrast-enhanced CT and (*B*) positron emission tomography/CT show an irregular cavitary lesion in the right upper lobe with standardized uptake value of 4.1 suspicious for a primary lung cancer. Biopsy revealed acute and chronic inflammation with confluent colonies of fungiform bacteria consistent with actinomyces. Note that infectious and inflammatory conditions can accumulate ^{18}F-labeled 2-deoxy-D-glucose and be misinterpreted as malignant.

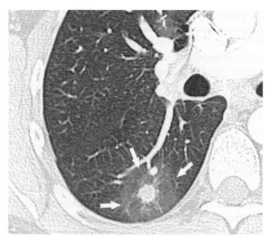

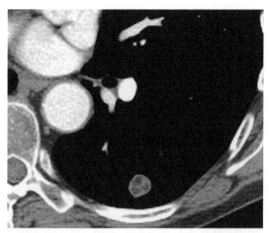

Fig. 3. Thirty-six-year-old man presenting with a cough. Contrast-enhanced CT shows a well-circumscribed right lower lobe nodule surrounded by a halo of ground-glass attenuation (*arrows*) and a satellite nodule anteriorly. Note that in patients with leukemia, the halo sign is highly suggestive of invasive aspergillus infection.

Fig. 5. Contrast-enhanced CT shows a well-circumscribed left lower lobe nodule. Low attenuation within the nodule (attenuation −46 Hounsfield units) is consistent with fat and is usually diagnostic of a hamartoma. Note that focal fat in a nodule can rarely be seen in liposarcoma metastases and lipoid pneumonia.

Described in cryptogenic organizing pneumonia[23] and paracoccidioidomycosis, the reverse halo sign is histologically due to a greater amount of inflammatory cells in the periphery of the lesion than in the center. In invasive fungal pneumonias, the reverse halo sign is due to infarcted lung with a greater amount of hemorrhage in the peripheral solid ring than in the center ground-glass region.[24]

Fat within a nodule is a characteristic finding of a hamartoma and is detected by CT in up to 50% of these neoplasms (**Fig. 5**).[25] Rarely, lung metastases in patients with liposarcomas or renal cell cancers can manifest as fat-containing nodules.[26]

Calcification patterns can be useful in determining benignity of a nodule and CT is considerably more sensitive than radiography for detecting calcification in a nodule.[18,27,28] However, partial volume averaging can be problematic when thicker sections are obtained, making calcification within a small nodule visually undetectable. In these cases, thin sections (1–3 mm) to improve spatial resolution should be performed to detect calcification. With the introduction of dual-energy CT, simultaneous 80-kV and 140-kV images can be obtained. It has been shown that measurement of CT attenuation values obtained at different kilovolt peaks may be useful in identifying areas of fat, calcium, bone, soft tissue, and iodinated contrast[29] and in evaluating tumor perfusion. However, a multi-institutional trial has shown that dual-energy CT is unreliable for distinguishing benign from malignant nodules.[30–32]

Common benign patterns of calcification include diffuse, central, laminated, and "popcorn." However, lung metastases from chondrosarcomas or osteosarcomas can present with "benign" patterns of calcification (**Fig. 6**).[26,33] Calcification can be detected in up to 13% of all lung cancers on CT, although the incidence in patients with lung cancer manifesting as nodules less than 3 cm is only 2%.[34–36] Calcification patterns, such as stippled, eccentric, or amorphous, are indeterminate in etiology as they can be seen in both benign and malignant conditions (**Fig. 7**).[36]

The widespread use of MDCT images has increased the detection of "subsolid" nodules containing a component of ground-glass

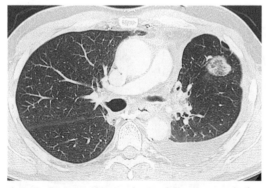

Fig. 4. Contrast-enhanced CT following radiofrequency ablation for a left upper lobe lung cancer shows a focal round area of ground-glass attenuation surrounded by a well-circumscribed region of consolidation (reverse halo sign). Note that the reverse halo sign is usually indicative of invasive fungal pneumonia in immunocompromised patients.

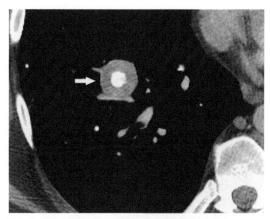

Fig. 6. Thirty-six-year-old man with a chondrosarcoma of the left proximal thigh. CT shows central calcification within the nodule in the right lower lobe (*arrow*). This appearance is highly suggestive of a benign calcified nodule secondary to granulomatous infection. However, knowledge of the clinical context must also be taken into account in establishing the diagnosis. Resection revealed metastatic chondrosarcoma.

attenuation. The "subsolid" category comprises pure ground-glass, as well as mixed solid and ground-glass (partly solid) lesions. In the ELCAP (Early Lung Cancer Action Project) study, 19% of positive results on the baseline screening were subsolid. Incidence of malignancy varies according to the degree of soft tissue attenuation. Henschke and colleagues[37] reported rates of malignancy for solid and subsolid nodules as 7% and 34%, respectively. Partly solid nodules had the highest incidence of malignancy (63%) (**Fig. 8**) while pure ground-glass nodules had an incidence of malignancy of 18%.

In terms of malignant potential, subsolid nodules have been associated with a spectrum of entities ranging from atypical adenomatous hyperplasia (a premalignant condition), to bronchioloalveolar carcinoma and invasive adenocarcinoma.[38] Atypical adenomatous hyperplasia (**Fig. 9**), a putative precursor to bronchioloalveolar carcinoma/adenocarcinoma, is defined by the World Health Organization as a

> …localized proliferation of mild to moderately atypical cells lining involved alveoli and sometimes respiratory bronchioles, resulting in focal lesions in peripheral alveolated lung, usually less than 5mm in diameter and generally in the absence of underlying interstitial inflammation and fibrosis.[39]

Ground-glass nodules less than 1 cm may represent atypical adenomatous hyperplasia or bronchioloalveolar carcinoma. Subsolid nodules greater than 1 cm are more likely to represent bronchioloalveolar carcinoma rather than atypical adenomatous hyperplasia. Noguchi and Shimosato[38] graded the spectrum of bronchioloalveolar carcinoma and invasive adenocarcinoma pathologically into types A through F, representing various degrees of aggressiveness. This grading system showed that the presence of solid component on CT in a ground-glass nodule is concerning for higher grades of adenocarcinoma.[40] In contradistinction, another study revealed that pure ground-glass opacities were less likely to have invasion and/or metastasis.[41]

Solid nodules have the lowest incidence of malignancy, as many infections, particularly mycoses and tuberculosis, have this appearance. However, despite the lower incidence of malignancy in solid nodules, most primary lung cancers and metastases present as solid nodules.[21]

Cavitation occurs in both infectious/inflammatory conditions as well as in primary and metastatic tumors. Up to 15% of primary lung malignancies cavitate and typically cavitation is seen in squamous cell histology (**Fig. 10**). Thick, irregular walls are typically seen in malignant cavitary nodules, whereas smooth, thin walls are seen in benign cavitary lesions.[19] It has been reported that 95% of cavitary nodules with a wall thickness greater than 16 mm are malignant and 92% with a wall thickness less than 4 mm are benign.[42,43] Although these measurements can add value in nodule evaluation, cavity wall thickness cannot be used to reliably differentiate benign and malignant nodules because of cavitary nodules with a wall thickness of 5 to 15 mm, 51% were found to be benign and 49% malignant.[43]

Additional morphologic imaging features that can be used in assessing the malignant or benign potential of solitary pulmonary nodules include the presence of internal lucencies, air bronchograms, and satellite nodules. Bronchioloalveolar carcinoma can also show small internal lucencies due to patent bronchi from lepidic growth of tumor cells (**Fig. 11**).[19] In one study, air bronchograms occurred more frequently in malignant nodules (30%) than in benign nodules (6%)[44]; and the differential diagnosis includes bronchioloalveolar carcinoma, lymphoma, and infection. Satellite nodules, small nodules adjacent to a dominant nodule, are more frequently associated with benign lesions. However, 6% to 16% of patients with lung cancer present with T4-satellite nodules.[45–47]

Nodule Growth

Nodule growth can be evaluated by reviewing prior films. Malignant nodules may double in volume

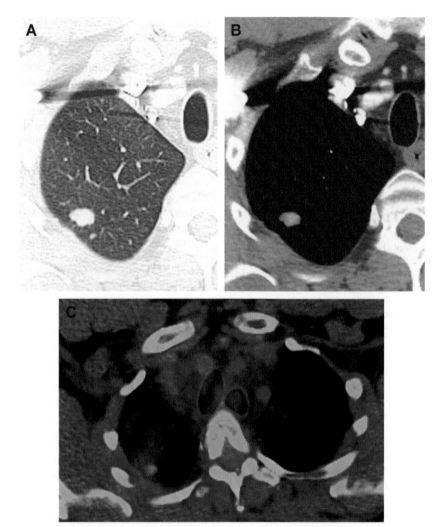

Fig. 7. Forty-seven-year-old man with a right upper lobe nodule with a lobular contour in (*A*) contrast-enhanced CT in lung windows, amorphous calcifications in (*B*) contrast-enhanced CT with mediastinal windows, and lack of ^{18}F-labeled 2-deoxy-D-glucose uptake in (*C*) positron emission tomography/CT. Despite the negative positron emission tomography, the lesion was biopsied because of the indeterminate calcification pattern and increase in size compared with 3 years earlier (not shown). Pathology revealed dense fibrosis, focal chronic inflammation, and no malignant cells.

between 30 and 400 days (**Fig. 12**).[48] Nodules that double in volume in less than 30 days are typically infectious or inflammatory in etiology but may also be seen in lymphoma or rapidly growing metastases (**Fig. 13**). Nodules that double in volume in greater than 400 days are usually benign neoplasms or sequelae of prior pulmonary infections. In general, the lack of growth over a 2-year period is reliable in determining benignity of a nodule.[49,50] This criterion does not apply to subsolid nodules because some well-differentiated adenocarcinoma and bronchioloalveolar carcinoma can have doubling times of up to 1346 days.[51] In a screening study analyzing the growth rates of small lung cancers, Hasegawa and

colleagues[52] found that approximately 20% (12 of 61) had volume-doubling time of greater than 2 years, typically seen with well-differentiated adenocarcinomas. Interestingly, the volume-doubling time was longer in nonsmokers than in smokers. Of small lung cancers, the longest doubling time was seen in nonsolid lesions, followed by partly solid lesions and, finally, solid lesions.[52]

Because nodule growth is an important consideration when assessing lesions for malignant potential, the accuracy of growth assessment needs to be addressed. For a nodule to double in volume, the change in nodule diameter is approximately 26%. For a small nodule, this small change in diameter may be difficult to detect. For

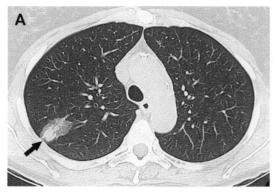 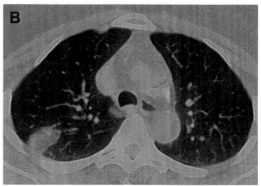

Fig. 8. Sixty-six-year-old man with a well-differentiated adenocarcinoma with bronchioloalveolar features manifesting as a partly solid right upper lobe nodule. (*A*) On CT, the nodule shows a solid component posteriorly (*arrow*). (*B*) Positron emission tomography/CT shows low metabolic activity with standardized uptake value of 3.3. Note that, compared with nonsolid and solid lesions, partly solid lesions have the highest likelihood of being malignant.

example, a 4-mm nodule will increase to only 5 mm in diameter after doubling in volume. Additionally, it has recently been shown that significant inter- and intraobserver variability in lesion measurement, particularly in lesions with spiculated margins, are confounding factors in determining growth.[53,54] It has been suggested that, for evaluating nodule size and growth, the measurement of volume is a more accurate and reproducible than the measurement of diameters, and that automated volume techniques are potentially useful for assessing growth.[55,56]

Nodule Enhancement and Metabolism

There are qualitative and quantitative differences in nodule perfusion and metabolism when comparing benign and malignant lesions. Contrast-enhanced CT has been shown in a multi-institutional trial to be useful in determining the likelihood of malignancy of nodules between 5 mm and 3 cm.[57] The intensity of nodule enhancement is directly related to the vascularity of the nodule, which is increased in malignant lesions.[57–59] Malignant lesions greater than 3 cm may show necrosis and fail to enhance, leading to a false-negative study. In the CT-enhancement protocol, 3-mm collimation images of the nodule are obtained before and after the intravenous administration of contrast (2 mL/s; 300-mg iodine/mL; 420-mg iodine/kg of body weight). Serial 5-second spiral acquisitions (3-mm collimation scans with 2-mm reconstruction intervals; 120 kVp, 280 mA, pitch of 1:1; standard reconstruction

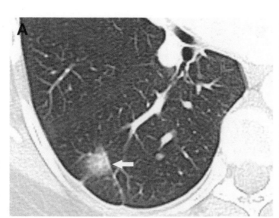 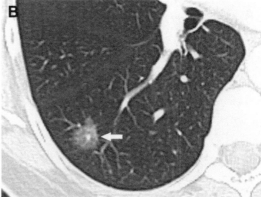

Fig. 9. Forty-five-year-old woman with thyroid cancer. (*A*) Contrast-enhanced CT shows a right lower lobe subsolid nodule (*arrow*) biopsy proven to be due to atypical adenomatous hyperplasia. (*B*) Contrast-enhanced CT 4 years later shows no change in nodule size and a decrease in nodule attenuation (*arrow*). Note that an exception to Fleischner's guidelines for evaluation of small pulmonary nodules is the nonsolid or partly solid nodule, for which reassessment may need to be continued beyond 2 years to exclude the risk of an indolent adenocarcinoma.

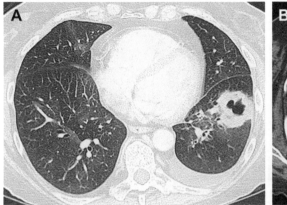
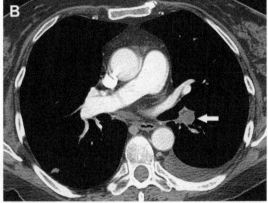

Fig. 10. Cavitary pulmonary infarction. (*A*) Contrast-enhanced CT shows a thick-walled cavitary nodule in left lower lobe suspicious for primary lung cancer. (*B*) Contrast-enhanced CT with mediastinal windows revealed clot in the left interlobar pulmonary artery consistent with pulmonary embolism (*arrow*).

algorithm; 15-cm field of view) are performed at 1, 2, 3, and 4 minutes after the onset of contrast injection. Enhancement is determined by subtracting the precontrast attenuation of the nodule from the peak nodule attenuation after contrast administration. To obtain measurements, the circular or oval region of interest is centered on the image closest to the nodule equator and should comprise roughly 70% of the diameter of a nodule. Region-of-interest measurements should be made on mediastinal window settings to minimize partial volume averaging. Careful inspection of the adjacent bronchovascular bundles to obtain region-of-interest measurements of the nodule at similar levels in the z-axis on serial scans is recommended. Typically, malignant nodules enhance more than 20 Hounsfield units (HU), while benign

nodules enhance less than 15 HU.[57] When a cutoff of 15 HU is used, the negative predictive value for malignancy is 96%.[57] There are, however, several potential limitations to clinical application of this technique. This technique should only be performed on nodules greater than 5 mm, relatively spherical in shape, and relatively homogeneous in attenuation (ie, without evidence of fat, calcification, cavitation, or necrosis). Because nodules that enhance less than 15 HU are almost certainly benign (sensitivity 98%, specificity 58%, accuracy 77%), the clinical utility of this technique, despite its limitations, does enable conservative management with serial imaging reassessment.

Recently, computer-aided diagnosis has been used to assist in differentiating benign from malignant nodules by examining vascular enhancement

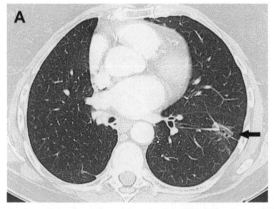
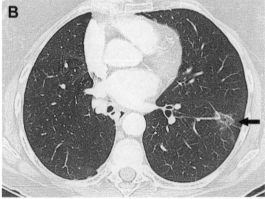

Fig. 11. Sixty-five-year-old woman with right lower lobectomy for lung cancer and left lower lobe subsolid nodule representing bronchioloalveolar carcinoma in (*A*) contrast-enhanced CT with small internal lucencies due to patent bronchi from lepidic growth of tumor cells (*arrow*). Comparison with a (*B*) contrast-enhanced CT 2 years earlier shows lack of growth (*arrow*). Note with small lung cancers, the longest doubling time is seen with nonsolid lesions, followed by partly solid lesions, and finally solid lesions.

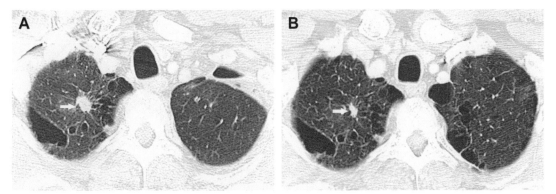

Fig. 12. Sixty-seven-year-old man with emphysema. (*A*) Contrast-enhanced CT shows a spiculated right apical lesion (*arrow*) has increased in size compared with (*B*) contrast-enhanced CT of 8 months earlier showing same lesion (*arrow*). Biopsy revealed a neuroendocrine carcinoma. Note that nodule growth is an important consideration when assessing lesions for malignant potential.

and nodule morphology. In a study by Shah and colleagues[60] a computer-aided diagnosis system used quantitative features to describe the nodule's size, shape, attenuation, and enhancement properties to differentiate benign from malignant nodules. This study showed that computer-aided diagnosis using volumetric and contrast-enhanced data from 35 CT data sets of solitary pulmonary nodules with a mean diameter of 25 mm (range 6–54 mm) is useful in assisting in the differentiation of benign and malignant solitary pulmonary opacities.

An alternative to CT enhancement to differentiate benign from malignant pulmonary nodules is functional imaging using ^{18}F-labeled 2-deoxy-D-glucose (FDG) positron emission tomography

(PET). The most common semiquantitative method of evaluation of pulmonary lesions using PET is FDG standardized uptake value (SUV_{max}). Metabolism of glucose is typically increased in malignancies and an SUV_{max} cutoff of 2.5 has been used to differentiate benign from malignant nodules.[61] PET has a sensitivity and specificity of approximately 90% for detection of malignancy in nodules 10 mm or greater in diameter.[62] To properly tailor patient management, FDG PET evaluations of solitary pulmonary nodules must be considered alongside such clinical risk factors as patient age, smoking history, and history of malignancy (**Fig. 14**). For instance, in a patient with a low pretest likelihood of malignancy (20%) being considered for serial imaging reassessment,

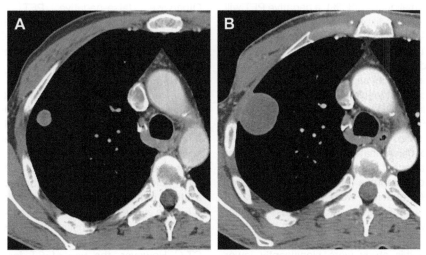

Fig. 13. Fifty-eight-year-old man with a pulmonary metastasis from a nasopharyngeal cancer. (*A*) Contrast-enhanced CT shows a small, well-circumscribed right upper lobe nodule. (*B*) Contrast-enhanced CT performed 28 days later shows a marked increase in size of right upper lobe lesion. Note that, although volume-doubling time of less than 30 days suggests infection, this can also be seen in lymphoma and rapidly growing metastases.

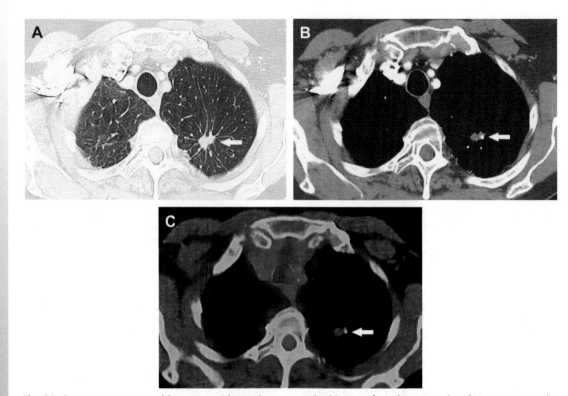

Fig. 14. Seventy-seven-year-old woman with emphysema and a history of smoking 3 packs of cigarettes per day for 40 years. (*A*) Contrast-enhanced CT with lung windows, (*B*) contrast-enhanced CT with mediastinal windows, and (*C*) PET/CT show a hypometabolic, spiculated left apical lung nodule with eccentric calcification (*arrow*). Despite the negative PET, further evaluation (biopsy or resection) is required because of the high clinical suspicion of malignancy owing to the age of the patient, smoking history, emphysema, and nodule characteristics of spiculation and eccentric calcification.

a negative PET will reduce the likelihood of malignancy to 1% and argues for conservative management.[62,63] However, in a patient with a high pretest likelihood of malignancy (80%), a negative PET will only reduce the likelihood of malignancy to 14%.[63,64] Accordingly, obtaining tissue for diagnosis with biopsy or resection would be recommended.

The high sensitivity and specificity of PET in the evaluation of solitary pulmonary nodules pertain to solid nodules of 10 mm or greater in diameter. However, FDG-uptake in malignant ground-glass and partly solid nodules is variable and cannot be used to differentiate benign from malignant lesions. In a recent study, 9 of 10 well-differentiated adenocarcinomas presenting as ground-glass nodular opacities were falsely negative on PET while 4 of 5 benign ground-glass nodular opacities were falsely positive.[65] The sensitivity (10%) and specificity (20%) for ground-glass opacities in this study were significantly lower than that for solid nodules (90% and 71%, respectively). Limitations in spatial resolution can also result in false-negative studies when lesions

smaller than 10 mm in diameter are evaluated.[65,66] With advances in PET technology, the evaluation of nodules of approximately 7 mm is possible.[67] Otherwise, false-negative PET results are uncommon, but may occur with carcinoid tumors and bronchioloalveolar carcinomas (**Fig. 15**).[68–70] The lower positive predictive value relates to the false-positive lesions due to infection and inflammation (**Fig. 16**).

The recent introduction of integrated PET/CT scanners has introduced the near-simultaneous acquisition of coregistered, spatially matched functional and anatomic data. The temporal and spatial fusion of these two data sets can be useful when used as the initial imaging modality in solitary pulmonary opacity characterization.[71] In a study comparing PET/CT and helical dynamic CT in the evaluation of solitary pulmonary nodules, PET/CT was more sensitive (96% vs 81%) and accurate (93% vs 85%) than helical dynamic CT.[71] However, the use of CT for attenuation correction of the PET images has introduced artifacts and quantitative errors that can affect the emission image and lead to misinterpretation.[72]

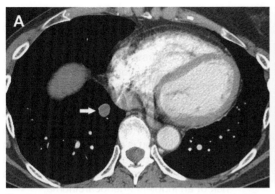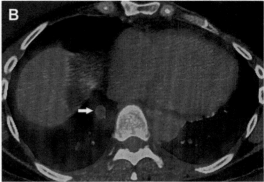

Fig. 15. Sixty-two-year-old woman with endometrial cancer and a right lung nodule detected on a preoperative chest radiograph. (*A*) Contrast-enhanced CT and (*B*) PET/CT show well-circumscribed hypometabolic nodule (*arrow*) in the right lower lobe. Transthoracic needle biopsy revealed a well-differentiated neuroendocrine tumor. Note that false-negative PET results may be seen with carcinoid and bronchioloalveolar carcinoma.

For instance, imaging during different stages of the patient's respiratory cycle may introduce a mismatch between the CT attenuation data obtained during breath-hold and the PET emission data obtained during quiet tidal breathing.[73,74] In addition to localization errors, this misregistration may also result in incorrect attenuation coefficients applied to the PET data that can affect the SUV_{max}, the most widely used parameter to quantify the intensity of FDG uptake.[73,75,76] Misregistration may lead to SUV_{max} being lower than expected and can potentially result in a false-negative study. Strategies to reduce the respiratory mismatch between the CT and PET images include obtaining the CT scan at end expiration, which most closely approximates the lung volumes during PET data acquisition at quiet tidal breathing. However, CT of the lungs at end expiration compromises anatomic detail and small nodules may be obscured. A more recent approach suggests the use of respiratory-averaged CT (CT cine images obtained over different portions of the respiratory cycle using four-dimensional CT techniques) to improve SUV_{max} quantification.[77] Respiratory-averaged CT used for attenuation correction of a PET scan has shown SUV_{max} differences of more than 50% in some lesions as compared with the standard method of CT attenuation using data obtained in the mid-expiratory phase.[77,78]

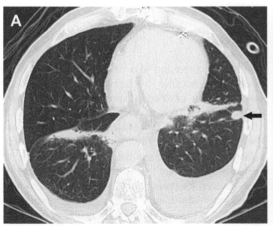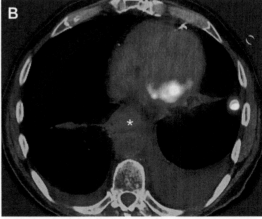

Fig. 16. Seventy-seven-year-old man with an esophageal cancer treated with chemoradiation. (*A*) CT and (*B*) PET/CT show a new well-circumscribed hypermetabolic left lower lobe nodule (*arrow* in *A*) with SUV_{max} of 9.3 suspicious for a metastasis. Asterisk in *B* shows esophageal cancer. Transthoracic needle aspiration biopsy revealed no malignant cells. Fungal elements morphologically consistent with *Cryptococcus* were identified. Note that infectious and inflammatory conditions with increased glucose metabolism can accumulate FDG and be misinterpreted as malignant.

DECISION ANALYSIS

Management algorithms for solitary pulmonary nodules are determined by patients' clinical risk factors as well as nodule characterization. Benign nodules, either because of their pattern of calcification or their stability over a long time, require no further evaluation. Nodules determined to be benign because of their pattern of calcification or their stability over a long time require no further evaluation. However, many nodules remain indeterminate in etiology after comprehensive noninvasive radiologic assessment. At this juncture in decision analysis, management options include observation with imaging reassessment, biopsy, or resection of the nodule. Detection of pulmonary nodules has increased with MDCT and many of these lesions are small (<7 mm) and benign. Multiple factors, including radiation exposure, cost, limited resources, patient anxiety, and the knowledge gleaned from the lung cancer CT screening trials have contributed to the recent release of guidelines for the management of pulmonary nodules discovered incidentally on routine and screening CT by the Fleischner Society[79] and more recently by the American College of Chest Physicians.[80] These guidelines take into consideration lesion size, morphology, and growth rate and patient age and smoking history.[79] In terms of size, small nodules (<4 mm) have a less than 1% chance of being a primary lung cancer, even in people who smoke, while the risk of malignancy increases to 10% to 20% in nodules in the 8-mm range.[79]

FLEISCHNER SOCIETY RECOMMENDATIONS

The following list gives the Fleischner Society's recommendations for an incidentally discovered nodule in an adult patient[79]:

A. Low-risk populations (little or no history of smoking, and no other risk factors)
   1. Nodule equal to or smaller than 4 mm: likelihood of malignancy very small and no reassessment is necessary.
   2. Nodule greater than 4 mm but less than or equal to 6 mm: reassessment CT at 12 months and, if stable, no further evaluation is required. The exception is the nonsolid or partly solid nodule, which may need to be reassessed to exclude the risk of an indolent adenocarcinoma.
   3. Nodule greater than 6 mm but less than or equal to 8 mm: reassessment CT at 6 to 12 months and, if stable, again at 18 to 24 months.
   4. Nodule greater than 8 mm: either reassessment CT scans at 3, 9, and 24 months to assess for stability in size or further evaluation with contrast-enhanced CT, PET/CT, or biopsy or resection.
B. High-risk populations (history of smoking, or other exposure or risk factor)
   1. Nodule equal to or smaller than 4 mm: reassessment at 12 months and, if stable, no further evaluation is required. The exception is the nonsolid or partly solid nodule, which may need to be reassessed to exclude the risk of an indolent adenocarcinoma.
   2. Nodule greater than 4 mm but less than or equal to 6 mm: Reassessment CT at 6 to 12 months and, if stable, again at 18 to 24 months.
   3. Nodule greater than 6 mm but less than or equal to 8 mm: reassessment CT at 3 to 6 months and, if stable, again at 9 to 12 months and at 24 months.
   4. Nodule greater than 8 mm: either reassessment CT at 3, 9, and 24 months to assess stability or perform contrast-enhanced CT, PET/CT, or biopsy or resection.

The Fleischner recommendations do not apply to patients with a history of malignancy, patients under 35 years with low risk of lung cancer, and in those patients with fever in which the nodules may be infectious.[79] For nodule reassessment, a noncontrast, thin-collimation, limited-coverage, low-dose CT scan is recommended by the Fleischner Society.[79] An example of a low-dose protocol is a 120-kilovolt (peak), 40–50-mAs algorithm reconstructed at 2.5 mm slice thickness with 2-mm intervals.

SUMMARY

With the increasing use of MDCT, more solitary pulmonary nodules are being detected. Although the majority of these lesions are benign, lung cancer constitutes an important consideration in the differential diagnosis of solitary pulmonary nodules. The goal of management is to correctly differentiate malignant from benign nodules to ensure appropriate treatment. Stratifying patients' risk factors for malignancy, including patient age, smoking history, and history of malignancy, is essential in the management of solitary pulmonary nodules. In terms of radiologic evaluation, obtaining prior films is important to assess for nodule growth. The detection of certain patterns of calcification and stability for 2 years or more have historically been the only useful findings for determining whether a nodule is or is not benign.

However, recent technological advances in imaging, including MDCT and PET/CT, have improved nodule characterization and surveillance. For solid nodules, CT enhancement of less than 15 HU and hypometabolism on PET (SUV_{max} <2.5) favor a benign etiology. Potential pitfalls in nodule enhancement and PET evaluation of solitary pulmonary nodules include infectious and inflammatory conditions. Stratified according to patient risk factors for malignancy and nodule size, recent guidelines for the management of incidentally detected small pulmonary nodules have been useful in decision analysis. An important exception to these guidelines is the evaluation and management of the subsolid nodule. These lesions are not suitable for CT enhancement studies and may show low metabolic activity on PET imaging. Due to their association with bronchioloalveolar carcinoma and adenocarcinoma, subsolid nodules require a more aggressive approach in terms of reassessing serial imaging and/or obtaining tissue diagnosis. As data from the low-dose CT lung cancer screening trials are analyzed and further studies with new imaging techniques are performed, management strategies for the imaging evaluation of the solitary pulmonary nodule will continue to evolve.

REFERENCES

1. Austin JH, Muller NL, Friedman PJ, et al. Glossary of terms for CT of the lungs: recommendations of the Nomenclature Committee of the Fleischner Society. Radiology 1996;200(2):327–31.
2. Swensen SJ, Jett JR, Hartman TE, et al. CT screening for lung cancer: five-year prospective experience. Radiology 2005;235(1):259–65.
3. American Cancer Society. Cancer facts and figures 2006. Atlanta (GA): American Cancer Society; 2006.
4. Viggiano RW, Swensen SJ, Rosenow EC III. Evaluation and management of solitary and multiple pulmonary nodules. Clin Chest Med 1992;13:83–95.
5. Mountain CF. Revisions in the international system for staging lung cancer. Chest 1997;111:1710–7.
6. Coakley FV, Cohen MD, Johnson MS, et al. Maximum intensity projection images in the detection of simulated pulmonary nodules by spiral CT. Br J Radiol 1998;71(842):135–40.
7. Gruden JF, Ouanounou S, Tigges S, et al. Incremental benefit of maximum-intensity-projection images on observer detection of small pulmonary nodules revealed by MDCT. Am J Roentgenol 2002;179:149–57.
8. Girvin F, Ko JP. Pulmonary nodules: detection, assessment, and CAD. Am J Roentgenol 2008; 191:1057–69.
9. Gurney JW, Lyddon DM, McKay JA. Determining the likelihood of malignancy in solitary pulmonary nodules with Bayesian analysis. Part II. Application. Radiology 1993;186:415–22.
10. Lee HJ, Im JG, Ahn JM, et al. Lung cancer in patients with idiopathic pulmonary fibrosis: CT findings. J Comput Assist Tomogr 1996;20(6):979–82.
11. Bailey-Wilson JE, Amos CI, Pinney SM, et al. A major lung cancer susceptibility locus maps to chromosome 6q2325. Am J Hum Genet 2004;75:460–74.
12. Ginsberg MS, Griff SK, Go BD, et al. Pulmonary nodules resected at video-assisted thoracoscopic surgery: etiology in 426 patients. Radiology 1999; 213(1):277–82.
13. Herder GJ, van Tinteren H, Golding RP, et al. Clinical prediction model to characterize pulmonary nodules: validation and added value of 18F-fluorodeoxyglucose positron emission tomography. Chest 2005;128(4):2490–6.
14. Seltzer SE, Judy PF, Adams DF, et al. Spiral CT of the chest: comparison of cine and film-based viewing. Radiology 1995;197(1):73–8.
15. Henschke CI, McCauley DI, Yankelevitz DF, et al. Early lung cancer action project: overall design and findings from baseline screening. Lancet 1999;354:99–105.
16. Kaneko M, Eguchi K, Ohmatsu H, et al. Peripheral lung cancer: screening and detection with low-dose spiral CT versus radiography. Radiology 1996;201:798–802.
17. Sone S, Takashima S, Li F, et al. Mass screening for lung cancer with mobile spiral computed tomography scanner. Lancet 1998;351(9111):1242–5.
18. Zerhouni EA, Stitik FP, Siegelman SS, et al. CT of the pulmonary nodule: a cooperative study. Radiology 1986;160:319–27.
19. Zwirewich CV, Vedal S, Miller RR, et al. Solitary pulmonary nodule: high-resolution CT and radiologic-pathologic correlation. Radiology 1991;179:469–76.
20. Heitzman ER, Markarian B, Raasch BN, et al. Pathways of tumor spread through the lung: radiologic correlations with anatomy and pathology. Radiology 1982;144(1):3–14.
21. Winer-Muram HT. The solitary pulmonary nodule. Radiology 2006;239(1):34–49.
22. Lee YR, Choi YW, Lee KJ, et al. CT halo sign: the spectrum of pulmonary diseases. Br J Radiol 2005;78:862–5.
23. Kim SJ, Lee KS, Ryu YH, et al. Reversed halo sign on high-resolution CT of cryptogenic organizing pneumonia: diagnostic implications. Am J Roentgenol 2003;180:1251–4.
24. Wahba H, Truong MT, Lei X, et al. Reversed halo sign in invasive pulmonary fungal infections. Clin Infect Dis 2008;46(11):1733–7.
25. Siegelman SS, Khouri NF, Scott WW Jr, et al. Pulmonary hamartoma: CT findings. Radiology 1986;160:313–7.

26. Muram TM, Aisen A. Fatty metastatic lesions in 2 patients with renal clear-cell carcinoma. J Comput Assist Tomogr 2003;27(6):869–70.

27. Siegelman SS, Khouri NF, Leo FP, et al. Solitary pulmonary nodules: CT assessment. Radiology 1986;160(2):307–12.

28. Siegelman SS, Zerhouni EA, Leo FP, et al. CT of the solitary pulmonary nodule. Am J Roentgenol 1980; 135:1–13.

29. Johnson TR, Krauss B, Sedlmair M, et al. Material differentiation by dual energy CT: initial experience. Eur Radiol 2007;17:1510–7.

30. Higashi Y, Nakamura H, Matsumoto T, et al. Dual-energy computed tomographic diagnosis of pulmonary nodules. J Thorac Imaging 1994;9(1):31–4.

31. Bhalla M, Shepard JA, Nakamura K, et al. Dual kV CT to detect calcification in solitary pulmonary nodule. J Comput Assist Tomogr 1995;19(1):44–7.

32. Swensen SJ, Yamashita K, McCollough CH, et al. Lung nodules: dual-kilovolt peak analysis with CT-multicenter study. Radiology 2000;214:81–5.

33. Seo JB, Im JG, Goo JM, et al. Atypical pulmonary metastases: spectrum of radiologic findings. Radiographics 2001;21(2):403–17.

34. O'Keefe ME, Good CA, McDonald JR. Calcification in solitary nodules of the lung. Am J Roentgenol 1957;77:1023–33.

35. Grewal RG, Austin JHM. CT demonstration of calcification in carcinoma of the lung. J Comput Assist Tomogr 1994;18:867–71.

36. Mahoney MC, Shipley RT, Corcoran HL, et al. CT demonstration of calcification in carcinoma of the lung. Am J Roentgenol 1990;154:255–8.

37. Henschke CI, Yankelevitz DF, Mirtcheva R, et al. CT screening for lung cancer: frequency and significance of part-solid and nonsolid nodules. Am J Roentgenol 2002;178:1053–7.

38. Noguchi M, Shimosato Y. The development and progression of adenocarcinoma of the lung. Cancer Treat Res 1995;72:131–42.

39. Colby TV, Wistuba II, Gazdar A. Precursors to pulmonary neoplasia. Adv Anat Pathol 1998;5: 205–15.

40. Yang ZG, Sone S, Takashima S, et al. High-resolution CT analysis of small peripheral lung adenocarcinomas revealed on screening helical CT. Am J Roentgenol 2001;176:1399–407.

41. Ohta Y, Shimizu Y, Kobayashi T, et al. Pathologic and biological assessment of lung tumors showing ground-glass opacity. Ann Thorac Surg 2006;81: 1194–7.

42. Woodring JH, Fried AM. Significance of wall thickness in solitary cavities of the lung: a follow-up study. Am J Roentgenol 1983;140:473–4.

43. Woodring JH, Fried AM, Chuang VP. Solitary cavities of the lung: diagnostic implications of cavity wall thickness. Am J Roentgenol 1980;135:1269–71.

44. Kui M, Templeton PA, White CS, et al. Evaluation of the air bronchogram sign on CT in solitary pulmonary lesions. J Comput Assist Tomogr 1996;20(6): 983–6.

45. Keogan MT, Tung KT, Kaplan DK, et al. The significance of pulmonary nodules detected on CT staging for lung cancer. Clin Radiol 1993;48(2):94–6.

46. Kunitoh H, Eguchi K, Yamada K, et al. Intrapulmonary sublesions detected before surgery in patients with lung cancer. Cancer 1992;70(7):1876–9.

47. Shimizu N, Ando A, Date H, et al. Prognosis of undetected intrapulmonary metastases in resected lung cancer. Cancer 1993;71(12):3868–72.

48. Lillington GA, Caskey CI. Evaluation and management of solitary multiple pulmonary nodules. Clin Chest Med 1993;14:111–9.

49. Good CA, Wilson TW. The solitary circumscribed pulmonary nodule. JAMA 1958;166:210–5.

50. Good CA. Management of patient with solitary mass in lung. Chic Med Soc Bull 1953;55:893–6.

51. Aoki T, Nakata H, Watanabe H, et al. Evolution of peripheral lung adenocarcinomas: CT findings correlated with histology and tumor doubling time. Am J Roentgenol 2000;174:763–8.

52. Hasegawa M, Sone S, Takashima S, et al. Growth rate of small lung cancers detected on mass CT screening. Br J Radiol 2000;73(876):1252–9.

53. Revel MP, Bissery A, Bienvenu M, et al. Are two-dimensional CT measurements of small noncalcified pulmonary nodules reliable? Radiology 2004;231(2): 453–8.

54. Erasmus JJ, Gladish GW, Broemeling L, et al. Interobserver and intraobserver variability in measurement of non-small-cell carcinoma lung lesions: implications for assessment of tumor response. J Clin Oncol 2003;21(13):2574–82.

55. Yankelevitz DF, Reeves AP, Kostis WJ, et al. Small pulmonary nodules: volumetrically determined growth rates based on CT evaluation. Radiology 2000;217(1):251–6.

56. Revel MP, Merlin A, Peyrard S, et al. Software volumetric evaluation of doubling times for differentiating benign versus malignant pulmonary nodules. Am J Roentgenol 2006;187(1):135–42.

57. Swensen SJ, Viggiano RW, Midthun DE, et al. Lung nodule enhancement at CT: multicenter study. Radiology 2000;214(1):73–80.

58. Yamashita K, Matsunobe S, Tsuda T, et al. Solitary pulmonary nodule: preliminary study of evaluation with incremental dynamic CT. Radiology 1995;194: 399–405.

59. Zhang M, Kono M. Solitary pulmonary nodules: evaluation of blood flow patterns with dynamic CT. Radiology 1997;205(2):471–8.

60. Shah SK, McNitt-Gray MF, Rogers SR, et al. Computer aided characterization of the solitary pulmonary nodule using volumetric and contrast

enhancement features. Acad Radiol 2005;12(10):1310–9.

61. Lowe VJ, Hoffman JM, DeLong DM, et al. Semiquantitative and visual analysis of FDG-PET images in pulmonary abnormalities. J Nucl Med 1994;35:1771–6.

62. Gould MK, Maclean CC, Kuschner WG, et al. Accuracy of positron emission tomography for diagnosis of pulmonary nodules and mass lesions: a meta-analysis. JAMA 2001;285(7):914–24.

63. Tan BB, Flaherty KR, Kazerooni EA, et al. American College of Chest Physicians. The solitary pulmonary nodule. Chest 2003;123(Suppl 1):89S–96S.

64. Gould MK, Ananth L, Barnett PG, et al. Veterans Affairs SNAP Cooperative Study Group. A clinical model to estimate the pretest probability of lung cancer in patients with solitary pulmonary nodules. Chest 2007;131(2):383–8.

65. Nomori H, Watanabe K, Ohtsuka T, et al. Evaluation of F-18 fluorodeoxyglucose (FDG) PET scanning for pulmonary nodules less than 3 cm in diameter, with special reference to the CT images. Lung Cancer 2004;45(1):19–27.

66. Lowe VJ, Fletcher JW, Gobar L, et al. Prospective investigation of PET in lung nodules (PIOPILN). J Clin Oncol 1998;16:1075–84.

67. Herder GJ, Golding RP, Hoekstra OS, et al. The performance of (18)F-fluorodeoxyglucose positron emission tomography in small solitary pulmonary nodules. Eur J Nucl Med Mol Imaging 2004;31:1231–6.

68. Erasmus JJ, McAdams HP, Patz EF Jr, et al. Evaluation of primary pulmonary carcinoid tumors using FDG PET. Am J Roentgenol 1998;170:1369–73.

69. Higashi K, Ueda Y, Seki H, et al. Fluorine-18-FDG PET imaging is negative in bronchioloalveolar lung carcinoma. J Nucl Med 1998;39(6):1016–20.

70. Sabloff BS, Truong MT, Wistuba II, et al. Bronchioalveolar cell carcinoma: radiologic appearance and dilemmas in the assessment of response. Clin Lung Cancer 2004;6(2):108–12.

71. Yi CA, Lee KS, Kim BT, et al. Tissue characterization of solitary pulmonary nodule: comparative study between helical dynamic CT and integrated PET/CT. J Nucl Med 2006;47(3):443–50.

72. Cook GJR, Wegner EA, Fogelman I. Pitfalls and artifacts in 18FDG PET and PET/CT oncologic imaging. Semin Nucl Med 2004;34(2):122–33.

73. Beyer T, Antoch G, Blodgett T, et al. Dual-modality PET/CT imaging: the effect of respiratory motion on combined image quality in clinical oncology. Eur J Nucl Med Mol Imaging 2003;30(4):588–96.

74. Osman MM, Cohade C, Nakamoto Y, et al. Respiratory motion artifacts on PET emission images obtained using CT attenuation correction on PET-CT. Eur J Nucl Med Mol Imaging 2003;30(4):603–6.

75. Goerres GW, Kamel E, Heidelberg TN, et al. PET-CT image co-registration in the thorax: influence of respiration. Eur J Nucl Med Mol Imaging 2002;29(3):351–60.

76. Goerres GW, Burger C, Kamel E, et al. Respiration-induced attenuation artifact at PET/CT: technical considerations. Radiology 2003;226(3):906–10.

77. Pan T, Mawlawi O, Nehmeh SA, et al. Attenuation correction of PET images with respiration-averaged CT images in PET/CT. J Nucl Med 2005;46(9):1481–7.

78. Truong MT, Pan T, Erasmus JJ. Pitfalls in integrated CT-PET of the thorax: implications in oncologic imaging. J Thorac Imaging 2006;21(2):111–22.

79. MacMahon H, Austin JH, Gamsu G, et al. Fleischner Society. Guidelines for management of small pulmonary nodules detected on CT scans: a statement from the Fleischner Society. Radiology 2005;237(2):395–400.

80. Gould MK, Fletcher J, Iannettoni MD, et al. American College of Chest Physicians. Evaluation of patients with pulmonary nodules: when is it lung cancer?: ACCP evidence-based clinical practice guidelines (2nd edition). Chest 2007;132(Suppl 3):108S–30S.

PET Versus PET/CT Dual-Modality Imaging in Evaluation of Lung Cancer

Lutz S. Freudenberg, MD, MA, MBA[a],*,
Sandra J. Rosenbaum, MD[a], Thomas Beyer, PhD[a],
Andreas Bockisch, PhD, MD[a], Gerald Antoch, MD[b]

KEYWORDS
- PET/CT • NSCLC • Lung cancer

Lung cancer is the leading cause of tumor-related deaths.[1] Although rates of bronchial carcinoma–related death in men have decreased on average by 1.8% annually during the past decade, the incidence of lung cancer in women is increasing.[1] Non–small cell lung cancer (NSCLC) accounts for approximately 80% of bronchogenic malignancies. Among the 150 factors that help determine NSCLC prognosis, the tumor stage, as defined by the American Joint Committee on Cancer is considered to be the most important.[2,3] Thus, the choice of therapy options, including surgery, radiation therapy, and chemotherapy—used alone or in combination[4,5]—is based on the tumor stage. Consequently, the accurate determination of tumor size, potential infiltration of adjacent structures, mediastinal lymph node involvement, and the detection of distant metastases are of central importance. Especially the diagnosis of contralateral lymph node metastases and distant metastases is crucial (stage IIIB and stage V) as these exclude a curative therapeutic approach.[6]

In general, morphological imaging with CT is the method of choice to define the extent of the primary tumor and to assess the tumor. However, one of the main limitations of CT is that it has a low accuracy when differentiating benign from malignant lymph nodes using a size criterion of 1 cm for mediastinal nodes and 7 mm for hilar nodes.[7–9] The limitations of this size-based node characterization system is well documented: up to 21% of nodes smaller than 10 mm are malignant, whereas 40% of nodes larger than 10 mm are benign.[8–11]

In contrast, metabolic imaging using fluorine-18-2-fluoro-2-deoxy-D-glucose (FDG) positron emission tomography (PET) has been shown to be substantially more sensitive and specific in the detection and characterization of metastases to mediastinal lymph nodes (**Fig. 1**). Several studies compared the accuracy of CT and FDG-PET:[6,11–14] in a meta-analysis on staging lung cancer with PET and CT, Dwamena and colleagues[11] concluded that FDG-PET was significantly more accurate than CT and reported sensitivity and specificity values of 79% and 91% for PET and 60% and 77% for CT, respectively. Weber and colleagues,[6] in a recent meta-analysis according to the Agency for Health Care Policy Research criteria, reported a significantly increased sensitivity and specificity of FDG-PET compared with CT in assessment of mediastinal lymph nodes and distant metastases with a sensitivity of 83% (95% CI: 75%–89%), and

This article originally appeared in *PET Clinics*, Volume 1, Issue 4, October 2006.
[a] Department of Nuclear Medicine, University of Duisburg, Hufelandstrasse 55 D-45122, Essen, Germany
[b] Department of Diagnostic and Interventional Radiology, University of Duisburg, Hufelandstrasse 55, D-45122 Essen, Germany
* Corresponding author.
E-mail address: lutz.freudenberg@uni-essen.de (L.S. Freudenberg).

Thorac Surg Clin 20 (2010) 25–30
doi:10.1016/j.thorsurg.2009.12.003
1547-4127/10/$ – see front matter

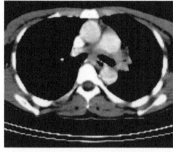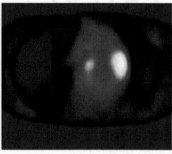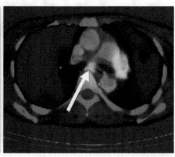

Fig. 1. CT (*left*), FDG-PET (*middle*), and FDG-PET/CT (*right*) of a 49-year-old male with diagnosis of NSCLC before neoadjuvant combined radiotherapy/chemotherapy. CT and FDG-PET clearly visualize a vital hilar metastasis. FDG-PET additionally shows additional tracer-uptake mediastinally. Exact localization is difficult due to little anatomic detail, CT alone is ambiguous. Integrated FDG-PET/CT allows diagnosis of a vital infracarinal metastasis (*arrow*).

96% (95% CI: 89%–99%), respectively. Based on FDG-PET findings, 18% of the patients received a different therapy compared with CT.[6]

On the other hand, limited anatomic information in FDG-PET images frequently renders localization of a lesion and its potential infiltration into adjacent organs difficult.[15,16] Thus, for maximal diagnostic benefit, functional data sets should be read in conjunction with morphologic images. Image fusion and side-by-side image evaluation of morphologic and functional data sets have been proposed.[17] However, differences in patient positioning and motion-induced data misregistration cause image fusion of separately acquired CT and PET image sets to be complex and often unsatisfactory.[18,19] This limitation can be overcome by collecting functional and morphologic data in one examination. The availability of dual-modality PET/CT tomographs provides the technical basis for intrinsically aligned functional and morphologic data sets.[19]

The purpose of this article is to summarize the accuracy of dual-modality FDG-PET/CT imaging in staging of NSCLC as compared with FDG-PET alone, and with FDG-PET as well as CT read side by side. Furthermore, an optimized PET/CT protocol for patients who have lung cancer is outlined.

FDG-PET/CT VERSUS FDG-PET

Several studies have reported a higher sensitivity of FDG-PET/CT compared with FDG-PET alone.

For tumor staging, the sole use of conventional FDG-PET is limited based on the limited anatomical data. Thus, tumor size and a potential infiltration may be difficult to assess on PET alone. It has been shown in recent studies that in tumor staging of patients who have lung cancer, analysis of integrated FDG-PET/CT images is superior to that of FDG-PET or CT images alone when assessing the tumor stage.[20–23] The integration of

morphologic CT and functional PET data sets particularly enables the most accurate differentiation of viable tumor tissue relative to all adjacent structures (eg, differentiation of tumor from atelectasis, detection of focal chest wall infiltration or mediastinal invasion) (**Fig. 2**).[20–22,24]

Furthermore, PET/CT resulted in further improvement of N staging compared with PET alone due to the ability to reveal the exact location of metastatic lymph nodes: accurate anatomic correlation is of benefit for exact localization of a solitary lymph node metastasis and thus allows exact classification as N1 or N2 disease, which is difficult but important.[25] Furthermore, FDG-PET/CT is important when identifying supraclavicular N3 disease (**Fig. 3**).[20,22,23,26] Results of recent studies with respect to the tumor–node–metastasis (TNM) system are summarized in **Table 1**. These studies reported significant advantages of FDG-PET/CT compared with FDG-PET alone.

It is generally concluded that dual-modality PET/CT represents the most efficient and accurate approach to NSCLC staging, with a profound effect on therapy and, hence, patient prognosis.[20,22,23,26,27] Antoch and colleagues[26] described that PET/CT findings led to a change

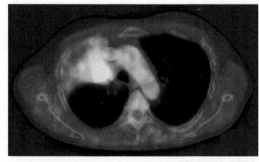

Fig. 2. FDG-PET/CT of a 47-year-old male with diagnosis of NSCLC before first treatment. Integrated FDG-PET/CT enables the most accurate differentiation of viable tumor tissue relative to atelectasis.

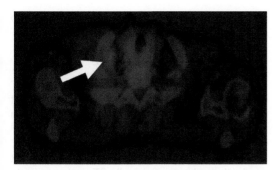

Fig. 3. FDG-PET/CT of a 54-year-old male with NSCLC (pancoast-tumor) showing a supraclavicular lymph node metastasis 0.5 cm in diameter not visible in CT alone and unambiguous in FDG-PET.

in tumor stage in 26% of patients compared with PET data alone, resulting in a change of treatment plans in 15%. Cerfolio and colleagues,[20] Lardinois and colleagues,[22] and Aquino and colleagues[23] likewise found tumor staging was significantly more accurate with integrated PET-CT than with PET alone, especially for stage I and stage II (see **Table 1**).[20,22,23,26,27]

In conclusion, dual-modality FDG-PET/CT data enabled more accurate staging of NSCLC than either FDG-PET or CT, reflecting the inherent limitations of these two imaging modalities when used alone. However, as Buell and colleagues[24] argue, the somewhat unrealistic comparisons of FDG-PET alone with integrated FDG-PET/CT must show an advantage for FDG-PET/CT. To allow for a more balanced study design that reflects clinical reality, FDG-PET/CT must be compared with a side-by-side evaluation of conventional FDG-PET and CT scans.

FDG-PET/CT VERSUS FDG-PET AND CT READ SIDE BY SIDE

In general, visual correlation of CT and FDG-PET improves interpretation of both datasets.[24,28] For image coregistration, computer-assisted support appears helpful. However, in clinical practice, routine acceptance of retrospective image fusion may be limited by the complexity of retrospective coregistration algorithms and their limited accuracy for aligning areas of interest in independently acquired scans. Nonlinear registration techniques are required to account for complex patient motion, especially in the thorax and upper abdomen.[29]

Several investigators have studied the impact of software image fusion in NSCLC showing significant improvement in staging of fused CT and FDG-PET data compared with FDG-PET alone.[21,23,24,30] However, Vansteenkiste and colleagues[30] reported no significant differences between image fusion of FDG-PET and CT data compared with visual correlation. Halpern and colleagues[21] as well as Buell and colleagues[24] describe advantages of software fusion with regard to the T stage and the N stage when compared with FDG-PET alone.

Lardinois and colleagues[22] reported significant advantages of FDG-PET/CT over FDG-PET and CT read side by side when examining 50 patients who have surgically staged NSCLC. They report a diagnostic accuracy for integrated FDG-PET/CT and visual correlation of FDG-PET and CT of 89% and 77%, respectively. This difference was statistically significant. Furthermore, they found additional information by FDG-PET/CT in 41%

Table 1
Sensitivity of FDG-PET versus FDG-PET/CT with respect to TNM and overall tumor staging (I–IV) according to American Joint Committee on Cancer

Study	Patients	TNM	FDG-PET	FDG-PET/CT	P Value
Cerfolio et al[20]	129	T	38%–70%	50%–100%	.001
		N	60%–80%	77%–92%	.008
		M	81%–82%	90%–92%	NS
		Overall staging	17%–83%	50%–94%	NR
Halpern et al[21]	36	T	67%	97%	<.05
		Overall staging	57%	83%	<.05
Lardinois et al[22]	50	N	49%	93%	.013
		Overall staging	40%	88%	.001
Aquino et al[23]	45	N	59%–76%	71%–76%	.01
		Overall staging	53%–62%	73%–76%	.002
Antoch et al[26]	27	Overall staging	74%	96%	<.05
Shim et al[27]	106	N	–	85%	–
Keidar et al[31]	42	Restaging	96%	96%	NS

Abbreviations: NR, not reported; NS, not significant.

of their patients. However, as Buell and colleagues[24] note, this advantage of PET/CT was achieved by evaluating a multitude of different parameters, some of which were only of limited clinical relevance. Keidar and colleagues[31] performed a study addressing the diagnostic value of FDG-PET/CT versus FDG-PET and CT read side by side in suspected lung cancer recurrence showing no differences in sensitivity. Although FDG-PET/CT performed better with respect to specificity and positive predictive values, these results did not reach the level of statistical significance.

Two recent studies evaluated the accuracy of PET/CT and included oncology patients who have different malignancies. Their results are of interest with respect to NSCLC, because patients who have lung cancer represent the largest patient cohort within both patient populations. Antoch and colleagues[32] evaluated FDG-PET/CT for tumor staging in 260 patients who have solid tumors (57 patients who have NSCLC) and conclude that FDG-PET/CT is able to detect significantly more lesions than FDG-PET or CT alone. Based on a change in the TNM stage, they reported a change in patient management in 6% of patients who have FDG-PET/CT compared with FDG-PET and CT evaluated side by side. Buell and colleagues[24] evaluated side-by-side analysis of CT and conventional FDG-PET in 733 patients (174 who have bronchial cancer) with respect to patient groups that may benefit the most from the integrated PET/CT scanners. They showed that side-by-side reading of FDG-PET and CT failed to yield conclusive data with regard to lesion characterization in only 7.4% of patients so FDG-PET/CT might have been helpful in these cases.

Until now, only one study has evaluated the differences of integrated FDG-PET/CT versus software-based image fusion in NSCLC. Halpern and colleagues[21] reported equal results with regard to the T stage and the N stage for image fusion and PET/CT in cases in which software fusion was successful. However, software fusion of separately obtained PET and CT studies was successful in only 68% of the patients and failed in 32%. As stated by the authors, the performance of software fusion can significantly be improved when including transmission PET scans to a success rate from approximately 70% to 95%.[33]

Further studies will have to evaluate the impact of integrated FDG-PET/CT versus software fusion keeping in mind that misregistration is not totally avoidable even with a combined PET/CT scanner.[34,35] Finally, the actual impact of more accurate tumor staging—beyond therapeutic decision making—on patient survival will have to be determined in future studies.

OPTIMIZED PET/CT PROTOCOL

Local misregistration between the CT and the PET in integrated PET/CT and the use of CT contrast media may bias the PET tracer distribution following CT-based attenuation correction.[36] Consequently, protocol requirements for PET/CT with diagnostic CT include alternative contrast application schemes to handle CT contrast agents appropriately. In addition, a special breathing protocol can avoid motion-induced artifacts in the area of the diaphragm. Using an optimized acquisition protocol significantly improves integrated PET/CT imaging and thus can further improve staging of NSCLC.

Breathing

The coregistration accuracy in combined PET/CT imaging is mainly impaired by respiration-induced mismatches between the CT and the PET. These artifacts are particularly severe when standard breath-hold techniques (eg, scanning at maximum inspiration) are transferred directly from clinical CT to combined PET/CT without further adaptation.[34] Goerres and colleagues[37] investigated the misregistration of pulmonary lesions with a combined PET/CT system and detected the mismatch between PET and CT to be most severe if the CT was performed during maximal inspiration of the patient. The registration error was found to be in the range of 5 to 33 mm in this setting.[37,38] Combined PET/CT scans during normal respiration go along with respiration artifacts in the majority of cases as well. To reduce potential misregistration from differences in the breathing pattern between two complementary PET and CT data sets, our protocol uses a limited breath-hold technique: patients are asked to hold their breath in normal expiration only for the time that the CT takes to cover the lower lung and liver, which is typically less than 15 seconds. Instructing the patient before the PET/CT examinations on the breath-hold command is essential in avoiding serious respiration artifacts.[39] When applying the limited breath-hold technique, the frequency of severe artifacts in the area of the diaphragm was reduced by half, and the spatial extent of respiration-induced artifacts can be reduced by at least 40% compared with the acquisition protocols without any breathing instructions.[39]

With the introduction of multirow CT technology of up to 64 detector rows into PET/CT designs, the incidence of respiration artifacts in PET/CT examinations can further be reduced. This applies also to patients who are unable to follow any breath-hold instructions. For PET/CT imaging of normally breathing patients, a substantial improvement of image quality can be expected from employing CT technology with six or more detector rows as respiration-induced artifacts are reduced in both magnitude and prominence.[38,40] In conclusion, special breathing protocols are effective and should be used for CT scans as part of combined imaging protocols in dual-modality PET/CT.

Contrast Agents

Standard application of intravenous CT contrast agents in combined PET/CT may lead to high-density artifacts on CT and attenuation-corrected PET.[35] To avoid associated diagnostic pitfalls, a special contrast injection protocol is needed. Comparing different protocols, Beyer and colleagues[41] found a reproducible high image quality in the CT image and in the attenuation-corrected PET image without high-density image artifacts when using a dual-phase injection (80 and 60 mL at 3 and 1.5 mL/s, respectively) of contrast agent in the caudocranial direction with a 50-second delay.

SUMMARY

Software coregistration of FDG-PET and CT datasets as well as integrated FDG-PET/CT enable significantly more accurate assessment of NSCLC staging than either modality alone. Integrated FDG-PET/CT has been shown to be more accurate in NSCLC staging than FDG-PET and CT read side by side. However, the benefits of anatometabolic imaging using FDG-PET/CT can only be fully exploited if optimized acquisition protocols are implemented.

REFERENCES

1. Jemal A, Thomas A, Murray T, et al. Cancer statistics, 2002. CA Cancer J Clin 2002;52:23–47.
2. Brundage MD, Davies D, Mackillop WJ. Prognostic factors in non-small cell lung cancer: a decade of progress. Chest 2002;122:1037–57.
3. Greene FL, Page DL, Fleming ID, et al. AJCC cancer staging manual. 6th edition. New York: Springer; 2002.
4. Smythe WR. Treatment of stage I and II non-small cell lung cancer. Cancer Control 2001;8:318–25.
5. Haura EB. Treatment of advanced nonsmall cell lung cancer: a review of current randomised clinical trials and an examination of emerging therapies. Cancer Control 2001;8:326–36.
6. Weber WA, Dietlein M, Hellwig D, et al. PET with (18)F-fluorodeoxyglucose for staging of non-small cell lung cancer. Nuklearmedizin 2003;42:135–44.
7. Glazer GM, Gross BH, Quint LE, et al. Normal mediastinal lymph nodes: number and size according to American Thoracic Society mapping. AJR Am J Roentgenol 1985;144:261–5.
8. Lowe VJ, DeLong DM, Hoffman JM, et al. Optimum scanning protocol for FDGPET evaluation of pulmonary malignancy. J Nucl Med 1995;36:883–7.
9. Deslauriers J, Gregoire J. Clinical and surgical staging of non-small cell lung cancer. Chest 2000; 117:96S–103S.
10. Staples CA, Muller NL, Miller RR, et al. Mediastinal nodes in bronchogenic carcinoma: comparison between CT and mediastinoscopy. Radiology 1988; 167:367–72.
11. Dwamena BA, Sonnad SS, Angobaldo JO, et al. Metastases from non-small cell lung cancer: mediastinal staging in the 1990s–meta-analytic comparison of PET and CT. Radiology 1999;213:530–6.
12. Adams S, Baum RP, Stuckensen T, et al. Prospective comparison of 18F-FDG PET with conventional imaging modalities (CT, MRI, US) in lymph node staging of head and neck cancer. Eur J Nucl Med 1998;25:1255–60.
13. Marom EM, McAdams HP, Erasmus JJ, et al. Staging non-small cell lung cancer with whole-body PET. Radiology 1999;212:803–9.
14. van Tinteren H, Hoekstra OS, Smit EF, et al. Effectiveness of positron emission tomography in the preoperative assessment of patients with suspected non-small-cell lung cancer: the PLUS multicentre randomised trial. Lancet 2002;359:1388–93.
15. Diederichs CG, Staib L, Vogel J, et al. Values and limitations of 18F-fluorodeoxyglucosepositron-emission tomography with preoperative evaluation of patients with pancreatic masses. Pancreas 2000; 20:109–16.
16. Weber WA, Avril N, Schwaiger M. Relevance of positron emission tomography (PET) in oncology. Strahlenther Onkol 1999;175:356–73.
17. Wahl RL, Quint LE, Cieslak RD, et al. "Anatometabolic" tumor imaging: fusion of FDG PET with CT or MRI to localize foci of increased activity. J Nucl Med 1993;34:1190–7.
18. Townsend DW. A combined PET/CT scanner: the choices. J Nucl Med 2001;42:533–4.
19. Beyer T, Townsend DW, Blodgett TM. Dual-modality PET/CT tomography for clinical oncology. Q J Nucl Med 2002;46:24–34.
20. Cerfolio RJ, Ojha B, Bryant AS, et al. The accuracy of integrated PET-CT compared with dedicated PET alone for the staging of patients with nonsmall cell lung cancer. Ann Thorac Surg 2004;78:1017–23.
21. Halpern BS, Schiepers C, Weber WA, et al. Presurgical staging of non-small cell lung cancer: positron

emission tomography, integrated positron emission tomography/CT, and software image fusion. Chest 2005;128:2289–97.

22. Lardinois D, Weder W, Hany TF, et al. Staging of non-small-cell lung cancer with integrated positron-emission tomography and computed tomography. N Engl J Med 2003;19:2500–7.

23. Aquino SL, Asmuth JC, Alpert NM, et al. Improved radiologic staging of lung cancer with 2-[18F]-fluoro-2-deoxy-D-glucose-positron emission tomography and computed tomography registration. J Comput Assist Tomogr 2003;27:479–84.

24. Buell U, Wieres FJ, Schneider W, et al. 18FDG-PET in 733 consecutive patients with or without side-by-side CT evaluation: analysis of 921 lesions. Nuklearmedizin 2004;43:210–6.

25. Asamura H, Suzuki K, Kondo H, et al. Where is the boundary between N1 and N2 stations in lung cancer? Ann Thorac Surg 2000;70:1839–45.

26. Antoch G, Stattaus J, Nemat AT, et al. Non-small cell lung cancer: dual-modality PET/CT in preoperative staging. Radiology 2003;229:526–33.

27. Shim SS, Lee KS, Kim BT, et al. Non-small cell lung cancer: prospective comparison of integrated FDG PET/CT and CT alone for preoperative staging. Radiology 2005;236:1011–9.

28. Reinartz P, Wieres FJ, Schneider W, et al. Side-by-side reading of PET and CT scans in oncology: which patients might profit from integrated PET/CT? Eur J Nucl Med Mol Imaging 2004;31:1456–61.

29. Hutton BF, Braun M. Software for image registration: algorithms, accuracy, efficacy. Sem Nucl Med 2003;33:180–92.

30. Vansteenkiste JF, Stroobants SG, Dupont PJ, et al. FDG-PET scan in potentially operable non-small cell lung cancer: do anatometabolic PET-CT fusion images improve the localisation of regional lymph node metastases? The Leuven Lung Cancer Group. Eur J Nucl Med 1998;25:1495–501.

31. Keidar Z, Haim N, Guralnik L, et al. PET/CT using 18F-FDG in suspected lung cancer recurrence:

diagnostic value and impact on patient management. J Nucl Med 2004;45:1640–6.

32. Antoch G, Saoudi N, Kuehl H, et al. Accuracy of whole-body dual-modality fluorine-18–2-fluoro-2-deoxy-D-glucose positron emission tomography and computed tomography (FDG-PET/CT) for tumor staging in solid tumors: comparison with CT and PET. J Clin Oncol 2004;22:4357–68.

33. Slomka PJ, Dey D, Przetak C, et al. Automated 3-dimensional registration of stand-alone (18)F-FDG whole-body PET with CT. J Nucl Med 2003;44:1156–67.

34. Beyer T, Antoch G, Muller S, et al. Acquisition protocol considerations for combined PET/CT imaging. J Nucl Med 2004;45(Suppl 1):25S–35S.

35. Cohade C, Osman M, Marshall LN, et al. PET-CT: accuracy of PET and CT spatial registration of lung lesions. Eur J Nucl Med Mol Imaging 2003;30:721–6.

36. Antoch G, Freudenberg LS, Egelhof T, et al. Focal tracer uptake: a potential artifact in contrast-enhanced dual-modality PET/CT scans. J Nucl Med 2002;43:1339–42.

37. Goerres GW, Burger C, Schwitter MR, et al. PET/CT of the abdomen: optimizing the patient breathing pattern. Eur Radiol 2003;13:734–9.

38. Goerres GW, Kamel E, Heidelberg TN, et al. PET/CT image co-registration in the thorax: influence of respiration. Eur J Nucl Med Mol Imaging 2002;29:351–60.

39. Beyer T, Antoch G, Blodgett T, et al. Dual-modality PET/CT imaging: the effect of respiratory motion on combined image quality in clinical oncology. Eur J Nucl Med Mol Imaging 2003;30:588–96.

40. Beyer T, Rosenbaum S, Veit P, et al. Respiration artifacts in whole-body (18)F-FDG PET/CT studies with combined PET/CT tomographs employing spiral CT technology with 1 to 16 detector rows. Eur J Nucl Med Mol Imaging 2005;32:1429–39.

41. Beyer T, Antoch G, Bockisch A, et al. Optimized intravenous contrast administration for diagnostic whole-body 18F-FDG PET/CT. J Nucl Med 2005;46:429–35.

Imaging of Tumors of the Trachea and Central Bronchi

G.R. Ferretti, MD, PhD[a,b,c,*], C. Bithigoffer, MD[b],
C.A. Righini, MD, PhD[b,c,d], F. Arbib, MD[e],
S. Lantuejoul, MD, PhD[b,c,f], A. Jankowski, MD[b]

KEYWORDS

- CT • Chest radiography • Trachea
- Main bronchi • Malignant tumor • Benign tumor

Primary tumors of the trachea and main bronchi are rare, accounting for 1% to 2% of all respiratory tract tumors.[1,2] In adults, most (60%–90%) of these tumors are malignant,[3,4] whereas benign tumors represent the majority of lesions in children. Among those tumors in adults, squamous cell carcinoma (SCC) and adenoid cystic carcinoma (ACC) are the most frequent, representing approximately 80% of all tumors of the trachea and main bronchi. Other tumors are less common, arising from epithelial or mesenchymal tissue, and constitute a large list of heterogeneous benign and malignant tumors (**Table 1**). Imaging plays a key role in depicting these tumors and assessing tumor extent within the lumen, airway wall, and surrounding structures before treatment planning.[2,5] Multidetector computed tomography (MDCT) has increased the quality of noninvasive imaging with the recent introduction of isotropic resolution and high quality two- and three-dimensional postprocessing.[6,7] Despite the high quality of CT, there is considerable overlap in CT appearance of most tumors; histologic evaluation is needed in nearly all cases.

CLINICAL PRESENTATION

Centrally located tumors of the airways present with a limited number of signs and symptoms generally related to the obstruction of the airways (eg, dyspnea, acute respiratory failure, wheezing, stridor, recurrent pneumonia, bronchiectasis, atelectasis), whereas other symptoms are not specific (eg, cough, expectoration, hemoptysis).[3] Clinical findings may erroneously suggest the presence of asthma or chronic obstructive lung disease.[1] In other cases, these tumors may be asymptomatic and the lesions are discovered incidentally. The mean duration of symptoms is shorter in patients with malignant tumors (4 months) compared to patients with benign neoplasms (8 months), with the exception of patients with ACCs (12 months).[3]

MULTIDETECTOR COMPUTED TOMOGRAPHY TECHNIQUE

MDCT technology has completely modified the diagnostic approach and the noninvasive planning of treatment in patients who present with central

This article originally appeared in *Radiologic Clinics of North America*, Volume 47, Issue 2, March 2009.
^a Clinique Universitaire de Radiologie et Imagerie Médicale, CHU Grenoble, 38043 Grenoble cedex, France
^b Université J Fourier, Clinique Universitaire de Radiologie et Imagerie Médicale, CHU Grenoble, 38043 Grenoble cedex, France
^c INSERM U 823, Institut A Bonniot, la Tronche, France
^d Clinique ORL, CHU Grenoble, 38043 Grenoble cedex, France
^e Clinique de Pneumologie, CHU Grenoble, 38043 Grenoble cedex, France
^f Pôle de biologie-Département d'Anatomie et Cytologie Pathologiques, CHU Grenoble, 38043 Grenoble cedex, France
* Corresponding author. Clinique universitaire de radiologie et imagerie médicale, CHU Grenoble, 38043 Grenoble cedex, France.
E-mail address: gferretti@chu-grenoble.fr (G.R. Ferretti).

Table 1
Classification of tracheal tumors

Epithelial Neoplasms	Mesenchymal Neoplasms
Surface epithelium	
Malignant	*Malignant*
SCC	Soft-tissue sarcomas
Adenocarcinoma	Chondrosarcoma
Large cell carcinoma	Lymphomas
Neuroendocrine tumors	*Benign*
Carcinoids (typical and atypical)	Lipoma
Large cell neuroendocrine tumor	Fibroma
Small cell carcinoma	Fibromatosis
Benign	Histiocytoma
Papilloma	Hemangioma
Papillomatosis	Hemangiopericytoma
	Chemodectoma
Salivary glands	Leiomyoma
Malignant	Granular cell tumor
Adenoid cystic carcinoma	Schwann cell tumors
Mucoepidermoid carcinoma	Chondroma
Carcinoma	Chondroblastoma
Benign	Secondary tumors
Adenoma, pleiomorphic	Invasion by adjacent malignancy (esophagus, thyroid, larynx, lung); hematogenous metastases
Adenoma, mucous gland	
Myoepithelioma	
Onconcytoma	

airway neoplasms.[6] Currently, MDCT enables acquisition of overlapped (30%–50%) thin section (<1 mm) images with voxels of almost cubic dimensions (isotropic resolution) of the entire airways in a single apnea of few seconds. Fast gantry rotation (<0.5 seconds) increases the temporal resolution of CT images. Contrast media administration is usually needed to analyze the relationships of tumors of the central airways with the surrounding anatomy and evaluate the contrast enhancement of the tumor. We typically inject 90 to 110 mL of nonionic contrast medium at a rate of 3 mL/s through a peripheral catheter. The natural high contrast between the airways and their environment allows reduction of radiation dose (80–120 kV, 70–160 mAs), particularly in children and young adults. Data should be reconstructed with a high spatial resolution kernel and a soft-tissue resolution kernel. Acquisition is usually performed at full inspiration but can be performed at the end of expiration or during expiration to study the dynamic of the airways and the impact of a tumor on the distal airways and lung parenchyma.[8] With isotropic images, the spatial resolution of images in any reformatted plane is equivalent to the resolution in the transaxial plane, which allows for the creation of excellent two- and three-dimensional reformatted images.[6]

POSTPROCESSING OF CT DATA

Postprocessing offers the opportunity to visualize the trachea and bronchi along their main axis, on external three-dimensional views, or on internal bronchoscopic images.[8–11] Multiplanar reformations in sagittal, coronal, or oblique planes create planar images that eliminate the known limitations of axial images, that is, the partial ability to detect subtle airway stenoses, the underestimation of longitudinal extent of narrowing, the inadequate representation of the airways oriented obliquely to axial plane, and the difficulty to display complex three-dimensional anatomy of the airways.[10] Adding high-quality three-dimensional reconstructions—whether the representation of the air cast[8] or the endoluminal view using virtual bronchoscopy (VB)[7,12]—may even enhance the detection of localized or diffuse diseases.

Three-dimensional surface rendering selects the surface of the column of air contained in the airways by thresholding. Most initial data are lost in the final reconstruction. Shading the surface creates the impression of depth. Although this technique offers an overview of the disease and allows for better understanding of extent of airway narrowing, it suffers from limitations, mainly because of the choice of threshold, which may artificially increase or decrease the size of airways.[6] With volume-rendering techniques, all the information contained in data acquisition is used in the final three-dimensional images. External three-dimensional volume rendering of the airways shows the surface of the airways and the adjacent anatomy, creating CT bronchographic images.[13] Such images enhance the detection of mild airway stenoses.[14]

Burke and colleagues[15] showed an excellent correlation between VB and conventional bronchoscopy regarding the description of stenotic shape and contour and stenosis-to-lumen ratio. Sensitivity of VB was 100% for detection of obstructive bronchogenic carcinoma and 83% for endoluminal non-obstructive neoplasms but 0% for mucosal abnormalities.[16] VB allows passing through high-grade airway stenosis to assess distal airways, which is impossible using classic bronchoscopy.[17] VB can provide a road map for bronchoscopy and guide transbronchial biopsy.[18] Main limitations of VB include false-positive results related to mucus or coagulated blood pseudotumors and the inability to visualize the mucosa or perform biopsy.

Thin slab maximum intensity projection should not be used to detect or characterize airway stenosis because selection of high-density voxels artificially increases the severity of stenosis in eliminating air-containing voxels and may even create artificial stenosis.[8] On the other hand, thin slab minimum intensity projection may artificially decrease the size of asymmetrical narrowing by specifically selecting air-containing voxels. Intraluminal growth of eccentric tumors is underestimated and may be completely ignored.[8] Viewing two- and three-dimensional images simultaneously on a workstation is beneficial for radiologists in increasing their diagnostic ability and confidence in their findings.[19] Two- and three-dimensional images facilitate the communication of information to colleagues who are not familiar with axial anatomy and improve preoperative planning of surgery and bronchoscopy and postprocedural noninvasive evaluation.[20]

CT BRONCHOSCOPIC CORRELATIONS

Lesions larger than 5 mm within the airways are usually detected using CT because of the excellent natural contrast between luminal air and soft-tissue density of lesions. Limitations of MDCT are well known: lesions smaller than 2 to 3 mm are not detected, whereas subtle irregularities of airway walls often result from prominent bronchial cartilage or volume averaging. CT is not able to separate between mucosal and submucosal lesions.

CLASSIFICATION OF MAIN AIRWAYS STENOSES

Surgery is the optimal therapy for malignant and benign tumors of central airways.[1,3,21] Radiation therapy is an option, as is endoluminal therapy.[4] MDCT is useful for detecting, describing, and grading airway stenosis. Description of the lesion should mention the precise location of the tumor, the distance from the cricoid cartilage to the upper limit of the tumor, the distance from the lower part of the lesion to the carina, and the craniocaudal length and its relationship to surrounding structures, including mediastinal vessels and esophagus. Using the same acquisition, enlarged lymph nodes, pulmonary metastases, and postobstructive complications can be described.

In order to standardize the therapeutic approach of airways stenoses, Freitag and colleagues[22] proposed a new classification system. This classification identified twp groups of airway stenoses (structural and dynamic); each structural stenosis is described according to the following categories:

1. *The type of the stenosis.* Type I: exophitic intraluminal tumor or granulation tissue; type II: extrinsic compression; type III: distortion, kinking, bending, or buckling; type IV: scarring or shrinking.
2. *The degree of stenosis* (0%, approximately 25%, approximately 50%, approximately 75%, approximately 90%, complete occlusion).
3. *The location of the stenosis.* Location I: upper third of the trachea; location II: middle third of the trachea; location III: lower third of the trachea; location IV: right main bronchus; location V: left main bronchus.
4. *The transition zone.* The transition zone or the abruptness of stenosis is relevant for treatment planning.

Most tumors of the trachea and main bronchi are type 1. Radiologists may use this classification in their reports to simplify communication with interventional pulmonologists, otorhinolaryngologists, or thoracic surgeons.

MALIGNANT TUMORS

Primary tracheal cancer is rare and its incidence is low compared to laryngeal or bronchial cancer.

It accounts for approximately 0.2% of malignant neoplasms of the respiratory tract.[21] It is more common in men in their 60s with a history of smoking. The prognosis of patients is poor, with the 5-year survival rate being 5% to 35%.[21] The distribution of histologic types of neoplasms may vary regarding the origin of data (surgical vs medical series). In surgical series, SCC accounts for approximately 50% of cases, ACC for approximately 30%, and carcinoid for approximately 10%.[3] The national Danish Cancer registry report (1978–1995) showed that SCC accounted for 63% of tracheal cancers and ACC for only 7% of cases.[23]

SQUAMOUS CELL CARCINOMA

SCC is the most frequent primary malignancy of the trachea, affecting predominantly men (sex ratio 4:1) between age 50 and 60. SCC is strongly associated with cigarette smoking and consequently with other smoking-related cancers of the upper and lower respiratory tract.[1] Macroscopically, SCC appears as a large mass within the central airways with either exophytic or ulcerative component. It can be multifocal in approximately 10% of patients. Regional extent into the esophagus or mainstem bronchi is frequent. The tumor often spreads to regional lymph nodes.

Chest radiography in patients with SCC is often considered unremarkable, but retrospective analysis usually shows focalized asymmetrical filling defect within the tracheal lumen. CT demonstrates a polypoid intraluminal mass of soft tissue density with irregular, smooth, or lobulated contours (**Fig. 1**).[2] The relationships of the tumor with the tracheal wall vary from localized eccentric pedunculated lesions to circumferential invasion. CT shows the extent to the adjacent anatomy. In some patients, the extent of SCC to the esophagus results in tracheoesophageal or bronchoesophageal fistulization.

ADENOID CYSTIC CARCINOMA

ACC is a low-grade malignancy formerly named cylindroma that is not associated with cigarette smoking.[21] It occurs in patients in their 40s; there is no sex predilection. ACC arises from the epithelium of the glands lining the mucosa of the airways and is the most common tumor of the mucosal glands. (It is also named sialadenoid tumor.)[24] In the central airways, ACC has a propensity to infiltrate the wall of the airways and spread along submucosal and perineural planes.[25] ACC grows slowly and is rarely associated with regional lymph node metastases. Distant metastases are rare and often are diagnosed late after the ACC but may present an intense fluorodeoxyglucose uptake.[26] Despite nonspecific signs or symptoms, early recognition of ACC may improve the surgical resectability and the prognosis of patients. Most of the tumors arise in the lower trachea or mainstem bronchi.

Unfortunately, chest radiography is often considered unremarkable; however, an intraluminal mass with smooth, irregular, or lobulated margins can be identified. CT shows a well-limited soft-tissue attenuating intraluminal mass that often infiltrates the airway wall (**Fig. 2**) and the surrounding mediastinal fat.[25] Other presentations include circumferential wall thickening of the trachea creating localized stenosis (**Fig. 3**) or multifocal narrowing.

MUCOEPIDERMOID CARCINOMA

This rare tumor originates from the minor salivary glands lining the tracheobronchial tree.[27] It usually occurs in patients younger than age 40 and affects

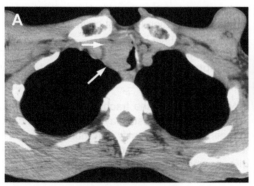
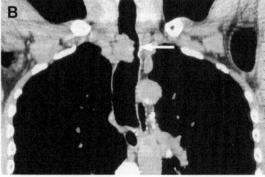

Fig. 1. Squamous cell carcinoma in a 63-year-old man. (*A*) Axial CT at the level of the upper trachea shows a lobulated, intraluminal mass extending to the cartilages of the trachea and to the mediastinal fat (*arrow*). (*B*) Coronal reformation of CT data shows the longitudinal extent of the tumor and the severity of the asymmetrical narrowing of the tracheal lumen (*arrow*).

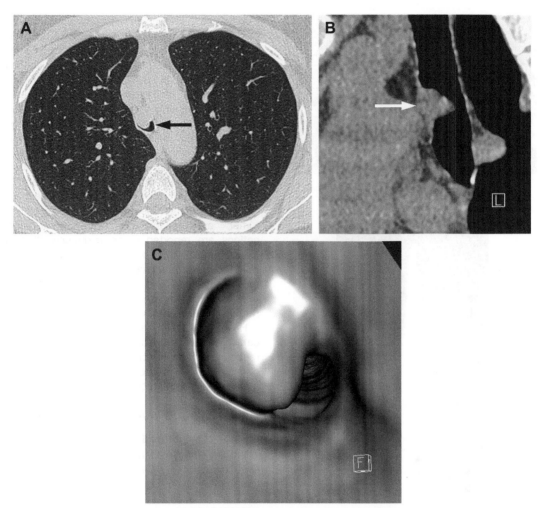

Fig. 2. Adenoid cystic carcinoma in a 36-year-old patient with clinical history of asthma. (*A*) Axial CT at the level of the aortic arch demonstrates severe narrowing of the lower trachea (*arrow*). (*B*) Sagittal reformation shows the large pedicle of the tumor and extraluminal component of the tumor (*arrow*). (*C*) Virtual endoscopy demonstrates the severity of the tracheal stenosis.

mainly the segmental bronchi,[28] creating airway obstruction. It is even rarer than ACC, representing 5% of sialadenoid tumors. Histologicaly, mucoepidermoid carcinoma associates variable proportions of squamous cells, mucus secreting cells, and intermediate cells with variable degree of mitoses, nuclear pleomorphism, and cellular necrosis, defining low- or high-grade malignancy (**Fig. 4**).[28]

Mucoepidermoid carcinoma shows the same CT pattern as bronchial carcinoid tumors. It presents as an endobronchial mass, often smoothly oval or lobulated with its long axis parallel to that of the airways containing the tumor, but contrast enhancement is usually mild.[28] Punctate calcifications within the tumor were present in 6 of 12 cases.[28] CT contrast enhancement of mucoepidermoid carcinoma has been differently

appreciated: mild enhancement was reported by Kim and colleagues,[28] whereas marked heterogeneous contrast enhancement was reported in four of five cases in a small series by Ishizumi and colleagues.[29] The presence of abundant microvessels at histopathology correlated with the CT findings.[29] Lymphadenopathy is rare.

CARCINOID TUMORS

Carcinoid tumors are rare thoracic neuroendocrine neoplasms that range from low-grade typical tumors to intermediate-grade atypical aggressive carcinoids and high-grade small cell carcinoma.[30] These tumors may secrete peptide hormones and neuroamines such as ACTH, serotonine, somatostatin, and bradikinin. Both sexes are affected in equal proportions, and patients are usually in their

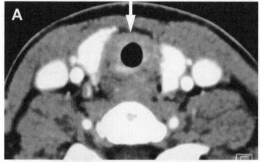

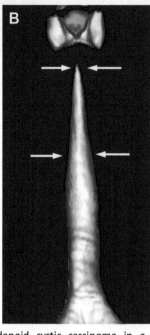

Fig. 3. Adenoid cystic carcinoma in a 50-year-old woman. (*A*) Axial CT after contrast media administration shows circumferential narrowing caused by circumferential wall thickening of the upper trachea (*arrow*). (*B*) Three-dimensional reconstruction of the trachea demonstrates the longitudinal extent of the tumor (*arrows*).

40s, whereas carcinoid is the most frequent bronchial tumor in childhood. No relation was found to cigarette smoking. Symptoms related to tracheobronchial obstruction and hemoptysis are by far more frequent than symptoms caused by ectopic secretion of hormones. In most cases (80%) these tumors are centrally located within the airways, affecting the main, lobar, and segmental bronchi. Tracheal involvement is exceptional. Carcinoid tumors classically appear as smooth, polypoid, cherry-red endobronchial masses at bronchoscopy. Although histologic diagnosis can be made with endoscopic biopsies, there is a high risk of hemoptysis.

Imaging presentation of centrally located carcinoids is similar for typical and atypical cases. In most cases, carcinoids are endobronchial but also can be partially encased in the bronchial wall, creating an iceberg growth pattern, which is nicely demonstrated using CT and multiplanar reconstructions. In some cases (up to 60%), CT demonstrates marked homogeneous early contrast enhancement of an endobronchial nodule that reflects the rich vascularity of the carcinoid tumor (**Fig. 5**).[31] This pattern is highly suggestive of bronchial carcinoid tumor but is not always present. Differential diagnosis of endobronchial tumors with marked contrast enhancement on early phase dynamic contrast-enhanced CT detects even rarer neoplasms, such as glomus tumor[32] and hemangioma.[33] Intratumoral calcifications are reported in approximately 25% of cases (**Fig. 6**).[31] In some cases, bronchial carcinoid tumors produce complete obstruction of the bronchial lumen and subsequent atelectasis of the distal lung. In case of partial obstruction, expiratory air trapping can be demonstrated.

Hilar or mediastinal enlargement of lymph nodes can be present and is often related to inflammatory reaction from recurrent pulmonary infection. Lymph node metastasis of carcinoid tumor also may occur, more frequently in atypical carcinoid tumors.

OTHER PRIMARY MALIGNANT NEOPLASMS

Other malignant neoplasms are listed in **Table 1**. Their imaging presentation is not specific except for chondrosarcoma, which shows foci of calcifications within a mass.

LYMPHOMA

Primary malignant lymphoma of the trachea is rare. It is usually related to the mucosa-associated lymphoid tissue, a low-grade malignancy.[34] Clinical presentation is nonspecific. CT can reveal focal tracheal narrowing caused by a solitary mass (**Fig. 7**) or polypoid thickening of the tracheobronchial wall caused by diffuse infiltration of the submucosa.

SECONDARY TRACHEAL MALIGNANCY

Direct invasion of the central airways by neoplasms of the thyroid, esophagus, lung, and larynx is much more frequent than hematogenous metastases. In case of massive direct invasion, CT demonstrates the primary neoplasm and its extension by contiguity to the main airways. The signs associated with tracheal invasion are evidence of an endoluminal mass, the destruction of the cartilage, or a tracheoesophageal or bronchoesophageal fistula (**Fig. 8**).[35] Many cancers have the potential to metastasize to the trachea and

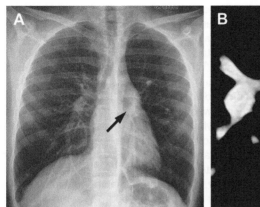
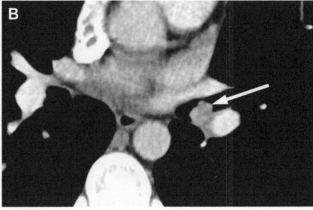

Fig. 4. Mucoiepidermoid carcinoma in a 23-year-old man who presented with hemoptysis. (*A*) Anteroposterior chest radiograph shows an endoluminal mass within the distal left mainstem bronchus (*arrow*). (*B*) Axial CT after contrast enhancement shows a 12-mm polypoid endobronchial mass slightly enhanced (*arrow*).

bronchi, such as breast, colorectal, renal, lung, ovarian, thyroid, uterine, and testicular and melanomas and sarcomas. The incidence of tracheal metastases in nonpulmonary malignancies is highly variable, ranging from 0.44% to 50%, according to their definition.[36] The overall incidence of tracheal metastasis in surgically resected non–small cell lung cancer was 0.44%; it was 0.77% in SCC and 0.18% in adenocarcinoma.[36] Endotracheal metastases of nonpulmonary cancers arise with a mean recurrence interval of 50.4 to 65.3 months[37] compared to a mean recurrence interval of 25.8 months in patients who present with lung malignancies. Endotracheal or endobronchial metastases appear as endotracheal nodules or eccentric thickening of the airway wall (**Fig. 9**) or soft-tissue density with contrast enhancement. Histopathologic examination of tracheal biopsy specimens demonstrates the diagnostic of metastasis.

BENIGN TUMORS

Benign tumors of the central airways are rare and account for less than 2% of all lung neoplasms.[4] They can be of epithelial, mesenchymal, neural, or composite origin.[38] These tumors appear in clinical practice as the differential diagnosis of malignant lesions that are much more common. Although fiberoptic bronchoscopy

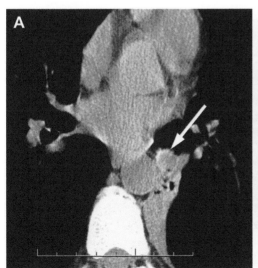
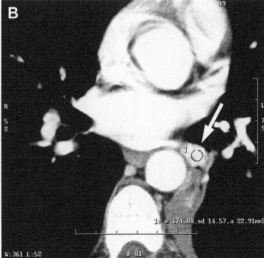

Fig. 5. Carcinoid tumor in a 14-year-old patient. (*A*) Unenhanced axial CT shows soft-tissue density (42 UH) nodule within the B6 bronchus and distal atelectasis (*arrow*). (*B*) Contrast-enhanced CT shows marked contrast enhancement of the nodule (174 UH) (*arrow*).

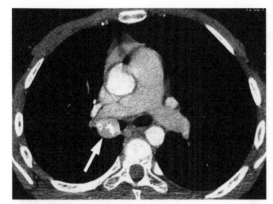

Fig. 6. Carcinoid tumor obstructing the right main stem bronchus. The tumor contains foci of calcifications and has an iceberg growth pattern (*arrow*).

identifieslesions within the airways, biopsies are often noncontributive because of severe inflammatory reaction in the periphery of the tumor. Chest radiography is usually unremarkable.[5] MDCT with thin collimation allows precise analysis of tissue attenuation of the lesions, enhancing in some cases the diagnostic capabilities of CT (**Box 1**). CT usually shows masses that are confined within the tracheobronchial lumen without evidence of invasion of surrounding structures.[39] Ko and colleagues[39] recently reported on a large series of 17 patients with pathologically proven benign tumors of the central airways.

HAMARTOMA

Hamartomas represent 3% to 10% of intrathoracic hamartomas.[40] These mesenchymal tumors are composed of a mixture of fat, cartilage, fibrous tissue, and an epithelial component. Endobronchial hamartomas arise more commonly in segmental bronchi;[41] tracheal location is unusual.[42] Radiologically, hamartomas are round, well-circumscribed lesions ranging from 0.5 to 3 cm in diameter. Demonstration of fat and calcifications within the lesion, which is considered diagnostic when present (**Fig. 10**),[43] is facilitated by using isotropic MDCT acquisitions with limited volume averaging effect. The fatty content or the calcifications may not be identified on CT, however,[42] and hamartoma appears as a nonspecific soft tissue mass. Goodman and colleagues[44] described a unique case of peripheral hamartoma arising from peripheral lung tissue with proximal extension and subsequent obstruction of the large airways. Because the tumor is slow growing, it may be responsible for bronchial obstruction and irreversible damage of the underlying lung. Hamartomas that develop within the airways require surgical treatment.

LIPOMA

Lipomas (0.1% of benign lung tumors) are often pedunculated and arise from the submucosal or interstitial adipose tissue of the central airways. Bronchial obstruction is frequent and responsible for atelectasis and postobstructive pneumonitis. As for other slow-growing endobronchial tumors, fiberoptic bronchoscopy is often nondiagnostic because of the fibrous capsule surrounding the lesions that may present with atypical inflammatory cells, leading to an incorrect diagnosis of

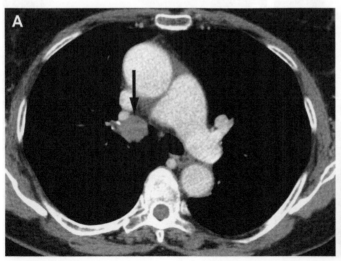
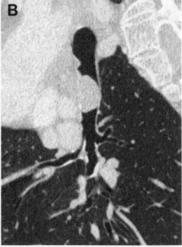

Fig. 7. Endobronchial mucosa-associated lymphoid tissue of the right main bronchus in an 80-year-old patient. (*A*) Axial CT after IV contrast media administration shows a 1.6-cm soft-tissue density mass (*arrow*). (*B*) Coronal oblique reformation of the tumor demonstrates the relationship with the bronchial tree.

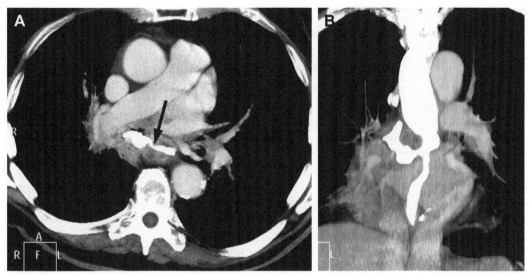

Fig. 8. Tracheoesophageal fistula in a patient with esophageal cancer extending to the right main bronchus. CT is acquired after contrast media opacification of the esophagus. (*A*) Axial CT shows the fistula between the esophagus and the right main bronchus (*arrow*). (*B*) Coronal maximum intensity projection provides a CT esophagogram, which shows the narrowed esophagus, the fistula, and the dilated esophagus above the cancer.

chronic inflammation or even bronchogenic carcinoma.[39] In those cases, CT is diagnostic when it shows the fatty density of the lesion without any calcification (**Fig. 11**).[45,46] A correct preoperative diagnosis may prevent lobectomy or pneumonectomy, because laser resection by means of bronchoscopy is the treatment of choice for endoluminal lipomas.

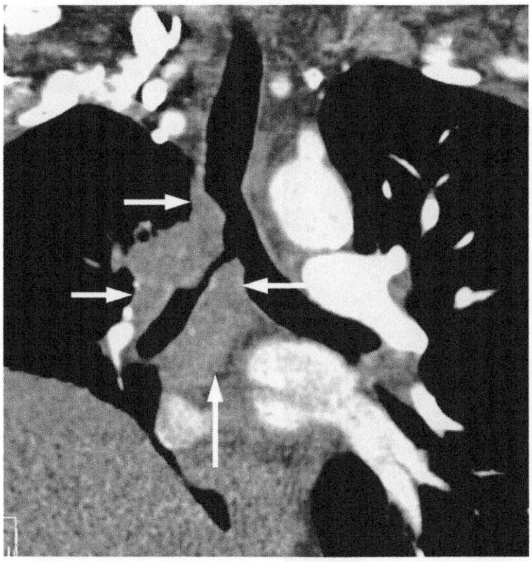

GRANULAR CELL TUMORS (ABRIKOSSOFF'S TUMOR OR MYOBLASTOMA)

Granular cell tumors are uncommon benign neoplasms of neuroectodermal origin that are mainly located in the head and neck region.[2] They are discovered in the fourth decade of life and are more common in women. Pathologically, these tumors show a characteristic appearance; the cells are polymorphic and are embedded in various amounts of connective or reticular tissues. Mitoses are uncommon. The tumors are circumscribed but not encapsulated. At the level of central airways, they appear as polypoid masses of soft tissue density that may totally obstruct bronchi. Differentiation of granular cell tumors from carcinomas on the basis of imaging findings is not possible.

PAPILLOMAS

Inflammatory papillomas or polyps are associated with chronic irritation of the airways and occur with endobronchial foreign bodies, broncholithiasis, or exposure to gases. Squamous cell papilloma is one of the most common benign neoplasms of the central airways. It involves the larynx, bronchi, and infrequently the trachea, predominantly in middle-aged men with a history of smoking. The tumor appears as a lobulated, well-limited

Fig. 9. Tracheobronchial metastasis of breast cancer in a 65-year-old woman. Coronal reformation shows soft-tissue density infiltration of the wall of the distal trachea extending to the right main bronchus (*arrows*), responsible for a severe narrowing of the right main bronchus lumen.

> **Box 1**
> **CT pathologic correlation in central airways neoplasms**
>
> Fat attenuation: lipoma, hamartochondroma
>
> Calcification: hamartoma, chondroma, carcinoid
>
> Fat and calcification: hamartoma
>
> High contrast-enhanced tumor: carcinoid, hemangioma, glomus tumor, fibroma

polypoid nodule within the airways without fatty content or calcification.[47]

Laryngotracheal papillomatosis is caused by infection with human papillomavirus. It can be contracted at birth or acquired through sexual transmission. The lesion arises in the larynx and spreads by seeding from the upper airways to the trachea in approximately 5% of cases.[48] Two

third of patients are diagnosed before age 5. Papillomas are cauliflower lesions that enlarge around a central fibrovascular core on the central airway mucosal surface. These strictly endoluminal lesions appear on CT as single or multiple nodular irregularities of soft-tissue density, 0.5 to 1.5 mm in diameter in the tracheal or bronchial lumen (**Fig. 12**).[49] When extended to the lung parenchyma (<1% of cases of laryngotracheal papillomatosis), papillomatosis produces nodules that may cavitate and form thin-walled cavities.[48] Lesions of papillomatosis are central and peripheral but with a predominance within the posterior half of the thorax. These lesions may transform into carcinoma and involve careful follow-up.

CHONDROMA

These rare benign cartilaginous tumors rarely develop in the trachea. CT may show foci of calcifications within a sharply defined polypoid lesion up

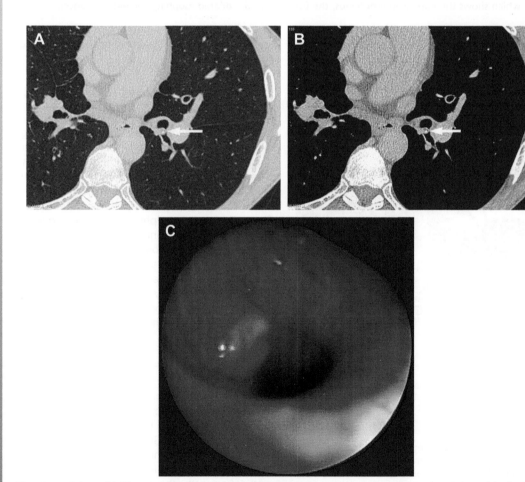

Fig. 10. Endobronchial hamartoma. (*A*) Axial CT without contrast shows an endoluminal nodule within the lumen of left B6 (*arrow*). (*B*) Axial CT (mediastinal window) shows fat and small calcifications within the lesion (*arrow*). (*C*) Bronchoscopy confirmed the diagnosis.

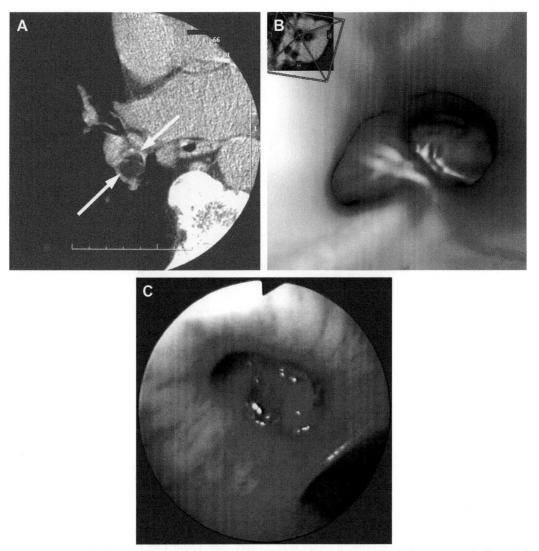

Fig. 11. Endobronchial lipoma. (*A*) Axial CT shows -90 HU rounded fatty mass (*arrow*) obstructing right lower lobe bronchus. VB (*B*) and real bronchoscopy (*C*) show excellent correlation.

to 3 cm in diameter.[50] Imaging is unable to differentiate a chondroma from a chondrosarcoma; however.

SCHWANNOMA

This neurogenic tumor is rare and may present at any age. It is composed of Schwann's cells of nerve sheath. Most cases occur in adults. They are typically unique encapsulated tumors attached to a nerve but contain no axon protruding within the airways.[51] On CT, schwannoma appears as a well-limited mass of low tissue density before contrast administration; the mass is homogeneously and strongly enhanced after contrast administration. Definitive diagnosis is demonstrated by biopsy under bronchoscopy.

ADENOMA

Pedonculated tracheobronchial adenoma (adenomatous polyp or mucous gland cystadenoma) arises from bronchial mucous glands and is rare. It appears as a solitary, spherical, soft-tissue density polypoid mass.[52]

LEIOMYOMA

This rare tumor accounts for approximately 2% of surgically resected benign lung tumors. Most leiomyomas are seen within the bronchi (70% of cases); 30% are detected in the trachea.[53]

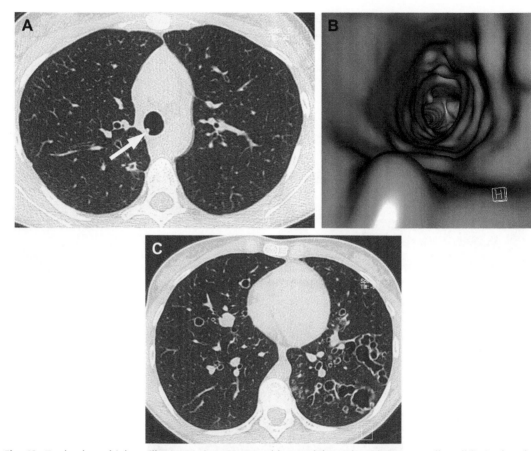

Fig. 12. Tracheobronchial papillomatosis in a 23-year-old man. (*A*) Axial CT shows a small, well-limited nodule (*arrow*). (*B*) Virtual endoscopy demonstrates multiple elevations of the tracheal wall caused by papillomas. (*C*) Axial CT at the level of lower lobes shows bilaterally distributed cysts. (*Courtesy of* D. Tack, MD, PhD, Baudour, Belgium.)

An iceberg tumor growth pattern with a large extraluminal component may be present on CT and should contraindicate bronchoscopic resection of these tumors. CT description of leiomyomas in the airways was reported by Kim and colleagues[53] in a series of 13 tumors: 2 were not depicted using CT because of their small size; 11 (84%) were identified using CT (9 as intraluminal nodules and 2 as iceberg tumors). Tumors are usually oval and are rarely lobulated or round. Obstructive pneumonia, atelectasis, or mucus plugging was present in 38% of cases. Calcifications are rare and are reported in less than 10% of cases. Most of these tumors appear as homogeneous nodules before contrast administration and become slightly enhanced after IV contrast injection.

OTHER BENIGN NEOPLASMS

Other neoplasms usually appear as smooth, polypoid, noncalcified nodules or masses limited to the airway wall. Histologic diagnosis is mandatory. See **Table 1** for more examples.

DIFFERENTIAL DIAGNOSIS
Mucoid Pseudotumor

Mucus is the most commonly encountered soft-tissue mass within the airways, creating a mucoid pseudotumor. In most cases, mucoid pseudotumor is easily identified because the lesion is of low tissue attenuation, does not enhance after contrast media administration, may contain small air bubbles, is located in the dependant portions of the airway, is not associated with disruption of the cartilaginous rings of the trachea, and is mobile after coughing. In rare cases, thick mucus does not contain air, adheres to the wall of the airway, is not mobile after coughing, and may be mistaken for a real tumor (**Fig. 13**). Such false-positive CT findings are diagnosed using fiberoptic bronchoscopy.

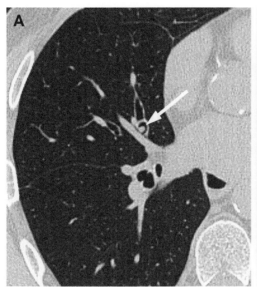

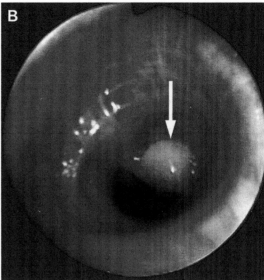

Fig. 13. Mucoid impaction mimicking endobronchial tumor. (*A*) Axial CT shows small, well-defined nodule within the right middle lobe bronchus (*arrow*). (*B*) Bronchoscopy demonstrates the mucous nature of the lesion (*arrow*).

Focal Infection

Focal infection may be responsible for tumor-like lesions when it produces granulation or endoluminal masses. Diagnosis is impossible with CT and requires fiberoptic bronchoscopy and microbacterial analysis. Specific pathogens include *Mycobacterium tuberculosis*, mucormycosis, *Klebsiella rhinoscleromatis*, and actinomycosis (**Fig. 14**).[54]

Broncholithiasis

Broncholithiasis may mimic a centrally located obstructive tumor on bronchoscopy. In these cases,

CT is more sensitive than bronchoscopy by identifying intraluminal and peribronchial calcifications distal to inflammatory airways stenosis.[55]

Tracheopathia Osteoplastica

Tracheopathia osteoplastica occurs almost exclusively in men over 50 years old; most patients are asymptomatic. This benign condition of unknown origin is characterized by multiple submucosal osteocartilaginous growths localized along the inner anterior and lateral walls of the trachea.[56] CT shows multiple irregular sessile nodules, 1 to 5 mm in diameter, that can be calcified protruding

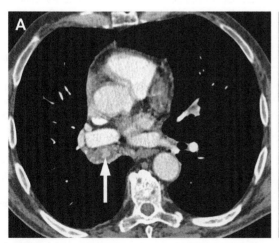

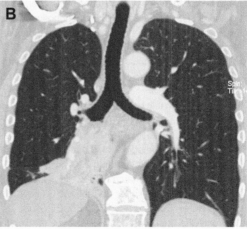

Fig. 14. Endobronchial actinomycosis mimicking endobronchial tumor. (*A*) Contrast-enhanced CT at the level of the right intermediate bronchus demonstrates complete occlusion of the bronchus (*arrow*). (*B*) Coronal reformation shows right lower lobe atelectasis. (*Courtesy of* D. Tack, MD, PhD, Baudour, Belgium.)

into the tracheal lumen. The posterior wall of the trachea is free of nodules.

Amyloidosis

Amyloidosis of the trachea is a rare condition that produces diffuse or focal irregular narrowing of the lower airways secondary to the deposits of extracellular amyloid within the submucosa. Deposits may be diffuse or multifocal with or without calcifications. Solitary amyloid pseudotumors are less common than diffuse disease.[57] CT shows concentric thickening of the tracheal wall that may extend up to the lobar bronchi with subsequent narrowing of the air column. Nodulation, plaques, and calcifications may be present.

REFERENCES

1. Grillo HC, Mathisen DJ. Primary tracheal tumors: treatment and results. Ann Thorac Surg 1990; 49(1):69–77.
2. McCarthy MJ, Rosado-de-Christenson ML. Tumors of the trachea. J Thorac Imaging 1995;10(3):180–98.
3. Regnard JF, Fourquier P, Levasseur P. Results and prognostic factors in resections of primary tracheal tumors: a multicenter retrospective study. The French Society of Cardiovascular Surgery. J Thorac Cardiovasc Surg 1996;111(4):808–13.
4. Macchiarini P. Primary tracheal tumours. Lancet Oncol 2006;7:83–91.
5. Kwong JS, Muller NL, Miller RR. Diseases of the trachea and main-stem bronchi: correlation of CT with pathologic findings. Radiographics 1992;12: 645–57.
6. Boiselle PM, Lee KS, Ernst A. Multidetector CT of the central airways. J Thorac Imaging 2005;20:186–95.
7. De Wever W, Vandecaveye V, Lanciotti S, et al. Multidetector CT-generated virtual bronchoscopy: an illustrated review of the potential clinical indications. Eur Respir J 2004;23(5):776–82.
8. Grenier PA, Beigelman-Aubry C, Fétita C, et al. New frontiers in CT imaging of airway disease. Eur Radiol 2002;12(5):1022–44.
9. Ferretti G, Bricault I, Coulomb M. Virtual tools for imaging the thorax. Eur Respir J 2001;18:1–12.
10. Ravenel JG, McAdams HP, Remy-Jardin M, et al. Multidimensional imaging of the thorax: practical applications. J Thorac Imaging 2001;16(4):269–81.
11. Luccichenti G, Cademartiri F, Pezzella FR, et al. 3D reconstruction techniques made easy: know-how and pictures. Eur Radiol 2005;15(10):2146–56.
12. Ferretti GR, Knoplioch J, Bricault I, et al. Central airway stenoses: preliminary results of spiral-CT-generated virtual bronchoscopy simulations in 29 patients. Eur Radiol 1997;7:854–9.
13. Remy-Jardin M, Remy J, Artaud D, et al. Tracheobronchial tree: assessment with volume rendering. Technical aspects. Radiology 1998;208(2):393–8.
14. Remy-Jardin M, Remy J, Artaud D, et al. Volume rendering of the tracheobronchial tree: clinical evaluation of bronchographic images. Radiology 1998; 208:761–70.
15. Burke AJ, Vining DJ, McGuirt WF Jr, et al. Evaluation of airway obstruction using virtual endoscopy. Laryngoscope 2000;110(1):23–9.
16. Finkelstein SE, Summers RM, Nguyen DM, et al. Virtual bronchoscopy for evaluation of malignant tumors of the thorax. J Thorac Cardiovasc Surg 2002;123(5):967–72.
17. Ferretti GR, Thony F, Bosson JL, et al. Benign abnormalities and carcinoid tumors of the central airways: diagnostic impact of CT bronchography. AJR Am J Roentgenol 2000;174:1307–13.
18. McAdams HP, Goodman PC, Kussin P. Virtual bronchoscopy for directing transbronchial needle aspiration of hilar and mediastinal lymph nodes: a pilot study. AJR Am J Roentgenol 1998;170:1361–4.
19. Boiselle PM, Reynolds KF, Ernst A. Multiplanar and three-dimensional imaging of the central airways with multidetector CT. AJR Am J Roentgenol 2002; 179:301–8.
20. Ferretti GR, Kocier M, Calaque O, et al. Follow-up after stent insertion in the tracheobronchial tree: role of helical computed tomography in comparison with fiberoptic bronchoscopy. Eur Radiol 2003;13:1172–8.
21. Honings J, van Dijck JA, Verhagen AF, et al. Incidence and treatment of tracheal cancer: a nationwide study in the Netherlands. Ann Surg Oncol 2007;14(2):968–76.
22. Freitag L, Ernst A, Unger M, et al. A proposed classification system of central airway stenosis. Eur Respir J 2007;30(1):7–12.
23. Licht PB, Friis S, Pettersson G. Tracheal cancer in Denmark: a nationwide study. Eur J Cardiothorac Surg 2001;19:339–45.
24. Kim TS, Lee KS, Han J, et al. Sialadenoid tumors of the respiratory tract: radiologic-pathologic correlation. AJR Am J Roentgenol 2001;177(5):1145–50.
25. Kwak SH, Lee KS, Chung MJ, et al. Adenoid cystic carcinoma of the airways: helical CT and histopathologic correlation. AJR Am J Roentgenol 2004;183(2): 277–81.
26. Campistron M, Rouquette I, Courbon F, et al. Adenoid cystic carcinoma of the lung: interest of 18FDG PET/CT in the management of an atypical presentation. Lung Cancer 2008;59(1):133–6.
27. Yousem SA, Hochholzer L. Mucoepidermoid tumors of the lung. Cancer 1987;60(6):1346–52.
28. Kim TS, Lee KS, Han J, et al. Mucoepidermoid carcinoma of the tracheobronchial tree: radiographic and CT findings in 12 patients. Radiology 1999;212(3): 643–8.

29. Ishizumi T, Tateishi U, Watanabe S, et al. Mucoepidermoid carcinoma of the lung: high-resolution CT and histopathologic findings in five cases. Lung Cancer 2008;60(1):125–31.

30. Jeung MY, Gasser B, Gangi A, et al. Bronchial carcinoid tumors of the thorax: spectrum of radiologic findings. Radiographics 2002;22(2):351–65.

31. Paillas W, Moro-Sibilot D, Lantuejoul S, et al. Bronchial carcinoid tumors: role of imaging for diagnosis and local staging. J Radiol 2004;85:1711–9.

32. Akata S, Yoshimura M, Park J, et al. Glomus tumor of the left main bronchus. Lung Cancer 2008;60(1): 132–5.

33. Rose AS, Mathur PN. Endobronchial capillary hemangioma: case report and review of the literature. Respiration 2008;76:221–4.

34. Fidias P, Wright C, Harris NL, et al. Primary tracheal non-Hodgkin's lymphoma: a case report and review of the literature. Cancer 1996;77(11):2332–8.

35. Rapp-Bernhardt U, Welte T, Budinger M, et al. Comparison of three-dimensional virtual endoscopy with bronchoscopy in patients with oesophageal carcinoma infiltrating the tracheobronchial tree. Br J Radiol 1998;71:1271–8.

36. Chong S, Kim TS, Han J. Tracheal metastasis of lung cancer: CT findings in six patients. AJR Am J Roentgenol 2006;186(1):220–4.

37. Kiryu T, Hoshi H, Matsui E, et al. Endotracheal/endobronchial metastases: clinicopathologic study with special reference to developmental modes. Chest 2001;119(3):768–75.

38. Shah H, Garbe L, Nussbaum E, et al. Benign tumors of the tracheobronchial tree: endoscopic characteristics and role of laser resection. Chest 1995;107(6): 1744–51.

39. Ko JM, Jung JI, Park SH, et al. Benign tumors of the tracheobronchial tree: CT-pathologic correlation. AJR Am J Roentgenol 2006;186:1304–13.

40. Arrigoni MG, Woolner LB, Bernatz PE, et al. Benign tumors of the lung: a ten-year surgical experience. J Thorac Cardiovasc Surg 1970; 60(4):589–99.

41. Cosío BG, Villena V, Echave-Sustaeta J, et al. Endobronchial hamartoma. Chest 2002;122(1):202–5.

42. Reittner P, Müller NL. Tracheal hamartoma: CT findings in two patients. J Comput Assist Tomogr 1999; 23(6):957–8.

43. Ahn JM, Im JG, Seo JW, et al. Endobronchial hamartoma: CT findings in three patients. AJR Am J Roentgenol 1994;163(1):49–50.

44. Goodman A, Falzon M, Gelder C, et al. Central airway obstruction caused by a peripheral hamartoma. Lung Cancer 2007;57(3):395–8.

45. Mata JM, Cáceres J, Ferrer J, et al. Endobronchial lipoma: CT diagnosis. J Comput Assist Tomogr 1991;15(5):750–1.

46. Raymond GS, Barrie JR. Endobronchial lipoma: helical CT diagnosis. AJR Am J Roentgenol 1999; 173(6):1716.

47. Naka Y, Nakao K, Hamaji Y, et al. Solitary squamous cell papilloma of the trachea. Ann Thorac Surg 1993; 55(1):189–93.

48. Kramer SS, Wehunt WD, Stocker JT, et al. Pulmonary manifestations of juvenile laryngotracheal papillomatosis. AJR Am J Roentgenol 1985;144(4):687–94.

49. Chang CH, Wang HC, Wu MT, et al. Virtual bronchoscopy for diagnosis of recurrent respiratory papillomatosis. J Formos Med Assoc 2006; 105(6):508–11.

50. Frank JL, Schwartz BR, Price LM, et al. Benign cartilaginous tumors of the upper airway. J Surg Oncol 1991;48(1):69–74.

51. Righini CA, Lequeux T, Laverierre MH, et al. Primary tracheal schwannoma: one case report and a literature review. Eur Arch Otorhinolaryngol 2005;262(2):157–60.

52. Newhause MT, Martin L, Kay JM, et al. Laser resection of a pedunculated tracheal adenoma. Chest 2000;118:262–5.

53. Kim YK, Kim H, Lee KS, et al. Airway leiomyoma: imaging findings and histopathologic comparisons in 13 patients. AJR Am J Roentgenol 2007;189(2): 393–9.

54. Naidich DP, Webb WR, Grenier PA, et al. Imaging of the airways: functional and radiologic correlations. Philadelphia: Lippincott Williams & Wilkins; 2005. p. 70–105.

55. Conces DJ, Tarver RD, Vix VA. Broncholithiasis: CT features in 15 patients. AJR Am J Roentgenol 1991;157:249–53.

56. Stark P. Radiology of the trachea. New York: Thieme Medical; 1991. p. 1–37.

57. Kirchner J, Jacobi V, Kardos P, et al. CT findings in extensive tracheobronchial amyloidosis. Eur Radiol 1998;8:352–4.

Nonneoplastic Tracheal and Bronchial Stenoses

Philippe A. Grenier, MD[a],*, Catherine Beigelman-Aubry, MD[a],
Pierre-Yves Brillet, MD, PhD[b]

KEYWORDS
- Tracheal stenosis • Bronchial stenosis
- Infectious tracheobronchitis • Relapsing polychondritis
- Wegener's granulomatosis • Tracheobronchial amyloidosis

Large airway diseases that may result in airway stenosis are neoplastic or nonneoplastic in origin. Tracheal and bronchial neoplasms are described in another article in this issue. Nonneoplastic diseases of central airways that may lead to airway lumen narrowing include iatrogenic strictures, infectious tracheobronchitis, systemic disease, saber sheath deformity of the trachea, tracheobronchopathia osteochrondroplastica, and broncholithiasis. Systemic diseases include amyloidosis, inflammatory bowel disease, relapsing polychondritis, sarcoidosis, and Wegener's granulomatosis. Tracheobronchomalacia that induces airway narrowing only during expiratory maneuver or cough is described in another article. Clinical recognition of tracheobronchial stenosis is notoriously difficult, especially early in its course. Clinical symptoms of airway obstruction are late and nonspecific. Earlier diagnosis is often possible with the advent of routine CT imaging.

Multidetector computed tomography (MDCT) is the imaging modality of choice for assessing such diseases.[1–4] It is important to be aware of the limitations of the axial plane for assessing airway stenosis. Subtle airway stenosis may be missed, and the craniocaudal extent of disease may be underestimated. By providing a continuous anatomic display of the airways, multiplanar reformations along and perpendicular to the central axis of the airways, and the three-dimensional reconstruction images help circumvent these limitations.[5–7] Such multiplanar and three-dimensional images help surgeons and interventional pulmonologists to select adequate procedures and determine response to treatment. The use of MDCT with thin collimation (0.6–1.5 mm) over the entire chest during a single breath hold at full inspiration allows acquisition of volumetric high resolution data sets. Reconstruction of axial overlapped thin slices permits multiplanar reformations of high quality and helps detect and characterize airway wall thickening and calcifications. Generally, intravenous contrast is not required for assessing nonneoplastic airway stenoses; however, it is recommended in cases in which there is a high likelihood of diseases in the adjacent lymph nodes and for cases in which neoplastic airway disease may be suspected.[8] Additional acquisition during dynamic expiration using low dose may be helpful to detect coexisting tracheal or bronchomalacia.[3,9]

When assessing airway narrowing, it is important to carefully assess the location and extent along the airways of the stenosis and characterize the presence, distribution, and type of airway wall thickening. Considering these factors in combination with associated features in the mediastinum, hilum, and lung parenchyma and pertinent clinical and laboratory data should allow radiologists to provide a limited number of differential diagnoses.

This article originally appeared in *Radiologic Clinics of North America*, Volume 47, Issue 2, March 2009.
[a] Hôpital Pitié-Salpêtrière, Assistance Publique-Hôpitaux de Paris (APHP), Université Pierre et Marie Curie, Service de Radiologie Polyvalente, Diagnostique et Interventionnelle, 47/83 boulevard de l'Hôpital, 75651 Paris cedex 13, Paris, France
[b] Hôpital Avicenne, Assistance Publique-Hôpitaux de Paris (APHP), Université Paris XIII, UPRES EA 2363, Service de Radiologie, 125, route de Stalingrad, 93009 Bobigny, France
* Corresponding author.
E-mail address: philippe.grenier@psl.aphp.fr (P.A. Grenier).

Thorac Surg Clin 20 (2010) 47–64
doi:10.1016/j.thorsurg.2009.12.005
1547-4127/10/$ – see front matter © 2010 Elsevier Inc. All rights reserved.

IATROGENIC STENOSIS

The most common iatrogenic airway stenoses are tracheal strictures secondary to intubation or tracheostomy and bronchial anastomosis stenosis after lung transplantation. Strictures of the trachea are usually secondary to damage from a cuffed endotracheal or tracheostomy tube. The prevalence of stenoses after endotracheal tube placement has decreased substantially to 1% since the introduction of low pressure cuff endotracheal tubes.[10] Conversely, the prevalence of tracheal stenosis after longstanding tracheostomy tube placement remains high, with a rate of approximately 30%.[11] Infection, mechanical irritation, steroid administration, use of positive pressure ventilation, and prolonged intubation may increase the risk of stenosis occurrence.

The principal site of stenosis after intubation is the subglottic region at the level of the endotracheal balloon. Strictures are believed to occur when the cuff pressure is high enough to impede local blood circulation, with resultant ischemic necrosis of the mucosa. The most susceptible portions of the trachea are those in which the mucosa overlies the cartilaginous rings, which subsequently soften and become fragmented with the risk of tracheomalacia. This phase is subsequently followed by granulation formation and fibrosis. Postintubation stenosis is characterized by eccentric or concentric tracheal wall thickening and associated luminal narrowing. The craniocaudal length usually ranges from 1.5 to 2.5 cm.[12] Posttracheostomy stenosis occurs most commonly at the stoma site or less commonly at the site where the tip of the tube has impinged on the tracheal mucosa. It involves 1.5 to 2.5 cm of tracheal wall.[12,13]

Patients with mild iatrogenic stenosis may be initially asymptomatic. When present, symptoms are often delayed several weeks after extubation and include dyspnea on exertion, stridor, or wheezing. MDCT is the imaging modality of choice for detecting and characterizing tracheal stenoses. On axial images, CT demonstrates eccentric or concentric soft-tissue thickening with associated luminal narrowing. Multiplanar and reformations along the long axis of the trachea and volume rendering reconstruction help assess the location and extent of the stenosis (**Fig. 1**). On longitudinal images, the focal and circumferential luminal narrowing may produce a characteristic "hourglass" configuration (**Fig. 2**).[8] Less commonly, tracheal or bronchial stenosis may present as a thin membrane or granulation tissue protruding into the airway lumen (**Fig. 3**). Interventional bronchoscopic (eg, balloon dilatation, stenting, or laser therapy) or surgical procedures (eg, resection and anastomosis) may be used to treat symptomatic tracheal stenosis.

After lung transplantation, bronchial anastomotic stenosis may occur in 10% to 15% of cases.[14,15] Risk factors include infection, rejection, and immunosuppression. Affected patients typically present with failure of anticipated improvements in symptoms in the first months after transplantation and decline in pulmonary function, especially the FEV_1. Severe stenosis may result in progressive airflow obstruction that is difficult to clinically differentiate from other causes of airflow limitation that may occur after lung transplantation, particularly obliterative bronchiolitis.[16] The diagnosis is obtained at bronchoscopy and shows a focal cicatricial narrowing at the anastomotic site. MDCT with multiplanar reformations and volume rendering techniques provides information on the length of the stenosis and the patency of the distal airways, which is important in planning treatment. CT findings consist of focal narrowing at the bronchial anastomotic site.[16] Virtual bronchoscopy assesses the grade of the stenosis with a good correlation with pulmonary function tests.[15] CT is also used to assess the patency of the airways distal to high-grade stenosis not traversable by the endoscope and assess the response to treatment in the follow-up. Treatment consists of balloon dilatation followed by placement of a stent.

TUBERCULOSIS

Tracheobronchial stenosis caused by tuberculosis may occur in the setting of acute infection or as late as 30 years after infection.[14] Endobronchial tuberculosis has been reported in 10% to 37% of patients with pulmonary tuberculosis, and a variable degree of stenosis has been reported to occur in 90% of cases.[14] Isolated tracheal involvement is likely a rare manifestation. Tuberculosis typically involves the distal trachea and proximal bronchi. Spread along peribronchial lymphatic channels seems to play a more important role than direct airway spread by infected sputum. Evidence supporting this hypothesis is that in many patients in whom the central airways biopsy is positive for tuberculosis, main tuberculous lesions are confined to the submucosa, with the mucosa either remaining intact or having only shallow ulceration.[17] Another mechanism is local extension from adjacent mediastinal tuberculosis lymphadenitis. The presence of lymphadenopathy contiguous to the tuberculous lesions in the trachea or main bronchi suggests that local extension is a probable mechanism (**Fig. 4**).[18]

Tuberculosis indirectly involves the bronchial wall, and the disease undergoes several evolutional

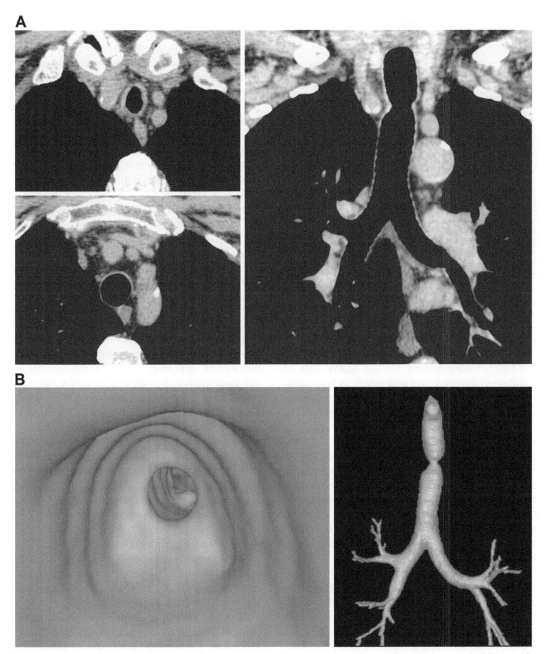

Fig. 1. Postintubation tracheal stenosis. (*A*) Transverse scans targeted on the trachea and coronal oblique reformat along the long axis and mainstem bronchi. (*B*) Descending virtual bronchoscopy and three-dimensional external rendering of the tracheobronchial tree. Presence of a short, concentric, and symmetric stenosis of the tracheal lumen at the level of the upper part of the intrathoracic portion of the trachea. Note on the transverse scan (*A*) a regular, concentric wall thickening at the level of the stenosis. Note calcifications of the aortic arch and right innominate artery.

stages, including early formation of tubercles in the submucosal layer, ulceration and necrosis of the mucosal wall, and healing with a variable degree of fibrosis or residual stenosis. Surprisingly, despite active infection, prebronchoscopic sputum samples produce negative results.[17] Endoscopic evaluation may not be diagnostic. Endobronchial biopsy has proven to be nonspecific in one third of the cases.[19] Although various stages of the disease may coexist in one patient, the prognosis is worse at the stage of fibrotic disease than in active disease. Not surprisingly, CT findings tend to reflect the stage of disease.[18–20] Stenosis in active disease occurs by hyperplastic changes

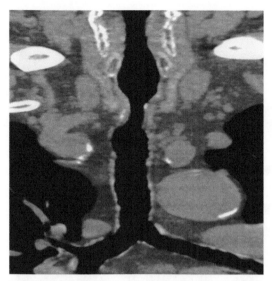

Fig. 2. Postintubation tracheal stenosis. Coronal obli-que reformation along the long axis of the trachea. Circumferential luminal narrowing extended along 2 cm associated with soft-tissue thickening, which produces the characteristic "hourglass configuration."

and inflammatory edema. On CT scans, loss of definition of the bronchial wall resulting from adja-cent lymphadenopathy, irregular luminal narrowing with wall thickening, contrast enhancement of the tracheal wall, and rim enhancement of enlarged mediastinal node are common findings.[18–20] Rarely tuberculous nodes are observed to cavitate, which results in communication with the adjacent airway (see **Fig. 4**). Nodobronchial fistula is depicted by the presence of gas in cavitated hila or mediastinal lymphadenopathy adjacent to the airway. Discrete visualization of the sinus tract between the bron-chial lumen and the hypertrophied cavitated lymph node can help plan therapy.

Stenosis in fibrotic disease occurs by fibroste-nosis, and tuberculomas are usually absent in the diseased bronchial wall. On CT scans, smooth narrowing of the tracheobronchial lumen with minimal wall thickening is typically seen (**Fig. 5**). The bronchial stenosis is concentric with uniform thickening of the bronchial wall and involvement of the long segment of the bronchus (>3 cm).[19] Unlike active infection, which involves the main-stem bronchi equally, fibrotic tuberculosis has been reported to involve the left mainstem bron-chus more often.

CT findings of central airway tuberculosis are nonspecific and need to be distinguished from bronchogenic carcinoma affecting the central airways. The differential diagnosis from broncho-genic carcinoma can be made by the longer segment of involvement, circumferential luminal narrowing, and absence of an intraluminal mass.

CT scans must always be supplemented by bron-choscopy and biopsy to confirm the diagnosis, however. On follow-up after medical treatment, CT findings of irregular airway narrowing, obstruc-tion, enlarged lymph nodes, and wall thickening, which are observed at the active stage of disease, are replaced by normal airways or smooth luminal narrowing with nearly normal wall thickness. In some patients, the airway disease progresses and residual fibrostenosis occurs. In fibrotic disease, usually there is no change in airway nar-rowing on follow-up CT studies. This disease form is resistant to medical treatment. Radiologic or surgical intervention is usually needed to restore the luminal patency.[14]

BRONCHIAL ANTHRACOFIBROSIS

Bronchial anthracofibrosis recently was defined as an inflammatory bronchial stenosis associated with anthracotic pigmentation on bronchoscopy without a relevant history of pneumoconiosis or smoking. Most patients with bronchial anthracosis have had no exposure to mining or industry and no history of smoking. A potential relationship between bronchial anthracosis and tuberculosis has been suggested, however. It has been hypoth-esized that the black pigments in the bronchial walls are derived from anthracotic material in the adjacent lymph nodes. The involved lymph nodes may perforate into the adjacent bronchi, and carbon particles in the lymph nodes may penetrate the bronchial wall as deep as the mucosa, result-ing in coloring of the bronchial mucosa. Subse-quently, healing with fibrotic response may occur and result in bronchial narrowing or obstruction with anthracotic pigmentation.[21,22]

Most patients are elderly women who usually present with cough, sputum, and dyspnea. On bronchoscopy, the right middle lobe bronchi is the most commonly involved site followed by the right upper, left upper, lingula division, right lower, and left lower lobe bronchi. Multiple site involve-ment may be seen in up to 50% of patients. On CT, a segmental collapse distal to the involved bronchi is the most commonly reported finding, with the right middle lobe being the most frequently involved lobe. The other findings include smooth bronchial narrowing accompanied by thickening of the wall and enlarged mediastinal or hilar lymph nodes adjacent to the involved bronchi (**Fig. 6**). Calcified nodes adjacent to the bronchi supplying the atelectatic lung are seen in more than 50% of patients. The CT findings are similar to those observed in bronchial tubercu-losis. Bronchial biopsy is required to eliminate malignancy.

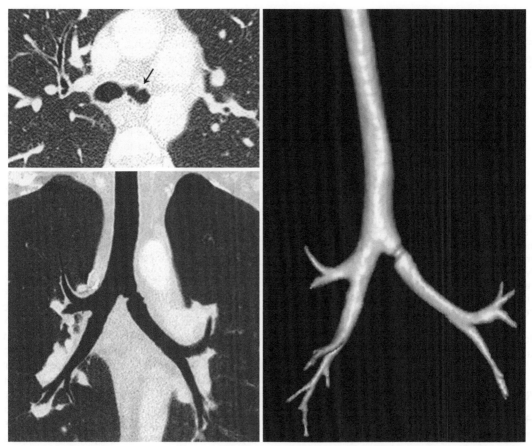

Fig. 3. Iatrogenic stenosis of the left mainstem bronchus occurred after a selective intubation. Transverse scan (*top left*), coronal oblique reformat of the tracheal lumen with minimum intensity projection (*bottom left*), and three-dimensional external rendering reformation of the tracheobronchial tree (*right*). The traumatic lesion occurred during intubation. Presence of nodular lesions along the inner surface of the left main bronchus (*arrow*) reflects granulation tissue and concentric narrowing of the origin of the left main bronchus.

RHINOSCLEROMA

Rhinoscleroma is a slowly progressive infectious granulomatous disease caused by *Klebsiella rhinoscleromatis,* a capsulated gram-negative bacterium that is endemic in tropical and subtropical areas.[23,24] Typically involving the upper respiratory tract, this organism also may involve the trachea and proximal bronchi. If left untreated, the infection progresses slowly over many years with alternating periods of remission and relapse. Pathologically in the granulomatous phase, nodules and masses cause partial obstruction of the involved airways (pseudoepitheliomatous hyperplasia). In the final sclerotic stage, the airway appears deformed, with stenosis developing secondary to fibrosis. The diagnosis is generally established by biopsy or positive culture results.

CT findings include diffuse nodular thickening of the proximal airway walls with luminal narrowing, nodularity of the tracheal mucosa, and concentric strictures of the trachea and bronchi. Mediastinal or hilar lymphadenopathy and postobstructive consolidation also may be present.[14] Antibiotherapy generally results in improvement, but advanced cases with fibrotic stenosis may benefit from interventional procedures.

FUNGAL TRACHEOBRONCHITIS

Acute tracheobronchitis caused by aspergillosis is uncommon and is usually restricted to the central airways. It usually occurs in severely immunocompromised individuals, especially persons with underlying malignancies or AIDS, or in individuals who have undergone bone marrow, lung, or heart transplantation.[25] Histologically, there is evidence of respiratory epithelial ulceration and submucosal inflammation. CT reveals nonspecific multifocal or diffuse tracheobronchial wall thickening, which results in either smooth or nodular luminal narrowing (**Fig. 7**).[26,27] Bronchial wall necrosis may lead

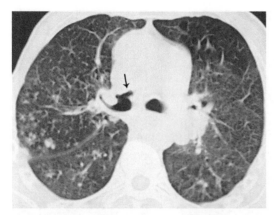

Fig. 4. Transverse scan in a patient with active tuberculosis. Nodobronchial fistula. There is direct communication between the anterior aspect of the right mainstem bronchus and the necrotic mediastinal lymphadenopathy (*arrow*). Multiple small, centrilobular, nodular opacities and nodules within the right upper lobe and, to a lesser extent, in the lower lobes represent endobronchial spread of tuberculosis.

to bronchial rupture, and associated rupture of the adjacent pulmonary artery may lead to death.[28]

RELAPSING POLYCHONDRITIS

Relapsing polychondritis is an unusual multisystemic disease of unknown origin that is

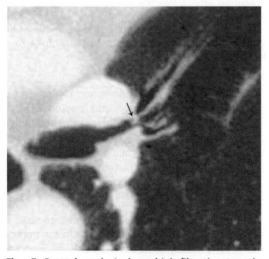

Fig. 5. Posttuberculosis bronchial fibrotic stenosis. Oblique reformat along the long axis of the left upper lobar bronchus. The bronchial stenosis visible at the origin of the lingular bronchus is short and has a nodular endoluminal appearance without any extrabronchial soft tissue mass (*arrow*). There is a distortion of the airways distal to the bronchial stenosis. (*From* Grenier PA. Imagerie thoracique de l'adulte. 3rd edition. Paris: Flammarion Médecine-Sciences; 2006; with permission.)

characterized by recurrent inflammation of the cartilaginous structures of the nose, external ear, peripheral joints, larynx, trachea, and bronchi.[29] Relapsing polychondritis is likely immune-mediated and considered to have an autoimmune pathogenesis. Although any age group may be affected, the peak of incidence of the disease is between the third and the sixth decades with a slight predominance in women. Airway involvement is present in up to 50% of patients and is a major cause of morbidity and mortality.[29,30] Rarely, it may occur as an isolated manifestation of the disease.[31] Airway involvement may be asymptomatic in early stages, but most patients with laryngotracheal involvement present with nonspecific respiratory tract symptoms, including cough, dyspnea, wheezing, aphonia, and hoarseness.[30]

The larynx and subglottic trachea are often the initial sites of involvement. As the disease progresses, the distal trachea and bronchi may be involved. The airway may be involved focally or diffusely. The distal bronchi may be involved to the level of the subsegmental bronchi. Pathologically, the disease is characterized by an acute inflammatory infiltrate in the cartilage and perichondrial tissue. Airway inflammation may result in luminal narrowing. Dissolution and fragmentation of the cartilage occur and may be followed by fibrosis.[32] In the late stages of the disease, this fibrosis-induced contraction of the airway may lead to severe luminal narrowing. Loss of structural cartilaginous support also may result in tracheobronchomalacia. The diagnosis of the disease is made on clinical criteria according to the lack of pathognomonic histologic or laboratory findings. Michet and colleagues[33] established major (auricular, nose, and laryngotracheal chondritis) and minor (ocular inflammation, hypoacousia, vestibular damage, seronegative inflammatory arthritis) criteria. The presence of two major criteria or one major criterion and two minor criteria permits the diagnosis.

The most common CT pattern is a combination of increased airway wall attenuation in association with smooth tracheal or bronchial wall thickening that characteristically spares the posterior membranous portion of the trachea (**Fig. 8**).[12–14,34] The degree of increased attenuation may range from subtle to a finding of frank calcification (see **Fig. 8**A, B).[34] Narrowing of airway lumen is more or less present (see **Fig. 8**C).[35] In advanced disease, circumferential wall thickening may be seen (**Fig. 9**). Gross destruction of the cartilaginous rings associated with fibrotic stenosis may occur. Important flaccidity of the airway wall may lead to considerable

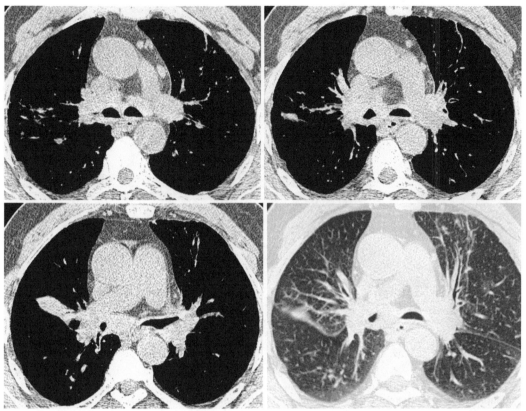

Fig. 6. Anthracofibrosis. Transverse nonenhanced CT scans. There is stenosis of the right upper lobar bronchus by a soft-tissue mass that extents medially into the mediastinum. Note thickening of the posterior wall of the right upper lobar and intermediate bronchi and narrowing and deformity of the lumen of the intermediate bronchus. Enlargement of the precarinal and subcarinal lymph nodes is visible.

collapse on expiratory CT images (see **Fig. 8**D). Using dynamic expiratory CT, Lee and colleagues[9] found malacia and expiratory air trapping in 13 and 17 of 18 patients, respectively, with relapsing polychondritis.

Differential diagnosis is easy when CT images depict the presence of characteristic smooth thickening of the anterior and lateral walls of the trachea, and a diagnosis of relapsing polychondritis can be made with a high degree of confidence. Tracheobronchopathia osteoplastica, which also spares the posterior membranous wall of the trachea, is easily distinguished from relapsing polychondritis by the presence of nodules arising from the submucosa of the tracheal lumen and protruding into the airway lumen.

Treatment is based on a combination of medications, including corticosteroids, immunosuppressive agents, and nonsteroidal anti-inflammatory drugs.[29] Although these drugs may temporarily decrease the severity of recurrences, disease usually progresses. CT may play a role in the follow-up to assess the response to therapy.[36] Tracheostomy, tracheal stenting, and tracheal

reconstruction may be used to provide long-term palliation.[37]

WEGENER'S GRANULOMATOSIS

Wegener's granulomatosis is a disease of unknown origin that is characterized by a necrotizing granulomatous vascularitis. Involvement of the large airways is a common manifestation of the disease. Its frequency was reported as 16% and 23% in two large series.[38,39] Although most often unassociated with symptoms or a late manifestation of well-established disease, tracheal or bronchial stenosis is occasionally responsible for the initial presentation.[40] Subglottic stenosis may occur in Wegener's granulomatosis without other evidence of pulmonary involvement. In one series, approximately 50% of tracheal stenoses occurred independently of other features of active Wegener's granulomatosis.[38]

Histologically, granulomatous inflammation and vascularitis typical of the disorder can be seen in the mucosa and submucosa in the early stage. Fibrosis is seen later. Endoscopic manifestations

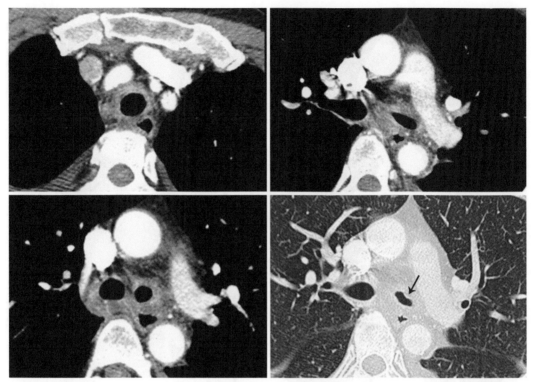

Fig. 7. Necrotizing aspergillosis of proximal airways in a young immunocompromised patient suffering from a B-lymphoma treated by chemotherapy and bone marrow transplantation. Transverse scans through the proximal airways. Diffuse and circumferential thickening of the tracheobronchial walls and soft tissue infiltration in the mediastinum fat around the trachea and mainstem bronchi are visible. There is regular narrowing of the left mainstem bronchus with a nodular appearance of the anterior inner surface of the left main bronchus (*arrow*).

include inflammatory tracheobronchial stenosis, ulcerating tracheobronchitis, and tracheobronchial stenosis without an inflammatory component. In a study of 77 patients with documented disease, Cordier and colleagues[41] found that 55% of patients in whom fiberoptic bronchoscopy was performed proved to have airway involvement. In another study by Daum and colleagues[42] that included 51 patients who underwent bronchoscopy, airway abnormalities were found in 59%, including subglottic stenosis in 17%, ulcerating tracheobronchitis in 60%, and tracheal or bronchial stenosis in 13%.

On CT, tracheal stenoses are most commonly subglottic (**Fig. 10**). In a study of ten patients with known tracheal involvement, Screaton and colleagues[43] noted that 90% of lesions were subglottic and identifiable as short segments of circumferential mucosal thickening. Usually tracheal stenosis presents as smooth or irregular circumferential narrowing approximately 2 to 4 cm long.[43,44] CT shows abnormal intratracheal soft tissue, which is often associated with thickening and calcification of the tracheal ring. Cartilaginous erosion also may be seen. CT studies have

demonstrated the high frequency of airway abnormalities on the more distal airways. For instance, Lee and colleagues[45] reported that central airway abnormalities could be identified in 30% of patients, whereas segmental and subsegmental bronchial wall thickening with or without luminal narrowing or obliteration was detectable in 73% of patients. Bronchial stenosis may result in distal collapse or consolidation of a lobe or lung.[41]

Virtual bronchoscopy may help detect subtle tracheal or bronchial stenosis. In a study of 18 virtual bronchoscopic examinations performed in 11 patients with Wegener's granulomatosis, 32 of 40 bronchoscopically visible stenoses, most in the lobar and intermediate bronchi, were identified on virtual bronchoscopy by at least one reading radiologist compared with only 22 on axial images.[46] According to the high prevalence of subglottic stenoses, this area always should be included in the imaging volume in patients with Wegener's granulomatosis.[8]

CT has proved valuable in follow-up of airway abnormalities. In the study by Lee and colleagues,[45] 20 patients had follow-up CT examinations. There was total resolution of previously

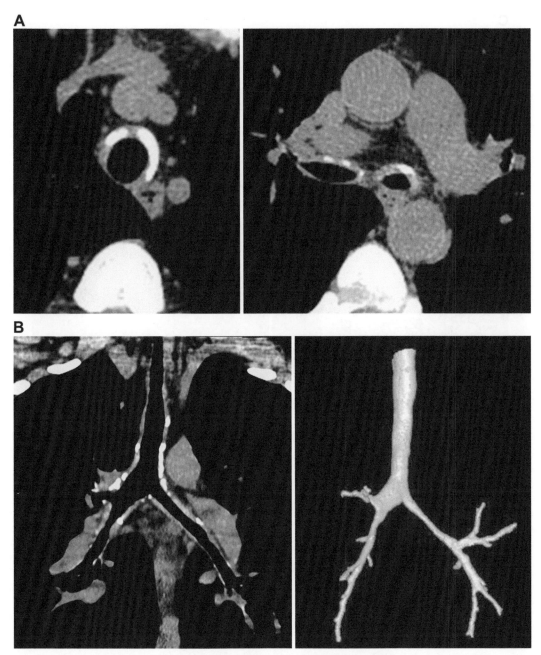

Fig. 8. Relapsing polychondritis. (*A*) Transverse scan through the trachea and mainstem bronchi. (*B*) Coronal oblique reformat along the proximal airways and three-dimensional external rendering of the tracheobronchial air content. (*C*) Transverse scan through the trachea and main and lobar bronchi. (*D*) Transverse scan of the carina at full inspiration (*top*) and during forced dynamic expiratory maneuver (*bottom*). There is diffuse and regular thickening of the anterior and lateral walls of the trachea and thickening of the anterior wall of the main and lobar bronchi. This wall thickening contains calcific deposits. Diffuse narrowing of the lumen of the mainstem and lobar bronchi is present. Tracheobronchomalacia with complete collapse of the mainstem bronchi during expiration was noted.

C

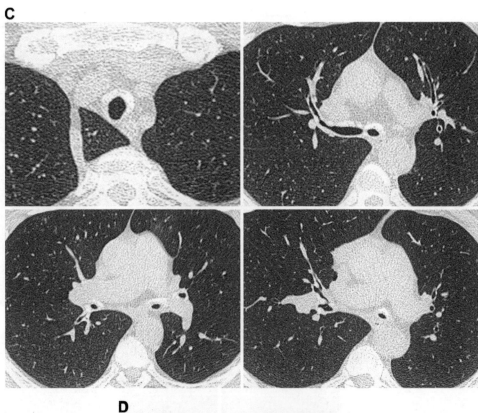

D

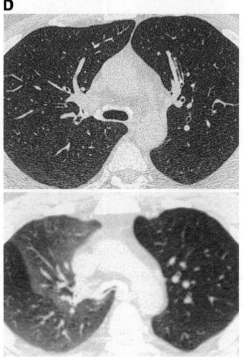

Fig. 8. (*continued*)

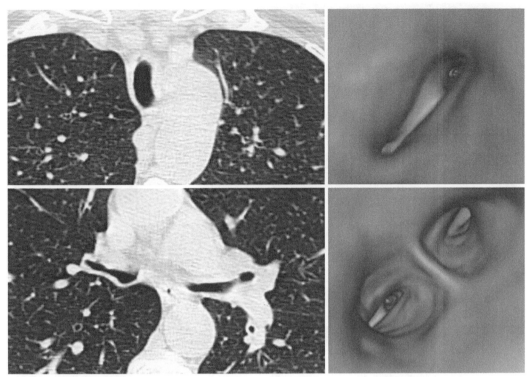

Fig. 9. Relapsing polychondritis in a patient with advanced disease. Transverse scan (*left*) and descending virtual endoscopic views (*right*). A circumferential wall thickening is present with narrowing and deformity of the tracheal and bronchial lumens.

identified airway abnormalities in 5 patients, lung parenchyma and airway lesions improved with partial disappearance in 12 patients, and 3 patients demonstrated evidence of recurrent disease. Tracheal stenosis is often unresponsive to systemic therapy, however, and local intervention is favored. Airway lesions may occur in the course of therapy, with symptomatic airway lesions occurring in the course of relapses.[47] CT may prove invaluable by demonstrating optimal sites for tracheostomy and by defining the true extent of disease when bronchial narrowing precludes complete bronchoscopic evaluation. Virtual bronchoscopy is particularly appreciated in this setting.[46] Park and colleagues[48] described MR findings of Wegener's granulomatosis stenosis. Abnormal soft tissue at the level of the stenosis is of intermediate signal on T1-weighted images, high signal on T2-weighted images, and enhances with contrast agent.

TRACHEOBRONCHIAL AMYLOIDOSIS

Deposition of amyloid in the tracheal bronchi may be seen in association with systemic amyloidosis or as an isolated manifestation.[49,50] Airway involvement may be focal, multifocal, or diffuse.

Diffuse involvement is most common. It may involve the larynx, trachea, main bronchi, and lobar or proximal segmental bronchi and often involves contiguous segments of the airway. Histologically the amyloid tends to be deposited initially in relation to tracheal gland acini and the walls of small blood vessels in the mucosa. As the amount of disease increases, the glands atrophy and the amyloid generates irregular plaques and nodules in the mucosa that are usually multifocal,or less commonly forms a single mass-like syndrome. The overlying mucosa is intact. Dystrophic calcification and ossification are frequently present at histologic examination.

Affected patients are often asymptomatic for a long time before diagnosis, which suggests that the disease progresses relatively slowly. In patients with proximal subglottic or laryngeal involvement, the disease manifests by hoarseness or stridor, whereas patients who have distal tracheal or bronchial involvement suffer from cough, wheezing, dyspnea, or hemoptysis.[49,50] In case of bronchial obstruction, patients may present with fever caused by obstructive pneumonitis. Endoscopic examination of the disease shows either submucosal plaques and nodules with a cobblestone appearance or a tumor-like

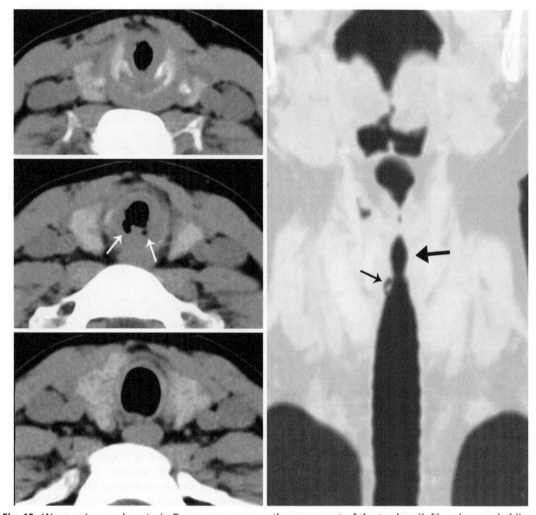

Fig. 10. Wegener's granulomatosis. Transverse scan over the upper part of the trachea (*left*) and coronal oblique reformat along the long axis of the trachea targeted on the larynx and cervical part of the trachea (*right*). Note short concentric stenosis of the subglottic area of the trachea (*large arrow*). Circumferential thickening of the tracheal wall at the level of the stenosis is visible. Note the presence of two small ulcerations within the posterior wall of the trachea (*small arrows*).

appearance or circumferential wall thickening. Endoscopic biopsies are diagnostic.[51]

On CT scans, amyloid results in circumferential tracheal or bronchial wall thickening caused by the submucosal deposition of nodules and plaques that induces a luminal narrowing (**Fig. 11**).[12,49,50,52–55] There may be multiple concentric or eccentric strictures. Mural calcifications are prominent features that have to be distinguished from calcified lymph nodes. Some patients with tracheobronchial amyloidosis have hilar or mediastinal calcified or noncalcified enlarged lymph nodes.[56] In patients with recurrent obstructive pneumonias, bronchiectasis also may be identified. Other patterns may be seen, such as eccentric strictures sparing the posterior membrane of the trachea.[50] Local lesions give rise to endoluminal masses (amyloidomas) that may be radiologically indistinguishable from neoplasms.[8]

There have been rare reports of concurrent tracheobronchial amyloidosis and tracheobronchopathia osteoplastica.[49,51] In most cases, however, these entities prove pathologically distinct. In patients with severe narrowing, the amyloid deposits may be removed by intermittent bronchoscopic resections using either forceps or laser.[57] Resection is not curative, however, and lesions often recur 6 to 12 months after treatment. Other options include stenting and radiation therapy.[58,59] Tracheostomies may be required in case of subglottic involvement.

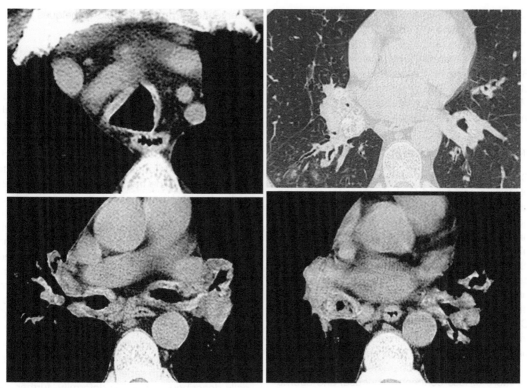

Fig. 11. Tracheobronchial amyloidosis as seen on transverse scans on the trachea and proximal bronchi. Thickening of the walls of the trachea is associated with tracheal lumen deformity. There is diffuse thickening of the bronchial walls containing calcific deposits. Luminal narrowing of the upper lobar and right intermediate bronchi and occlusion of the lumen of the right middle and lower lobar bronchi is visible.

SARCOIDOSIS

Involvement of the trachea is rare, and when it occurs, it is usually associated with laryngeal involvement.[60] The proximal and distal parts of the trachea may be affected, and the appearance of the stenosis may be smooth, irregular and nodular, or even mass-like. Bronchial involvement is much more common as a manifestation of sarcoidosis.[61] It was reported in 65% of 60 patients with sarcoidosis in a study by Lenique and colleagues[62] using high resolution computed tomography. The most common findings are regular or nodular bronchial wall thickening of the lobar, segmental, or subsegmental airways. The thickening likely reflects the presence of granulomas and fibrous tissue in the peribronchial interstitium. This bronchial wall thickening may result in smooth or irregular luminal narrowing, as was observed in 23% of patients by Lenique and colleagues (**Fig. 12**).[62] The luminal narrowing correlates with the presence of mucosal thickening at bronchoscopy and presumably reflects prominent inflammation in this location. Recognition of these abnormalities may be diagnostically important, because endobronchial biopsy of an abnormal site is likely to yield granulomas.

Obstruction of lobar or segmental bronchi may occur as a result of airway wall fibrosis and granulomas or peribronchial lymph node compression

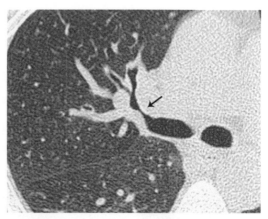

Fig. 12. Sarcoidosis. Transverse scan targets the right upper lobe. Stenosis of the distal part of the right upper lobar bronchus extending to the anterior segmental bronchus is visible (*arrow*).

and conglomerate fibrosis or some combination of these phenomena.[63] Lobar or segmental atelectasis remains an uncommon manifestation, occurring in approximately 1% of cases of sarcoidosis.[64] Bronchial stenosis caused by sarcoidosis may clear spontaneously or with steroid treatment.[65] Mechanical dilatation or stenting may be proposed in case of refractory stenosis.[66,67]

INFLAMMATORY BOWEL DISEASE

Chronic inflammatory bowel diseases, including ulcerative colitis and Crohn's disease, occasionally may demonstrate extraintestinal manifestations. Among them, airway disease is relatively uncommon and may take several forms, including ulcerative tracheitis and tracheobronchitis, bronchiectasis, and small airway disease, most commonly obliterative bronchiolitis.[68–70] Tracheobronchial complications are rare and occur more often in association with ulcerative colitis than Crohn's disease. In most—but not all—cases, the diagnosis of inflammatory bowel disease precedes the presence of airway disease.

Tracheobronchitis is characterized histologically by more or less concentric mucosal and submucosal fibrosis and chronic inflammation. Ulceration and luminal narrowing may be evident. The cartilaginous plates may be calcified but are not destroyed. Affected patients present with nonspecific symptoms of airway obstruction, including stridor, dyspnea, and cough. CT findings are nonspecific.[14] The tracheobronchial walls are thickened and produce irregular luminal narrowing. Bronchial wall thickening and bronchiectasis also may be present with or without mucoid impaction. If medical therapy (intravenous steroids and cyclosporine) fails to resolve symptoms, interventional bronchoscopic techniques may be considered.[8]

SABER SHEATH TRACHEA

Sabear sheath trachea is a relatively uncommon deformity of the trachea characterized by reduction in coronal diameter and elongation of the sagittal diameter. It is defined by a coronal diameter equal to or less than one-half its sagittal diameter, measured at 1 cm above the top of the aortic arch.[71,72] This deformity affects only the intrathoracic portion of the trachea, with abrupt widening of the tracheal lumen above the thoracic inlet. It may extend downward on the mainstem bronchi. This deformity is almost always associated with chronic obstructive pulmonary disease and has been described exclusively in men.[71] It has been postulated to be the consequence of abnormal pattern and magnitude pressure changes related to hyperinflated lungs.[13] The deformity is often detected incidentally on chest radiograph or CT (**Fig. 13**). The inner contour of the trachea is often smooth but occasionally has a nodular contour. Calcification of tracheal cartilage is frequently evident.[73] Although saber sheath trachea is classically described as a static deformity, further narrowing of the tracheal lumen can be documented when patients are examined during forced expiration, reflecting excessive collapsibility of lateral walls (tracheomalacia).[74]

TRACHEOBRONCHOPATHIA OSTEOCHONDROPLASTICA

This rare disorder is characterized by the presence of multiple submucosal cartilaginous or bony nodules projecting into the tracheobronchial lumen.[12–14,75] It is a benign disease of unknown

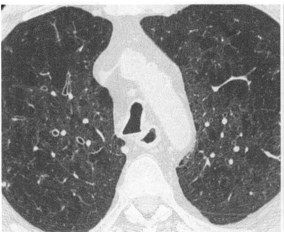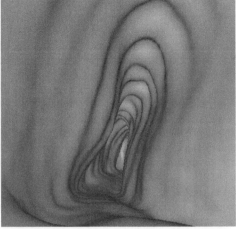

Fig. 13. Saber sheath trachea in a patient with severe chronic obstructive pulmonary disease. Transverse scan (*left*) and descending virtual endoscopy view (*right*). Characteristic deformity of the tracheal lumen is present.

origin. Men are more frequently involved than women, and most patients are older than age 50. Several potential causes or associations have been postulated, including amyloidosis, hereditary factors, chemical irritation, and infection. Most cases are asymptomatic, but patients may present with chronic cough, hoarseness, stridor, or wheezing that is sometimes confused with asthma. It has been reported to cause hemoptysis.[76] Histologically, the nodules are recognized as submucosal osteocartilaginous growths. The mucosal surface is intact, and a connection between the nodule and the perichondrium of the tracheal cartilaginous ring is frequently identified. Because it contains no cartilage, the posterior wall of the trachea is spared.

CT is the imaging modality of choice for this condition.[75,77–79] It demonstrates a pattern of multiple calcified nodules arising from the anterior and lateral walls of the trachea and protruding into the lumen. The nodules typically range in size from 3 to 8 mm. They result in diffuse luminal narrowing and are associated with thickening and deformity of the tracheal rings. The posterior membranous portion of the trachea is spared. The differential diagnoses include amyloidosis and tuberculosis, but these diseases do not respect the posterior wall. Relapsing polychondritis also affects the posterior wall, but the thickening of the wall is not nodular in appearance. In most patients, the disease progresses slowly. Therapy is requisite only when the tracheal or bronchial lumens become compromised. Therapeutic options include surgical or laser resection, radiation therapy, and stent placement.

BRONCHOLITHIASIS

Broncholithiasis is a condition in which calcified lymph nodes distort and erode into the tracheobronchial tree, and patients may expectorate or aspirate the calcified material.[80] Most broncholiths are composed of fragments of calcified material that were originally located in a peribronchial lymph node. Broncholithiasis is considered as a late complication of granulomatous lymphadenitis caused by *Mycobacterium tuberculosis* or fungi such as *Histoplasma capsulatum*. Pathologically the airway is fibrotic and distorted, and erosion by calcified lymph nodes may be apparent. Bronchial wall fibrosis and obstruction pneumonitis may be present. Identification of calcified material within an acute inflammatory exudate or granulation tissue is key for diagnosis on bronchoscopic biopsy specimen. The diagnosis may be made at CT by identifying a focus of calcified material within the bronchial lumen without any mass (**Fig. 14**).[80–82] Peribronchial

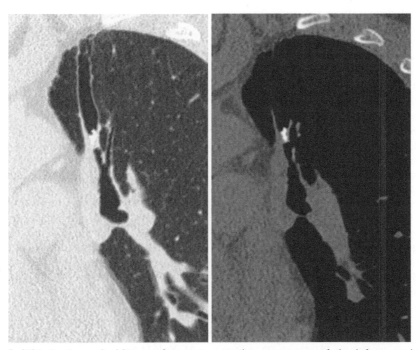

Fig. 14. Broncholithiasis. Coronal oblique reformat targets the upper part of the left upper lobe. There is complete obliteration of the lumen of the subsegmental bronchus by endoluminal calcified material, complicated by postobstructive bronchiectasis.

lymph node calcification is commonly seen. Post-obstructive abnormalities are often present, including bronchiectasis, obstructive consolidation, and air trapping.

SUMMARY

MDCT using thin collimation and postprocessing techniques, such as multiplanar reformations along and perpendicular to the central axes of the central airways, and volume rendering techniques, such as virtual bronchoscopy and virtual bronchography, has become the imaging modality of choice for the diagnosis of nonneoplastic tracheal and bronchial stenoses. It may ensure accurate assessment of the location and extent of the stenosis and good characterization of the presence, distribution, type, and calcification of airway wall thickening. The consideration of these abnormalities in combination with associated CT findings observed in the mediastinum, hilum, or lung parenchyma and available clinical and laboratory data help the radiologist to shorten the list of different diagnoses. The role of MDCT is also to guide surgical and interventional endoscopic procedures and assess response to treatment.

REFERENCES

1. Boiselle PM, Ernst A. Recent advances in central airway imaging. Chest 2002;121(5):1651–60.
2. Boiselle PM, Reynolds KF, Ernst A. Multiplanar and three-dimensional imaging of the central airways with multidetector CT. AJR Am J Roentgenol 2002; 179(2):301–8.
3. Grenier PA, Beigelman-Aubry C, Fetita C, et al. New frontiers in CT imaging of airway disease. Eur Radiol 2002;12(5):1022–44.
4. Salvolini L, Bichi Secchi E, Costarelli L, et al. Clinical applications of 2D and 3D CT imaging of the airways: a review. Eur J Radiol 2000;34(1):9–25.
5. Naidich DP, Gruden JF, McGuinness G, et al. Volumetric (helical/spiral) CT (VCT) of the airways. J Thorac Imaging 1997;12(1):11–28.
6. Remy-Jardin M, Remy J, Artaud D, et al. Volume rendering of the tracheobronchial tree: clinical evaluation of bronchographic images. Radiology 1998; 208(3):761–70.
7. Remy-Jardin M, Remy J, Artaud D, et al. Tracheobronchial tree: assessment with volume rendering: technical aspects. Radiology 1998;208(2):393–8.
8. Boiselle PM, Castena J, Ernst A, et al. Tracheobronchial stenosis. In: Boiselle PM, Lynch DA, editors. CT of the airways. Totowa (NJ): Humana Press; 2008. p. 121–49.
9. Lee KS, Ernst A, Trentham DE, et al. Relapsing polychondritis: prevalence of expiratory CT airway abnormalities. Radiology 2006;240(2):565–73.
10. Stauffer JL, Olson DE, Petty TL. Complications and consequences of endotracheal intubation and tracheotomy: a prospective study of 150 critically ill adult patients. Am J Med 1981;70(1):65–76.
11. Norwood S, Vallina VL, Short K, et al. Incidence of tracheal stenosis and other late complications after percutaneous tracheostomy. Ann Surg 2000; 232(2):233–41.
12. Webb EM, Elicker BM, Webb WR. Using CT to diagnose nonneoplastic tracheal abnormalities: appearance of the tracheal wall. AJR Am J Roentgenol 2000;174(5):1315–21.
13. Marom EM, Goodman PC, McAdams HP. Focal abnormalities of the trachea and main bronchi. AJR Am J Roentgenol 2001;176(3):707–11.
14. Prince JS, Duhamel DR, Levin DL, et al. Nonneoplastic lesions of the tracheobronchial wall: radiologic findings with bronchoscopic correlation. Radiographics 2002;22:S215–30.
15. Shitrit D, Valdsislav P, Grubstein A, et al. Accuracy of virtual bronchoscopy for grading tracheobronchial stenosis: correlation with pulmonary function test and fiberoptic bronchoscopy. Chest 2005;128(5): 3545–50.
16. McAdams HP, Palmer SM, Erasmus JJ, et al. Bronchial anastomotic complications in lung transplant recipients: virtual bronchoscopy for noninvasive assessment. Radiology 1998;209(3):689–95.
17. Lee JH, Park SS, Lee DH, et al. Endobronchial tuberculosis: clinical and bronchoscopic features in 121 cases. Chest 1992;102(4):990–4.
18. Kim Y, Lee KS, Yoon JH, et al. Tuberculosis of the trachea and main bronchi: CT findings in 17 patients. AJR Am J Roentgenol 1997;168(4):1051–6.
19. Choe KO, Jeong HJ, Sohn HY. Tuberculous bronchial stenosis: CT findings in 28 cases. AJR Am J Roentgenol 1990;155(5):971–6.
20. Moon WK, Im JG, Yeon KM, et al. Tuberculosis of the central airways: CT findings of active and fibrotic disease. AJR Am J Roentgenol 1997; 169(3):649–53.
21. Chung MP, Lee KS, Han J, et al. Bronchial stenosis due to anthracofibrosis. Chest 1998; 113(2):344–50.
22. Kim HY, Im JG, Goo JM, et al. Bronchial anthracofibrosis (inflammatory bronchial stenosis with anthracotic pigmentation): CT findings. AJR Am J Roentgenol 2000;174(2):523–7.
23. Amoils CP, Shindo ML. Laryngotracheal manifestations of rhinoscleroma. Ann Otol Rhinol Laryngol 1996;105(5):336–40.
24. Yigla M, Ben-Izhak O, Oren I, et al. Laryngotracheobronchial involvement in a patient with nonendemic rhinoscleroma. Chest 2000;117(6):1795–8.

25. Miller WT Jr, Sais GJ, Frank I, et al. Pulmonary aspergillosis in patients with AIDS: clinical and radiographic correlations. Chest 1994;105(1):37–44.

26. Franquet T, Muller NL, Oikonomou A, et al. Aspergillus infection of the airways: computed tomography and pathologic findings. J Comput Assist Tomogr 2004;28(1):10–6.

27. Franquet T, Serrano F, Gimenez A, et al. Necrotizing aspergillosis of large airways: CT findings in eight patients. J Comput Assist Tomogr 2002; 26(3):342–5.

28. Taouli B, Cadi M, Leblond V, et al. Invasive aspergillosis of the mediastinum and left hilum: CT features. AJR Am J Roentgenol 2004;183(5):1224–6.

29. Trentham DE, Le CH. Relapsing polychondritis. Ann Intern Med 1998;129(2):114–22.

30. Letko E, Zafirakis P, Baltatzis S, et al. Relapsing polychondritis: a clinical review. Semin Arthritis Rheum 2002;31(6):384–95.

31. Tsunezuka Y, Sato H, Shimizu H. Tracheobronchial involvement in relapsing polychondritis. Respiration 2000;67(3):320–2.

32. Tillie-Leblond I, Wallaert B, Leblond D, et al. Respiratory involvement in relapsing polychondritis: clinical, functional, endoscopic, and radiographic evaluations. Medicine (Baltimore) 1998; 77(3):168–76.

33. Michet CJ Jr, McKenna CH, Luthra HS, et al. Relapsing polychondritis: survival and predictive role of early disease manifestations. Ann Intern Med 1986;104(1):74–8.

34. Behar JV, Choi YW, Hartman TA, et al. Relapsing polychondritis affecting the lower respiratory tract. AJR Am J Roentgenol 2002;178(1):173–7.

35. Kilman WJ. Narrowing of the airway in relapsing polychondritis. Radiology 1978;126(2):373–6.

36. Im JG, Chung JW, Han SK, et al. CT manifestations of tracheobronchial involvement in relapsing polychondritis. J Comput Assist Tomogr 1988;12(5): 792–3.

37. Sarodia BD, Dasgupta A, Mehta AC. Management of airway manifestations of relapsing polychondritis: case reports and review of literature. Chest 1999; 116(6):1669–75.

38. Langford CA, Sneller MC, Hallahan CW, et al. Clinical features and therapeutic management of subglottic stenosis in patients with Wegener's granulomatosis. Arthritis Rheum 1996;39(10): 1754–60.

39. McDonald TJ, Neel HB 3rd, DeRemee RA. Wegener's granulomatosis of the subglottis and the upper portion of the trachea. Ann Otol Rhinol Laryngol 1982;91(6 Pt 1):588–92.

40. Stein MG, Gamsu G, Webb WR, et al. Computed tomography of diffuse tracheal stenosis in Wegener granulomatosis. J Comput Assist Tomogr 1986; 10(5):868–70.

41. Cordier JF, Valeyre D, Guillevin L, et al. Pulmonary Wegener's granulomatosis: a clinical and imaging study of 77 cases. Chest 1990;97(4):906–12.

42. Daum TE, Specks U, Colby TV, et al. Tracheobronchial involvement in Wegener's granulomatosis. Am J Respir Crit Care Med 1995;151(2 Pt 1):522–6.

43. Screaton NJ, Sivasothy P, Flower CD, et al. Tracheal involvement in Wegener's granulomatosis: evaluation using spiral CT. Clin Radiol 1998;53(11): 809–15.

44. Cohen MI, Gore RM, August CZ, et al. Tracheal and bronchial stenosis associated with mediastinal adenopathy in Wegener granulomatosis: CT findings. J Comput Assist Tomogr 1984;8(2):327–9.

45. Lee KS, Kim TS, Fujimoto K, et al. Thoracic manifestation of Wegener's granulomatosis: CT findings in 30 patients. Eur Radiol 2003;13(1):43–51.

46. Summers RM, Aggarwal NR, Sneller MC, et al. CT virtual bronchoscopy of the central airways in patients with Wegener's granulomatosis. Chest 2002;121(1):242–50.

47. Aberle DR, Gamsu G, Lynch D. Thoracic manifestations of Wegener's granulomatosis: diagnosis and course. Radiology 1990;174(3 Pt 1):703–9.

48. Park KJ, Bergin CJ, Harrell J. MR findings of tracheal involvement in Wegener's granulomatosis. AJR Am J Roentgenol 1998;171(2):524–5.

49. Georgiades CS, Neyman EG, Barish MA, et al. Amyloidosis: review and CT manifestations. Radiographics 2004;24(2):405–16.

50. Kim HY, Im JG, Song KS, et al. Localized amyloidosis of the respiratory system: CT features. J Comput Assist Tomogr 1999;23(4):627–31.

51. Piazza C, Cavaliere S, Foccoli P, et al. Endoscopic management of laryngo-tracheobronchial amyloidosis: a series of 32 patients. Eur Arch Otorhinolaryngol 2003;260(7):349–54.

52. Kirchner J, Jacobi V, Kardos P, et al. CT findings in extensive tracheobronchial amyloidosis. Eur Radiol 1998;8(3):352–4.

53. Ozer C, Nass Duce M, Yildiz A, et al. Primary diffuse tracheobronchial amyloidosis: case report. Eur J Radiol 2002;44(1):37–9.

54. Pickford HA, Swensen SJ, Utz JP. Thoracic cross-sectional imaging of amyloidosis. AJR Am J Roentgenol 1997;168(2):351–5.

55. Urban BA, Fishman EK, Goldman SM, et al. CT evaluation of amyloidosis: spectrum of disease. Radiographics 1993;13(6):1295–308.

56. Crestani B, Monnier A, Kambouchner M, et al. Tracheobronchial amyloidosis with hilar lymphadenopathy associated with a serum monoclonal immunoglobulin. Eur Respir J 1993;6(10):1569–71.

57. Flemming AF, Fairfax AJ, Arnold AG, et al. Treatment of endobronchial amyloidosis by intermittent bronchoscopic resection. Br J Dis Chest 1980;74(2): 183–8.

58. Kalra S, Utz JP, Edell ES, et al. External-beam radiation therapy in the treatment of diffuse tracheobronchial amyloidosis. Mayo Clin Proc 2001;76(8):853–6.

59. Yang S, Chia SY, Chuah KL, et al. Tracheobronchial amyloidosis treated with rigid bronchoscopy and stenting. Surg Endosc 2003;17(4):658–9.

60. Brandstetter RD, Messina MS, Sprince NL, et al. Tracheal stenosis due to sarcoidosis. Chest 1981; 80(5):656.

61. Miller A, Brown LK, Teirstein AS. Stenosis of main bronchi mimicking fixed upper airway obstruction in sarcoidosis. Chest 1985;88(2):244–8.

62. Lenique F, Brauner MW, Grenier P, et al. CT assessment of bronchi in sarcoidosis: endoscopic and pathologic correlations. Radiology 1995;194(2): 419–23.

63. Olsson T, Bjornstad-Pettersen H, Stjernberg NL. Bronchostenosis due to sarcoidosis: a cause of atelectasis and airway obstruction simulating pulmonary neoplasm and chronic obstructive pulmonary disease. Chest 1979;75(6):663–6.

64. Freundlich IM, Libshitz HI, Glassman LM, et al. Sarcoidosis: typical and atypical thoracic manifestations and complications. Clin Radiol 1970;21(4): 376–83.

65. Corsello BF, Lohaus GH, Funahashi A. Endobronchial mass lesion due to sarcoidosis: complete resolution with corticosteroids. Thorax 1983;38(2):157–8.

66. Fouty BW, Pomeranz M, Thigpen TP, et al. Dilatation of bronchial stenoses due to sarcoidosis using a flexible fiberoptic bronchoscope. Chest 1994;106(3): 677–80.

67. Mayse ML, Greenheck J, Friedman M, et al. Successful bronchoscopic balloon dilation of nonmalignant tracheobronchial obstruction without fluoroscopy. Chest 2004;126(2):634–7.

68. Camus P, Colby TV. The lung in inflammatory bowel disease. Eur Respir J 2000;15(1):5–10.

69. Ulrich R, Goldberg R, Line WS. Crohn's disease: a rare cause of upper airway obstruction. J Emerg Med 2000;19(4):331–2.

70. Wilcox P, Miller R, Miller G, et al. Airway involvement in ulcerative colitis. Chest 1987;92(1):18–22.

71. Greene R. "Saber-sheath" trachea: relation to chronic obstructive pulmonary disease. AJR Am J Roentgenol 1978;130(3):441–5.

72. Trigaux JP, Hermes G, Dubois P, et al. CT of saber-sheath trachea: correlation with clinical, chest radiographic and functional findings. Acta Radiol 1994; 35(3):247–50.

73. Rubenstein J, Weisbrod G, Steinhardt MI. Atypical appearances of "saber-sheath" trachea. Radiology 1978;127(1):41–2.

74. Gamsu G, Webb WR. Computed tomography of the trachea: normal and abnormal. AJR Am J Roentgenol 1982;139(2):321–6.

75. Restrepo S, Pandit M, Villamil MA, et al. Tracheobronchopathia osteochondroplastica: helical CT findings in 4 cases. J Thorac Imaging 2004;19(2): 112–6.

76. Briones-Gomez A. Tracheopathie osteoplastica. J Bronchol 2000;7:301–5.

77. Bottles K, Nyberg DA, Clark M, et al. CT diagnosis of tracheobronchopathia osteochondroplastica. J Comput Assist Tomogr 1983;7(2):324–7.

78. Mariotta S, Pallone G, Pedicelli G, et al. Spiral CT and endoscopic findings in a case of tracheobronchopathia osteochondroplastica. J Comput Assist Tomogr 1997;21(3):418–20.

79. Onitsuka H, Hirose N, Watanabe K, et al. Computed tomography of tracheopathia osteoplastica. AJR Am J Roentgenol 1983;140(2):268–70.

80. Conces DJ, Tarver RD, Vix VA. Broncholithiasis: CT features in 15 patients. AJR Am J Roentgenol 1991;157(2):249–53.

81. Kowal LE, Goodman LR, Zarro VJ, et al. CT diagnosis of broncholithiasis. J Comput Assist Tomogr 1983;7(2):321–3.

82. Shin MS, Ho KJ. Broncholithiasis: its detection by computed tomography in patients with recurrent hemoptysis of unknown etiology. J Comput Tomogr 1983;7(2):189–93.

MDCT of Trachea and Main Bronchi

Cylen Javidan-Nejad, MD

KEYWORDS

- Tracheobronchial imaging • Trachea • Central airway
- Tracheomalacia

Diseases of the trachea and main bronchi are rare and present insidiously with nonspecific symptoms of dyspnea, cough, wheezing, and stridor. They commonly are misdiagnosed as asthma.[1]

Early recognition of tracheal disease is difficult, because the imaging findings are easily missed on imaging, such that the trachea has been regarded as the blind spot of the chest.[2] Timely diagnosis is further hampered, because symptoms of tracheal obstruction manifest only when the lesion occludes more than 75% of the tracheal lumen. At such point, the disease usually has advanced where similar therapeutic measures may not be feasible. If a tumor causes hemoptysis, it is discovered at an earlier stage.[3]

Once suspected, traditionally, many of these patients are evaluated by bronchoscopy, given its ability to directly visualize, biopsy, and sometimes treat lesions of the main airways. Bronchoscopy, however, is not well-tolerated by all patients, and it is associated with many complications, which can include minor ones, such as vasovagal reactions, nausea and vomiting, arrhythmias. More serious complications include sudden rise of intracranial pressure, pulmonary edema, laryngospasm, bronchospasm, and oxygen desaturation.[4] Furthermore, bronchoscopy is limited in evaluating the airway lumen beyond severe stenoses.[5] Therefore, for purposes of routine screening and treatment planning, a noninvasive method such as computed tomography (CT) is very helpful. With the advent and increased availability of multidetector CT, which allows fast volumetric image acquisition in a single breath hold and easy creation of two- and three-dimensional reformatted images of excellent quality, CT has become the imaging modality of choice for evaluating diseases of the trachea and main bronchi.[6,7]

MDCT TECHNIQUE

The inherent natural contrast of the lung parenchyma renders diagnostic imaging without use of intravenous contrast, at relatively lower radiation doses (110 to 140 kV and 50 to 80 mAs). The thinnest detector collimation is used when scanning. The newer multidetector scanners of 64 rows of detectors or more use detector collimators as thin as 0.625 mm. The images are reconstructed at a slice thickness of 1 mm, with 50% overlap, in the transaxial plane. A collimation of 0.625 mm creates a near-isometric resolution voxel of 0.4 mm.[8]

Imaging is performed twice, from the pharynx to the level of the first or second branching of the main bronchi, first at suspended end-inhalation, followed by scanning during active exhalation. The latter is performed only if there is a concern for tracheobronchomalacia. The advantage of active or forced exhalation is that it increases the sensitivity in diagnosis of subtle tracheobronchomalacia (**Fig. 1**).[9] Scanning should be performed only after coaching the patient with breathing instructions. For the dynamic exhalation portion of the examination, one should stress that the patient exhales without pursing his or her lips, because doing so artificially increases the intraluminal tracheal pressure, which may prevent manifestation of subtle tracheomalacia.[10]

To prevent scanning after the patient has finished active exhalation, it is imperative to know the fixed scan delay of the particular CT scanner being used. This is the time that lapses

This article originally appeared in *Radiologic Clinics of North America*, Volume 48, Issue 1, January 2010.
Section of Cardiothoracic Imaging, Department of Radiology, Washington University School of Medicine, 510 South Kingshighway Boulevard, Box 8131, St Louis, MO 63110, USA
E-mail address: javidanc@mir.wustl.edu

Thorac Surg Clin 20 (2010) 65–84
doi:10.1016/j.thorsurg.2009.12.006

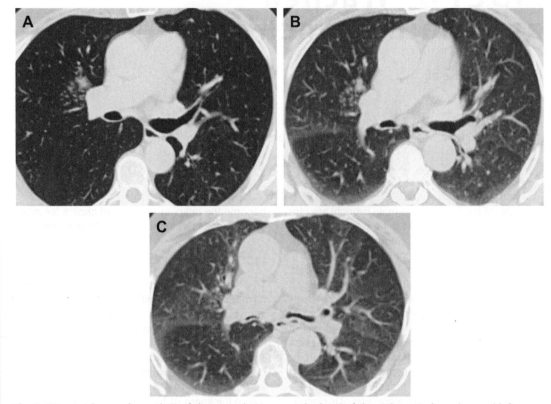

Fig. 1. Transaxial nonenhanced CT of the central airways at the level of the right main bronchus and left upper lobe bronchus in 49 year old man with chronic shortness of breath, not responding to treatment. The patient was imaged three times, per dynamic airway protocol, once at suspended end-inhalation (*A*), next at suspended end-expiration (*B*), and lastly during dynamic exhalation (*C*). The airways maintain normal caliber during suspended end-inhalation and end-expiration. However, when scanning was performed during active, forceful exhalation (*C*), marked narrowing of the lumina due to bronchial wall collapse is noted, diagnostic of bronchomalacia.

between when the technologist initiates the scan, and when the detectors rotate and imaging actually begins. Because forced exhalation only lasts 4 to 6 seconds, the scanning sequence should be as follows:

> The patient is told to take a deep breath
> The scanning is initiated
> Command to exhale is given only after that fixed time has transpired

The technologist must not use the automated patient instruction recording but should verbalize the command to exhale.[11]

The inherent motion artifact in the images of the lung parenchyma during active exhalation makes it difficult to use such images to diagnose coexisting small airway disease. For this reason, in the author's institution, the patient is scanned a third time, using a low-dose technique, from the thoracic inlet to the lung bases, at suspended end-exhalation to detect mosaic attenuation and air trapping.

Intravenous contrast is useful if tracheal stenosis is caused by a highly vascular mass such as a paraganglioma, or by extrinsic compression by a vessel, such as a pulmonary sling. Contrast use also improves visualization of segmental intraluminal bronchial masses, such as carcinoid tumors, which when arising in the segmental bronchi, cause postobstructive lung collapse and pneumonia, and may be obscured by the surrounding consolidated lung, unless intravenous contrast is used (**Fig. 2**).[8,11]

INTERPRETATION AND IMAGE AFTER PROCESSING

Interpretation should begin with viewing the transaxial images, with attention to the trachea and bronchial lumina and walls, and the surrounding mediastinal and hilar tissues. This initial screening allows a quick overview to identify disease, thereby directing the kind of postprocessed image to be created, to better display the abnormality.

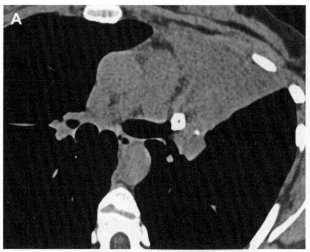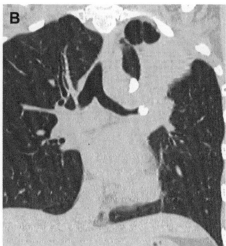

Fig. 2. Transaxial (*A*) and coronal (*B*) MPR images of nonenhanced CT of the chest in a 42-year old woman with chronic hemoptysis. A densely calcified broncholith, caused by erosion of calcified hilar lymph nodes into the airway lumina, obstructs the left upper lobe bronchus, causing complete collapse. The inherent dense calcification of this lesion makes it easily visible without use of intravenous contrast.

Multiplanar two- and three-dimensional reconstructed images not only provide a more anatomically meaningful portrayal of the airways, with use of such images, but also augment the identification of subtle and short segment airway stenosis. The relationship of mediastinal structures to the airways, depiction of the branching airways that have an oblique course relative to the transaxial plane, and understanding the craniocaudal extension of disease, are all understood better when employing such reformations.[11,12]

Two-dimensional multiplanar reformations (MPRs) in the coronal, sagittal, or oblique planes, can be created easily at the imaging PACS, or at a remote postprocessing station. These images display a section of single-voxel thickness, approximating 0.6 to 0.8 mm.[5,8] By creating an oblique coronal image aligned along the long axis of the trachea, to include the vocal cords and carina, one can create a single image of the trachea and main bronchi beyond what is visible with a laryngoscope (**Fig. 3**).[5]

Curved MPR is useful in measuring distances in a structure that has a nonlinear or curved axis. It involves straightening of that structure along its long axis and measuring distances between two points. It is also useful in obtaining a true cross-sectional diameter or area of that structure. It is crucial to create such images when stenosis or a lesion is measured in a bent or kinked trachea, which can be a normal tracheal alignment in older individuals. It also is used when a lesion or stenosis is located in a segmental bronchus or along a bronchial bifurcation, and accurate measurements of the lesion length, luminal narrowing, and distance from the carina need to be determined, for planning bronchoscopic stent placement or surgery.[7]

Three-dimensional multiplanar volume reformations display the combined information of a slab of chosen thickness in any given plane. If in such reformations, only the lowest attenuation pixels are projected in the chosen slab, a minimum intensity projection (MinIP) is created. This is useful for quickly displaying the distribution of air trapping and emphysema in the lung parenchyma. Its drawback in depicting airway disease is that it commonly underestimates the severity of asymmetric stenosis, to the extent that the intraluminal growth of a tumor can be missed. It is also very vulnerable to partial volume-averaging effects, leading to artificial decreased depiction of airway caliber, such that a severe stenosis can appear as airway total occlusion (**Fig. 4**).[7,8,12]

Creating volume-rendered reformatted images is based on isolating the surface of the luminal air column, by applying a segmentation threshold. If shading is applied to the other surface of these segmented data, a three-dimensional image of the entire tracheobronchial tree is generated. Such images are useful in providing an overview of pathology in the longitudinal plane. These images, similar to two- and three-dimensional MPRs, are subject to partial volume and stair step artifacts, and the degree of stenosis can be depicted inaccurately based on the threshold chosen for segmentation. CT bronchoscopy is a volume-rendered image where coloring similar to normal mucosa is applied to the segmented data as it is viewed from within. Many

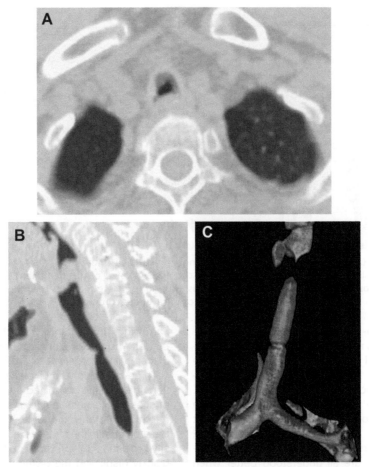

Fig. 3. Patient with history of prior intubation has stridor. Nonenhanced trachea CT shows a membrane-like soft-tissue extending into the tracheal lumen in the transaxial image (*A*). The sagittal reformatted image (*B*) best demonstrates that it has a shelf-like configuration and is located in the mid trachea, causing focal stenosis, due to prior intubation. Volume rendering (*C*) with arbitrary copper coloring, displays the waist-like short segment narrowing of the trachea. This technique involves post-processing where the surrounding lung parenchyma is segmented out to create an image only displaying the central airways. In this image the lung parenchyma posterior to the distal trachea and bilateral main bronchi have not been segmented out.

postprocessing engines allow navigating through the tracheal and bronchial lumina of these images, simulating a bronchoscopic experience **(Fig. 5)**.[7,12]

It is of utmost importance that one should not overlook the transaxial CT images in favor of the postprocessed CT ones. The axial images are important to identify motion artifacts and various normal structures, which can easily simulate disease on postprocessed reformations. They are also valuable in evaluating the mediastinum and neighboring lung parenchyma.

CT OF NORMAL TRACHEA

The normal trachea measures approximately 10 to 12 cm in length, 2 to 4 cm of which are extrathoracic and the remaining 6 to 8 cm in the thorax. The upper limits of normal for the trachea in the coronal and sagittal dimensions are 25 mm and 27 mm for men and 21 mm and 23 mm for women, respectively. The lower limit of normal in both coronal and sagittal planes is 13 mm for men and 11 mm for women. Pathologic widening or narrowing of the trachea refers to tracheal dimensions greater or less than these values, respectively.[13]

The tracheal wall gains its support through the horseshoe-shaped rings of hyaline cartilage, which uphold the anterior and lateral walls. A thin membrane comprises the posterior wall and is composed of smooth muscle and fibrous tissue.[14] The transaxial configuration of the trachea on CT is varied; it is usually round or oval in shape on inspiration, but it also can appear horseshoe-, triangular-, or pear-shaped.[15] On expiration, the posterior membrane flattens or bows anteriorly,

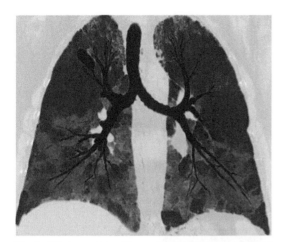

Fig. 4. Minimum intensity projection (MinIP) reformat of nonenhanced CT of a chest in a man who has undergone lung transplantation and suffers from chronic dyspnea. There are patchy areas of varying density. The low density areas represent air trapping and bronchiolitis obliterans (obliterative bronchiolitis), due to chronic rejection.

such that it decreases the sagittal diameter up to 30% in normal individuals.[14] Tracheal course in the chest can range from straight and vertical, to kinked and angled, where the trachea appears bent in more than one location, without focal narrowing.

The cartilaginous portion of the tracheal wall should not exceed 2 mm in thickness in normal individuals. Its posterior membrane is thinner and commonly imperceptible, detectable only because of the surrounding fat or obscured by the esophagus. Calcification of the tracheal cartilage is common in older individuals or patients receiving Coumadin (**Fig. 6**).[16]

TRACHEOBRONCHIAL DISEASES

Diseases of the central airways can be classified into two groups: those that cause luminal narrowing and those that cause luminal widening. Such grouping can be subdivided further, based on their extent of involvement, into localized or focal

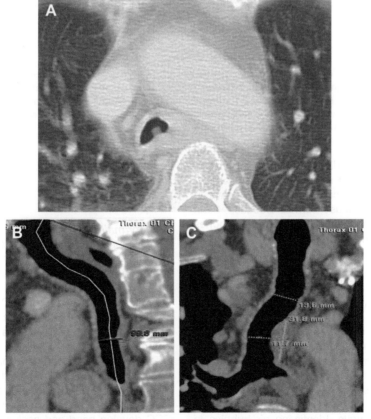

Fig. 5. Transaxial (A), curved MPR (B) and coronal reformatted images of CT of the airway shows a small lesion arising from that posterior wall of the trachea (A). Curved MPR helps measure the distance of this lesion from the carina (B) and creates a straightened image of the trachea, allowing the entire trachea to be seen on the coronal reformatted image (C). Biopsy revealed squamous cell carcinoma.

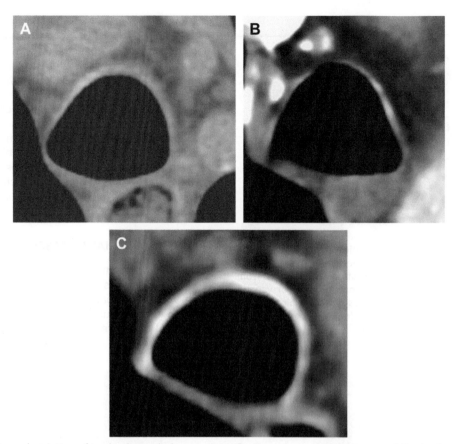

Fig. 6. Normal variation of tracheal morphology and calcification – Transaxial CT images of the trachea of three different people taken at suspended end-inhalation. Trachea can have an oval shape on cross-sectional imaging, where the cartilaginous portion of the wall is non-calcified (*A*). A triangular configuration with minimal calcification of the left lateral wall is also a normal appearance (*B*). Dense uniform calicification in a horse-shoe shaped trachea of an older woman, also a normal variation (*C*).

and long-segment or diffuse diseases. It is important to recognize that such grouping is arbitrary, as certain diseases can involve the airways in both focal and diffuse forms. Because most central airway diseases fall in the two categories of focal narrowing and diffuse narrowing, in this article, the discussion is limited to these two groupings.

FOCAL NARROWING

Short-segment luminal narrowing most commonly is caused by malignant or benign neoplasms arising from the airway, or by stenoses in the setting of prior trauma and medical intervention such as tracheostomy or endotracheal intubation. In daily practice, the most common intraluminal mass seen is mucus. Identifying air bubbles in this pseudolesion can help distinguish it from a polyp. Sometimes it is necessary to repeat the scan after the patient coughs to assess for

a change in morphology, to differentiate mucus from a mass (**Fig. 7**).[17]

Neoplasms

Primary malignant neoplasms

Primary tumors of the trachea and main bronchi are rare and represent only 1% of tracheobronchial neoplasms. Ninety percent of such tumors are malignant, and of those, 86% are caused by squamous cell carcinoma (SCC) and adenoid cystic carcinoma (ACC). Carcinoid and mucoepidermoid tumors occur with less frequency in the central airways.[3]

SCC is the most common primary malignancy of the central airways. It arises from the surface epithelium and is strongly associated with smoking. Forty percent of patients with airway SCC develop head and neck or lung cancers at a point in their lives. SCC affects men two to four times more often than women, and it frequently presents between the ages of 50 and 60. It is

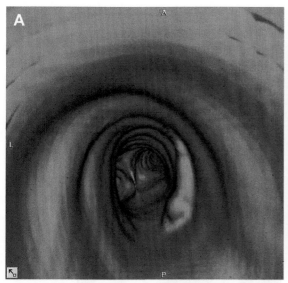

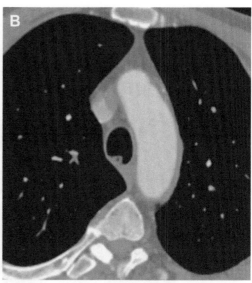

Fig. 7. Virtual bronchoscopy volume rendering of non-enhanced CT of the trachea (*A*) demonstrates a focal polyp-like lesion arising from the right inferolateral wall of the trachea. When the original transaxial CT image of the trachea (*B*) is viewed at that same level, the lesion appears to have bubbles of air within it. It is not a neoplasm, it is mucus.

commonly infiltrative, with a large exophytic component at the time of diagnosis. Mediastinal lymphadenopathy and pulmonary metastases are common. These lesions have high uptake on FDG-positron emission tomography (PET) imaging (**Fig. 8**).[18,19]

ACC is the most common lung cancer that arises from the salivary glands in the airway, and it is the second most common primary malignancy of the trachea. It is not associated with smoking and occurs with equal frequency among men

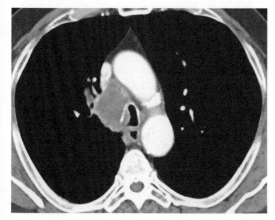

Fig. 8. Fifty six year old man with long history of smoking has hemoptysis. Non-enhanced transaxial CT of chest reveals a mass arising from the right tracheal wall, growing both into the lumen and exophytically, infiltrating the mediastinum.

and women. Its age of occurrence is at a younger age than SCC, most commonly in the fourth decade of life. It occurs mostly in the trachea and proximal bronchi. ACC appears as an intraluminal focal mass on bronchoscopy and even CT, but because it grows along the submucosa of the airway, there is circumferential wall thickening of the airway with infiltrative growth along a long craniocaudal segment, best appreciated on coronal and sagittal MPR images. ACC grows slowly and rarely is associated with regional lymphadenopathy or distant metastases. It shows variable FRG uptake on PET imaging, where the higher the grade of the tumor, the more avid the FDG uptake (**Fig. 9**).[18,19]

Mucoepidermoid carcinoma (MEC) and carcinoid tumors are other primary malignancies of the airways and relative to SCC and ACC, they arise in the more distal airways, most commonly in the lobar and segmental bronchi. MEC is a tumor arising from the minor salivary glands, but it is more rare than ACC. Carcinoid tumors are neuroendocrine neoplasms that can excrete hormones and neuroamines, such as corticotropin (ACTH), serotonin, somatostatin, and bradykinin. Based on the mitotic activity of the tumor cells, its grading ranges from low-grade typical tumors, to intermediate-grade atypical locally aggressive tumors, to high-grade small cell carcinoma.[18,19]

MEC and carcinoid tumors have many common features. Both present with hemoptysis and symptoms of lung collapse and repeated infections, and

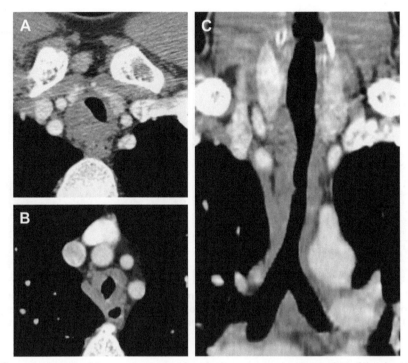

Fig. 9. Thirty five year old man with several months of stridor has a contrast-enhanced CT of the chest to further evaluate the cause. Transaxial image of the trachea at the level of the thoracic inlet (*A*) shows a large mass arising from the right posterolateral tracheal wall, obstructing more than half the luminal area. There is circumferential tracheal wall thickening, seen both at the level of the mass and on the transaxial image of trachea lower in the chest (*B*), at the level of the great vessels of the superior mediastinum. Coronal reformation (*C*) best demonstrates the craniocaudal growth of this tumor along the tracheal wall, which upon biopsy was proven to be adenoidcystic carcinoma.

neither is associated with smoking or shows gender predilection. On CT and bronchoscopy, they appear as smooth-margined or lobulated, oval or round endoluminal masses (**Fig. 10**). Both can have internal calcifications. CT shows that these masses arise from the airway wall, causing focal wall thickening, which helps differentiate such lesions from benign airway tumors, which lack wall invasion. Postobstructive atelectasis, mucus plugging, and repeated pneumonia are frequent features. Because both lesions are vascular, they demonstrate enhancement with contrast. The degree of enhancement is variable (**Fig. 11**).[18,19]

Metastases

Metastases to the trachea and main bronchi are commonly caused by local invasion, such as thyroid, laryngeal, esophageal, and lung cancers. More rarely endoluminal metastases are caused by hematogenous spread from primary malignancies such as colorectal, breast, and renal cell carcinoma, sarcomas, melanoma, and hematogenous malignancies such plasmacytoma and granulocytic carcinoma or chloroma. Such metastases are diagnosed, on average, 4 years after the

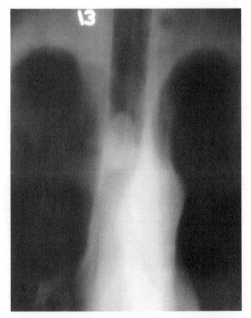

Fig. 10. Coronal tomogram of trachea shows an oblong-shaped mass growing endoluminally in the lower trachea, which was a mucoepidermoid carcinoma. Before the widespread availability of CT, such tomograms were routinely used in evaluating the trachea.

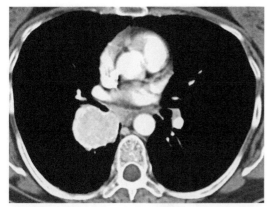

Fig. 11. Forty one year old woman with hemoptysis and chronic cough is further evaluated by contrast-enhanced CT of the chest. Transaxial image at the level of the lower lobe bronchi shows a large enhancing mass arising from the left lower lobe bronchus.

primary malignancy has been discovered. Hemoptysis and coughing are the most common presenting symptoms. CT can detect such metastases and direct bronchoscopy for biopsy.[20]

Metastatic lesions are usually solitary, but they may be multiple. They could have imaging features simulating primary tracheal malignancies such as squamous cell and adenoidcystic carcinoma. If they occur in the main bronchi, they can present with lobar collapse. A prior history of extratracheal malignancy is most helpful in determining the etiology of such lesions (**Fig. 12**).[1,19]

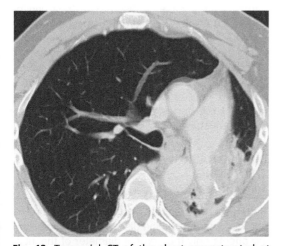

Fig. 12. Transaxial CT of the chest reconstructed at lung window settings in a patient with known history of melanoma shows a mass occupying the entire lumen of the left main bronchus, causing near-complete collapse of the left lung with marked shift of the mediastinum into the left hemithorax.

Benign neoplasm

Benign neoplasms of the trachea are much less common than malignant ones, and they have the common appearance of focal, well-defined intraluminal lesions that do not invade the tracheal wall or adjacent mediastinum. Of these, squamous cell papillomas and polyps are the most common.[21]

Squamous cell papillomas are benign neoplasms, and they have two forms: multiple or juvenile laryngotracheal papillomatosis, and solitary, which is less frequent and occurs in adults. The multiple form, or laryngotracheal papillomatosis, is caused by infection with human papillomavirus types 6 and 11, acquired by birth or by sexual transmission. It most commonly presents in children younger than 4 years of age, and it begins as a laryngeal mass. In a fraction of such children, especially if incompletely treated, multiple trachea and bronchial polyps develop later in adolescence or young adulthood, as a result of endobronchial dissemination. When the distal airways are involved, these lesions manifest as pulmonary nodules that usually cavitate. Such patients can present with repeated infections and symptoms of airway obstruction. Medical management and surgical management are aimed at slowing the rate of papilloma growth using antiviral and cytotoxic agents, and excision of endoluminal lesions using electrocautery, cryotherapy, and CO_2 laser. The high risk of malignant transformation of such lesions warrants continued surveillance by CT and bronchoscopy, especially when pulmonary nodules have developed.[21,22]

The term polyp is attributed to the solitary form of squamous cell papillomas. They are also called inflammatory, or fibroepithelial polyps and are more common in middle-aged smokers. They are believed to be caused by chronic mucosal irritation, either by hot or corrosive gases, endobronchial foreign bodies, or by broncholiths. These lesions usually regress after removal of the caustic agent and do not have a high tendency for malignant transformation (**Fig. 13**).[21]

Non-neoplastic Etiologies

Iatrogenic and post-traumatic stenoses

Strictures most commonly are caused by iatrogenic means, where the inflated cuff of an endotracheal or tracheostomy tube inserts local pressure on the tracheal mucosa and cartilage of the subglottic trachea and impedes blood flow. This leads to ischemic necrosis and eccentric or circumferential intimal hyperplasia and luminal stenosis. Less commonly, similar stenosis is located several centimeters above the carina, caused by the tip of the endotracheal tube or tracheostomy tube

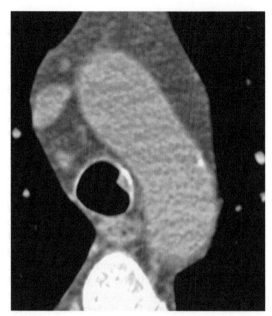

Fig. 13. Transaxial image of nonenhanced CT of the airway of a smoker reveals a solitary polyp arising from the left lateral wall of the lower trachea. Benign lesions have the common feature of being well-circumscribed and do not cause tracheal wall thickening or extend into the mediastinum.

damaging the tracheal wall, causing focal mucosal and cartilage ischemia and damage. Tracheostomy tubes, at the site of the stoma, permanently damage the anterior arc-like cartilaginous ring along the midline, resulting in inward collapse of the lateral walls of the trachea with associated focal scarring and irregular wall thickening. Regardless of the cause, the stenosis can develop/or manifest much later than the traumatic event. The location of stenosis, history of endotracheal intubation or tracheostomy, and in stomal injury, the typical morphology of the cartilaginous ring deformity, help one correctly identify the iatrogenic etiology of the stenosis (Fig. 14).[23]

Traumatic injury of the airway is caused, either by perforation of the tracheal wall at the time of intubation, by blunt trauma to the trachea, or by shearing injury to the main stem bronchi located where the bronchi are anchored to the hilar pleura. These injuries heal with strictures, commonly creating an hourglass configuration of the airway lumen.[1,23,24]

CT imaging depicts the site, morphology, length, and location of the tracheal narrowing. Because the wall thickening is sometimes thin and web-like, coronal, sagittal, and curved MPRs are needed to detect it, given the increased sensitivity of such techniques in revealing subtle stenoses. They are also necessary to accurately

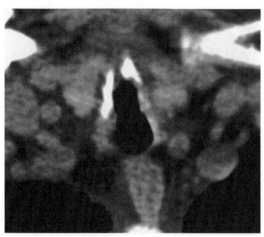

Fig. 14. Nonenhanced transaxial CT of the trachea of a patient with history of prior tracheostomy and stridor, shows narrowing of the tracheal lumen a few centimeter below the vocalcords. The lateral walls of the trachea have collapsed inward and there is a defect along the anterior midline of the tracheal arc-like cartilage.

measure luminal dimensions, length of stenosis, and distance from the vocal chords or carina; all information needed for treatment planning. The narrowing is typically less than 3 cm in length and is either symmetric or eccentric, causing an hourglass-shaped stenosis.[24]

DIFFUSE NARROWING

Narrowing of the airway beyond a length of 3 cm is considered long-segment narrowing.[24] There are many causes of diffuse tracheobronchial luminal narrowing. For ease of discussion, they can be categorized into two groups, based on the absence or presence of airway wall thickening. It is important to note that many of the inflammatory, infiltrative, and infectious diseases of the airway that cause narrowing associated with diffuse smooth or nodular wall thickening become fibrotic in their later stages, causing cicatricial stenosis without much wall thickening.

DIFFUSE NARROWING WITHOUT WALL THICKENING
Saber Sheath Trachea

Saber sheath trachea occurs in the setting of chronic obstructive lung disease. Luminal narrowing affects only the coronal diameter of the intrathoracic trachea, sparing the extrathoracic portion. It is usually asymptomatic and an incidental finding on chest radiographs and CT. Sometimes mild tracheomalacia on expiratory images is discovered (see Fig. 13).[14]

Tracheobronchomalacia

Tracheobronchomalacia is another cause of diffuse narrowing without associated airway wall thickening. The diffuse pattern, best diagnosed with dynamic expiratory imaging, can manifest as either inward collapse of the tracheal cartilage or exaggerated anterior collapse of the posterior membrane, and it can be associated with abnormal cross-sectional morphology of trachea, where the coronal diameter exceeds that of the sagittal diameter, creating a flattened, frown-shaped appearance of the trachea on CT.[15,25] Commonly, a decrease of 50% of the cross-sectional area is used as the criteria for diagnosis; however, Boiselle and colleagues[26] have demonstrated a wide range of airway collapsibility in normal individuals. They therefore suggested applying a threshold of 75% of decreased cross-sectional luminal area for more specificity (**Fig. 15**).

Tracheobronchomalacia can be seen in chronic obstructive pulmonary disease. In such situations, the luminal narrowing is caused by exaggerated anterior bowing of the posterior membrane, rather than collapse of the cartilaginous wall.[27] If focal, malacia is more likely caused by focal congenital partial or complete absence of a cartilaginous ring, or as the sequelae of trauma or focal infection. Vascular rings are associated with focal tracheobronchomalacia, possibly because of chronic airway compression.[28]

Mounier-Kuhn disease, or congenital tracheobronchomegaly, is associated with diffuse tracheomalacia in its moderate and severe forms. It is caused by congenital abnormality of the connective tissue of the airway cartilage and membranes between the cartilaginous rings, which manifests relatively later in life, especially if the individual is a smoker. Although this entity is usually discussed as a cause of diffuse luminal widening, it is mentioned here in cases where the tracheomalacia is severe and CT imaging is performed at end-expiration; the airway collapses, and it appears diffusely narrowed. CT taken on inspiration is diagnostic in displaying that abnormally enlarged caliber of the central airways (**Fig. 16**).[29,30]

DIFFUSE NARROWING WITH WALL THICKENING
Acute Inflammation

Airway wall thickening causing long-segment luminal narrowing can be seen with acute tracheal inflammation. This can be caused by inhalation of noxious fumes but is more commonly caused by an acute or subacute infection. In children, such tracheal swelling most commonly is caused by parainfluenza virus, resulting in layngotracheobronchitis (croup).[31] Ventilator-associated tracheobronchitis is a common nosocomial infection of adults hospitalized in the intensive care unit. It predominantly is caused by gram-negative

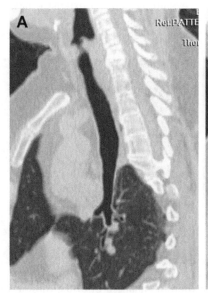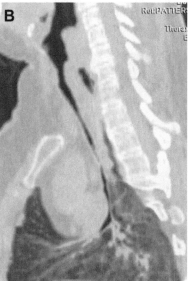

Fig. 15. Fifty one year old woman with chronic cough and wheezing. Coronal multiplanar reformats of CT of chest performed at suspended end inhalation (A) and during forced exhalation (B), according to the dynamic trachea protocol, shows marked exaggerated relaxation of the posterior membrane of the entire intrathoracic trachea, causing severe diffuse narrowing, with areas of complete luminal obliteration.

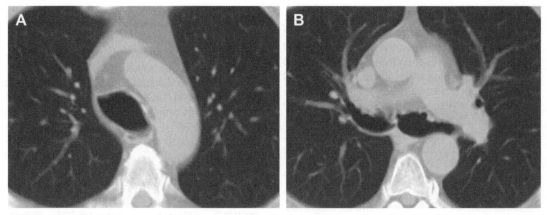

Fig. 16. Transaxial CT images of the chest, at the levels of the trachea (*A*) and main bronch (*B*) demonstrate marked enlargement of the lumina of the trachea and main bronchi in patient with Mounier-Kuhn syndrome. The configuration of the trachea on cross sectional is such that the coronal diameter exceeds the sagittal diameter, a morphology indicative of tracheomalacia.

bacteria, and it is associated with fever, cough, increased sputum production, and associated lower respiratory tract inflammation, in the absence of pneumonia. CT and bronchoalveolar lavage with cultures are most helpful in diagnosis.[32]

Invasive tracheal aspergillosis is a rare and highly fatal cause of progressive airway obstruction in immunocompromised patients. Ulcerative tracheobronchitis after lung transplantation initially is limited to the anastomosis sites of the main bronchi, due to the relative ischemia, but it can spread to involve the trachea also. Ulceration, necrosis, and pseudomembrane formation are pathologic features. On CT, nonspecific diffuse wall thickening of the central airways is noted; however, generally diagnosis is made by

bronchoscopy. Treatment is debridement of the affected mucosa, in addition to oral antifungal therapy (**Fig. 17**).[33–35]

Chronic Infection

Rhinoscleroma is a chronic granulomatous infection caused by *Klebsiella rhinoscleromatis*. It is an endemic disease in Guatemala, El Salvador, Egypt, India, Indonesia, Poland, Hungary, and Russia. It usually affects the nasal mucosa, but can involve the larynx, and much less commonly, the tracheobronchial tree. It progresses slowly if untreated, with periods of remissions and relapse, eventually causing extensive airway destruction. CT findings are subglottic stricture and nodular wall thickening of the trachea and central bronchi,

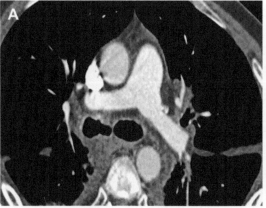
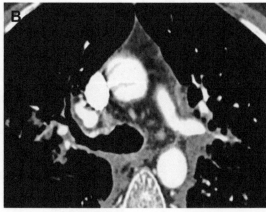

Fig. 17. Thirty nine year old man hospitalized after bilateral lung transplantation has low grade fevers. No pneumonia was identified, however on transaxial images of contrast-enhanced CT of the chest at the levels of the main bronchi (*A*) and right upper lobe bronchus (*B*) diffuse wall thickening of the airway is noted, causing luminal narrowing, especially of the right main bronchus. The surround fat planes are indistinct due to inflammatory changes. Biopsy revealed aspergillus in the airway wall, with mucosal ulceration, consistent with invasive tracheobronchial aspergillosis.

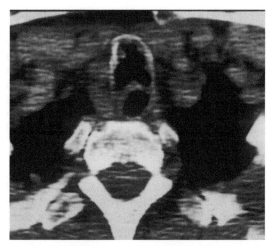

Fig. 18. Young immigrant woman with chronic cough. Transaxial image of CT of chest shows multiple noncalcified nodules arising from the tracheal wall. Biopsy revealed Klebsiella rhinoscleroma infection of the airways.

leading to concentric narrowing of their lumens. There is no associated calcification. The involvement can be localized or diffuse. The mainstay of treatment is surgical debridement and prolonged antibiotic therapy (**Fig. 18**).[24,36,37]

Tuberculosis (TB) of the tracheobronchial tree is seen much less frequently with current improved antibiotic treatment regimens. The stenosis caused by TB can manifest in the setting of acute infection or several years later. It typically involves the distal trachea and main bronchi. It spreads to the central airways by peribronchial lymphatic pathways and by local extension from adjacent TB lymphadenitis.[23] The disease begins as edema and lymphocytic infiltration of the airway submucosa and tubercle formation. The granulation tissue destroys and replaces the mucosa, leading to fibrosis and airway stenosis. In the acute phase, the disease involves the main bronchi symmetrically; however, late, fibrotic TB is more common in the left mainstem bronchus. Mediastinal

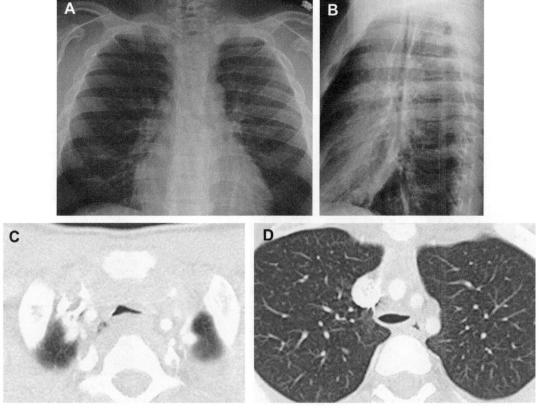

Fig. 19. Transaxial CT images of the chest at the levels of extrathoracic (*A*) and intrathoracic trachea (*B*) of a 21 year old man with chronic cough and repeated pneumonia shows diffuse tracheomalacia where the trachea appears flattened (*C, D*).

lymphadenopathy is common. On CT, there is diffuse circumferential thickening of distal tracheal and bronchial walls, with irregular luminal narrowing and peribronchial soft tissue thickening, involving a long segment of the airway.[38,39]

Diffuse laryngeotracheobronchial papillomatosis can have numerous polypoid lesions involving the airway mucosa, causing nodular wall thickening and luminal narrowing. The lesions are not calcified. Parenchymal cavitary nodules are common when there is extensive disease.[24]

Relapsing Polychondritis

Relapsing polychondritis (RP) is a rare multisystem disorder characterized by recurrent inflammation and destruction of cartilage. Fifty percent of patients with RP develop respiratory tract involvement at some point of their disease. Airway involvement is a poor prognostic sign and is the leading cause of death. Its cause is unknown; however, an immune-mediated mechanism is postulated. It can develop at any age, but most commonly is diagnosed in the fourth and fifth decades of life. It is more frequent in whites and shows no gender predilection.[40]

The most common findings on inspiratory CT are smooth and diffuse airway wall thickening, sparing the posterior membrane, and increased airway wall attenuation, which ranges from a subtle increase to frank calcification. Progressive cartilage calcification frequently is seen over serial

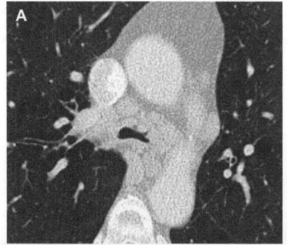

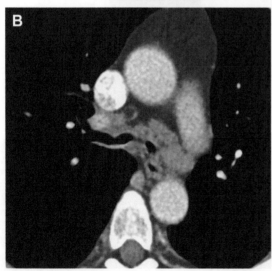
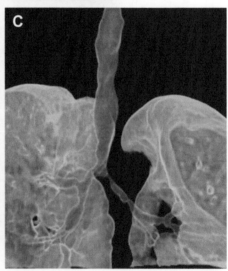

Fig. 20. Nonenhanced CT images of a woman with chronic cough and known diagnosis of C-ANCA positive granulomatosis of the lungs, shows nodular non-calcified soft tissue thickening around the airways at the level of the carina (*A*), causing luminal narrowing as evidenced on the transaxial image of the trachea (*B*). Volume rendered post-processed image (*C*) in the coronal plane shows marked nodular wall narrowing of the distal trachea, bilateral main and lobar bronchi.

imaging. Both the trachea and main bronchi are involved equally. Luminal narrowing is diffuse, but not always the predominant feature. Although the wall thickening is most commonly smooth, nodular thickening can sometimes occur. Tracheobronchomalacia is considered a key feature of this disease, and may be the only airway abnormality detected on CT, early in the process. If appropriate dynamic expiratory CT is performed, tracheomalacia and air trapping are detected in over 90% of such patients. Fixed airway narrowing occurs when fibrosis sets in after chronic inflammation (**Fig. 19**).[41,42]

Wegener Granulomatosis

Wegener or C-ANCA positive granulomatosis is characterized by necrotizing granulomatous inflammation and necrotizing vascultis affecting the small arteries, veins and capillaries. It has a predilection for the upper respiratory tract, such as the sinuses and nasal mucosa, the kidneys, and the lungs. Tracheobronchial involvement occurs in 50% of patients, usually in conjunction with disease manifestation elsewhere. Subglottic stenosis is the most frequent airway manifestation. Sometimes the airway involvement is isolated, leading to delayed diagnosis. Occasionally after successful remission with immunosuppressive therapy of other manifestations of disease elsewhere, the airway involvement either is diagnosed for the first time or continues to progress to scarring and stenosis (**Fig. 20**).[24,43]

Patients younger than 30 years old are more prone to having airway involvement. Common symptoms are dyspnea, wheezing, and hemoptysis, usually from concomitant pulmonary disease with alveolar hemorrhage. CT shows focal or long segments of circumferential mass-like wall thickening of the trachea and bronchi, associated with thickening and calcification of the cartilaginous rings. Mucosal ulceration noted on bronchoscopy may be hard to identify on CT. Bronchiectasis and peribronchial thickening of small airways are common. Airway lesions demonstrate partial or complete improvement with treatment. Tracheomalacia or bronchomalacia can occur as a result of the chronic inflammation.[43]

Amyloidosis

Tracheobronchial amyloidosis (TBA) is a rare disease that results from abnormal extracellular deposition of amyloid and autologous fibrillar proteins in a beta-pleated sheet configuration, which leads to formation of submucosal plaques or nodules. It can be associated with systemic disease, or isolated to the trachea. Patients present with nonspecific symptoms of chronic cough or wheezing, and diagnosis is based on biopsy, which shows green birefringence of Congo-red stained deposits when viewed under polarized light. TBA is more common in men,

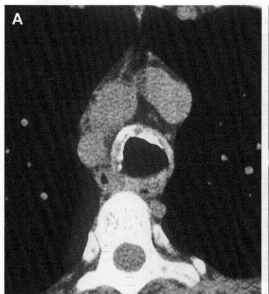
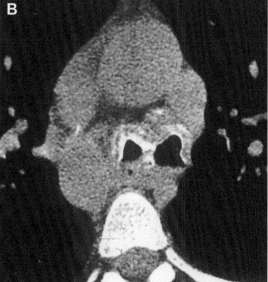

Fig. 21. Amyloidosis of the airway causing diffuse calcification and wall thickening of the trachea (*A*) and bilateral main bronchi (*B*) on transaxial images of nonenhanced CT of the chest.

most commonly first presenting in the fifth and sixth decades of life.[24,44,45]

CT findings include focal or diffuse irregular and asymmetric wall thickening, with mural calcifications, causing luminal narrowing. Concentric or eccentric structuring is a possible associated finding. It can involve anywhere from the trachea to the segmental bronchi in contiguous segments.[24] Nodular thickening can occlude the airway lumen, causing atelectasis, postobstructive pneumonia, or air trapping. Magnetic resonance imaging (MRI) can be helpful, where the amyloid deposits show intermediate T1-signal intensity and low T2-signal intensity (**Fig. 21**).[44]

There is no established treatment for TBA. Resection is not curative, and lesions recur 6 to 12 months after surgery.[24] External-beam radiation therapy has been shown to improve pulmonary function, with visible improvement on CT and bronchoscopy.[45]

Sarcoidosis

Tracheal and bronchial stenosis in association with sarcoidosis is unusual. Airway involvement can occur in the absence of lung parenchymal manifestations of sarcoidosis. The larynx and lobar bronchi are affected more commonly than the trachea. When it occurs, tracheal stenosis is a late manifestation of disease. The progressive luminal stenosis with smooth or nodular wall thickening may be treated with prolonged courses of corticosteroids and repeated tracheal dilations.[24,31,46]

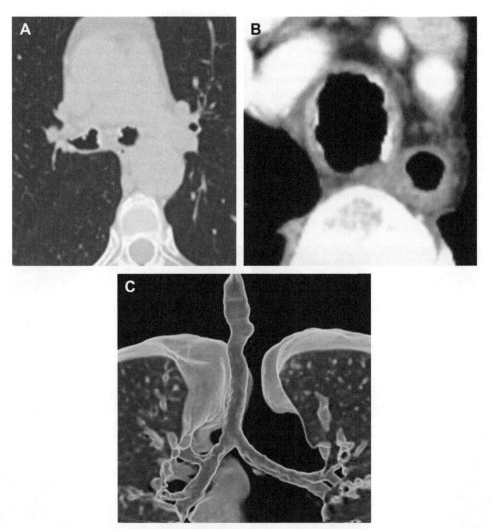

Fig. 22. Tracheobronchopathia osteochondroplastica causing calcified nodules protruding into the tracheal lumen (*A*) and causing luminal narrowing of the main bronchi (*B*) on transaxial CT images of the chest. Volume-rendered post-processed image (*C*) shows the distribution of disease.

Tracheobronchopathia Osteochondroplastica

Tracheobronchopathia osteochondroplastica (tracheopathia osteoplastica TPOP) is a disease of the distal trachea and mainstem and lobar bronchi, causing nodular narrowing of the airway lumina. It is caused by benign proliferation of bone and cartilage, creating numerous 1 to 3 mm nodules in the submucosa of the cartilaginous portion of the airway wall. It spares the posterior membranous wall of the trachea. On pathologic specimens in the submucosa, cartilaginous and osseous islands of tissue with close association to the perichondrium are found. Foci of bone marrow with active hematopoiesis also are identified. One theory of its histogenesis is that the nodules are ecchondroses and exosostoses of the cartilaginous rings.[47]

It usually is discovered incidentally in adults in their fourth and fifth decades of life. Women and men are affected equally, and there is no association with smoking. The presence or lack of symptoms depends on the degree of luminal narrowing. Symptoms range from none to coughing, hoarseness, wheezing, and hemoptysis. A superimposed infection may spur on the onset of symptoms. The disease sometimes is discovered because of difficult intubation.[48]

On chest radiography, nodular, long-segment narrowing of the trachea is noted on the frontal radiograph only. CT best demonstrates the dense or calcified nodules protruding into the airway lumen, narrowing it along the coronal diameter. The presence of nodules in TPOP differentiates it from saber-sheath trachea, which also narrows

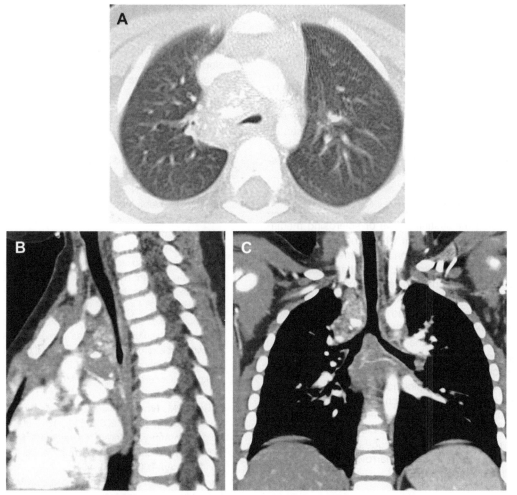

Fig. 23. Sixteen-year-old girl with chronic shortness of breath and past history of histoplasmosis causing mediastinal lymphadenopathy several years ago, has a CT of chest to evaluate the cause. Transaxial image at the level of the trachea (*A*) shows luminal narrowing by external compression of the anterior wall. Sagittal (*B*) and coronal (*C*) double-oblique reformatted images show a long segment of tracheal narrowing by a large calcified mediastinal mass due to fibrosing mediastinitis.

the coronal diameter, but has no wall thickening (**Fig. 22**).[47,48]

The main differential diagnosis consists of amyloidosis, Wegener granulomatosis, and lymphoma, which also can have submucosal nodules. These entities do not spare the posterior wall of the trachea. Occasionally pathology is necessary to confirm the diagnosis.

TPOP is easily differentiated from tracheobronchial papillomatosis, as the latter lacks calcification of the submucosal nodules and is associated with parenchymal nodules. In TPOP, the mediastinal fat is intact, thereby differentiating it from mediastinal fibrosis, which also can calcify. Nodular wall thickening in RP is rare. Another entity easily confused with TPOP is diffuse tracheobronchial chondrocalcification, which is normal in older individuals, but can be seen prematurely with warfarin use. This form of chondral calcification can be discontinuous, simulating nodules. The calcifications, however, never protrude into the lumen to cause narrowing (**Fig. 23**).[47,48]

The goal of treatment is to provide symptomatic relief and varies from patient to patient.

Severe conditions that are complicated by bleeding, severe obstructive symptoms, or recurrent infections require more aggressive intervention. Bronchoscopic therapeutic methods can be used, which include endobronchial Nd:YAG laser photoevaporation, coring through rigid bronchoscopy, and stenting.[47,48]

Fibrosing Mediastinitis

Fibrosing mediastinitis (FM) or sclerosing mediastinitis is rare condition where there is excessive fibrous tissue deposition in the mediastinum. Its exact cause is unknown, and it has been postulated that it is caused by an immunologic reaction to an infection or other allergens. CT demonstrates localized or diffuse and confluent soft tissue, commonly calcified, in the mediastinum and hila, which obliterate the normal fat planes and compress the neighboring vessels and airways. If associated with histoplasmosis and other granulomatous diseases, calcified mediastinal lymph nodes also are seen. Tracheobronchial narrowing occurs in severe cases, where vascular involvement is already present. The cicatricial and infiltrative nature of the disease process causes localized or long-segment airway narrowing with irregular wall thickening.[49,50]

Other Non-neoplastic Causes

Inflammatory bowel disease, such as Crohn and ulcerative colitis, and other inflammatory diseases such as Behcet syndrome rarely can cause tracheobronchitis.[14,24] Ulcerative colitis is the most common frequent of these to involve the airways. Almost always the airway involvement is discovered after the gastrointestinal manifestations have developed. The mechanism of wall thickening is mucosal ulceration, diffuse and chronic submucosal inflammation, leading to fibrosis and irregular wall thickening and luminal stenosis.[51]

SUMMARY

Tracheobronchial imaging has undergone a major revolution since the advent of MDCT. The improved spatial and temporal resolution not only allows reformatting images that enhance the comprehension of disease before bronchoscopy or surgery, it has introduced newer techniques such as dynamic expiratory imaging to evaluate for tracheomalacia, which can be a subtle, but a confounding entity for patients and clinician alike. Tracheobronchial diseases can be arbitrarily divided into those that cause focal and diffuse narrowing and widening. Such groupings can help develop a practical approach in evaluating diseases of the central airways.

REFERENCES

1. Kwong JS, Muller NL, Miller RR. Diseases of the trachea and main-stem bronchi: correlation of CT with pathologic findings. Radiographics 1992;12:645–57.
2. Berkmen YM. The trachea: the blind spot in the chest. Radiol Clin North Am 1984;22:539–62.
3. Naidich DP, Webb WR, Grenier PA, et al. Imaging of the airways—functional and radiologic correlations. Philadelphia: Lippincott Williams Wilkins; 2005. p. 70–105.
4. British Thoracic Society Bronchoscopy Guidelines Committee. British Thoracic Society guidelines on diagnostic flexible bronchoscopy. Thorax 2001; 56(Suppl 1):1–21.
5. Koletsis EN, Kalogeropoulou C, Prodromaki E, et al. Tumoral and nontumoral trachea stenoses: evaluation with three-dimensional CT and virtual bronchoscopy. J Cardiothorac Surg 2007;2:18.
6. Prokop M. General principles of MDCT. Eur J Radiol 2003;45:S4–10.
7. Boiselle PM, Ernst A. Recent advances in central airway imaging. Chest 2002;121(5):1651–60.
8. Beigelman-Aubry C, Brillet PY, Grenier PA. MDCT of the airways: technique and normal results. Radiol Clin North Am 2009;47:185–201.
9. Baroni RH, Feller-Kopman D, Nishino M, et al. Tracheobronchomalacia: comparison between end-expiratory and dynamic expiratory CT for evaluation of central airway collapse. Radiology 2005;235(2):635–41.
10. Bankier AA, O'Donnell CR, Boiselle PM. Quality initiatives—respiratory instructions for CT

examinations of the lungs: a hands-on guide. Radiographics 2008;28:919–31.

11. Boiselle PM, Lee KS, Ernst A. Multidetector CT of the central airways. J Thorac Imaging 2005;20(3):186–95.

12. Grenier PA, Beigelman-Aubry C, Fetita C, et al. New frontiers in CT imaging of airway disease. Eur Radiol 2002;12:1022–44.

13. Breatnach E, Abbott GC, Fraser AG. Dimensions of the normal human trachea. AJR Am J Roentgenol 1984;142:903–6.

14. Webb EM, Elicker BM, Webb WR. Pictorial essay-using CT to diagnose non-neoplastic tracheal abnormalities: appearance of the tracheal wall. AJR Am J Roentgenol 2000;174:1315–21.

15. Boiselle PM, Ernst A. Tracheal morphology in patients with tracheomalacia: prevalence of inspiratory lunate and expiratory "frown" shapes. J Thorac Imaging 2006;21(3):190–6.

16. Joshi A, Berdon WE, Ruzal-Shapiro C, et al. CT detection of tracheobronchial calcification in an 18-year-old on maintenance warfarin sodium therapy: cause and effect? AJR Am J Roentgenol 2000;175(3):921–2.

17. Westra D, Verbeeten B Jr. Some anatomical variants and pitfalls in computed tomography of the trachea and mainstem bronchi. I. Mucoid pseudotumors. Diagn Imaging Clin Med 1985;54(5):229–39.

18. Park CM, Goo JM, Lee HJ, et al. Tumors in the tracheobronchial tree: CT and FDG PET features. Radiographics 2009;29:55–71.

19. Ferretti GR, Bithigoffer C, Righini CA, et al. Imaging of tumors of the trachea and central bronchi. Radiol Clin North Am 2009;47:227–41.

20. Durdun AB, Demirag F, Sokak ME, et al. Endobronchial metastases: a clinicopathological analysis. Respirology 2005;10(4):510–4.

21. Ko JM, Jung JI, Park SH, et al. Benign tumors of the tracheobronchial tree: CT–pathologic correlation. AJR Am J Roentgenol 2006;186:1304–13.

22. Bondaryev A, Makris D, Breen DP, et al. Airway stenting for severe endobronchial papillomatosis. Respiration 2009;77:455–8.

23. Grenier PA, Beigelman-Aubry C, Brillet PY. Nonneoplatic tracheal and bronchial stenosis. Radiol Clin North Am 2009;47:243–60.

24. Prince JS, Duhamel DR, Levin DL, et al. Nonneoplastic lesions of the tracheobronchial wall: radiologic findings with bronchoscopic correlation. Radiographics 2002;22:S215–30.

25. Carden KA, Boiselle PM, Waltz DA, et al. Tracheomalacia and tracheobronchomalacia in children and adults. Chest 2005;127:984–1005.

26. Boiselle PM, O'Donnell CR, Bankier AA, et al. Tracheal collapsibility in healthy volunteers during forced expiration: assessment with multidetector CT. Radiology 2009;252(1):255–62.

27. Sverzellati N, Rastelli A, Chetta A, et al. Airway malacia in chronic obstructive pulmonary disease: prevalence, morphology and relationship with emphysema, bronchiectasis and bronchial wall thickening. Eur Radiol 2009;19(7):1669–78.

28. Lee EY, Boiselle PM. Tracheobronchomalacia in infants and children: multidetector CT evaluation. Radiology 2009;252(1):7–22.

29. Giannoni S, Benassai C, Allori O, et al. Tracheomalacia associated with Mounier-Kuhn syndrome in the Intensive Care Unit: treatment with Freitag stent. A case report. Minerva Anestesiol 2004;70(9):651–9.

30. Menon B, Aggarwal B, Iqbal A. Mounier-Kuhn syndrome: report of 8 cases of Tracheobronchomegaly with associated complications. South Med J 2008;101(1):83–7.

31. Muller NL, Miller RR, Ostrow DN, et al. Clinico-radiologic-pathologic conference diffuse thickening of the tracheal wall. J Can Assoc Radiol 1989;40: 213–5.

32. Nseir S, Ader F, Marquette CH. Nosocomial tracheobronchitis. Curr Opin Infect Dis 2009;22:148–53.

33. Kramer MR, Denning DW, Marshall SE, et al. Ulcerative tracheobronchitis after lung transplantation. A new form of invasive aspergillosis. Am Rev Respir Dis 1991;144:552–6.

34. Warman M, Lahav J, Feldberg E, et al. Invasive tracheal aspergillosis treated successfully with voriconazole: clinical report and review of the literature. Ann Otol Rhinol Laryngol 2007;116(10):713–6.

35. Franquet T, Muller NL, Oikonomou A, et al. Aspergillus infection of the airways: computed tomography and pathologic findings. J Comput Assist Tomogr 2004;28(1):10–6.

36. Verma G, Kanawaty D, Hyland R. Rhinoscleroma causing upper airway obstruction. Can Respir J 2005;12(1):43–5.

37. Simons ME, Granato L, Oliveira RCB, et al. Rhinoscleroma: case report. Braz J Otorhinolaryngol 2006;72(4):568–71.

38. Smati B, Boudaya MS, Ayadi A, et al. Tuberculosis of the trachea. Ann Thorac Surg 2006;82:1900–1.

39. Kim Y, Lee KS, Yoon JH, et al. Tuberculosis of the trachea and main bronchi: CT findings in 17 patients. AJR Am J Roentgenol 1997;168:1051–6.

40. Faix LE, Branstetter BF. Uncommon CT findings in relapsing polychondritis. AJNR Am J Neuroradiol 2005;26:2134–6.

41. Behar JV, Choi YW, Hartman TA, et al. Relapsing polychondritis affecting the lower respiratory tract. AJR Am J Roentgenol 2002;178:173–7.

42. Lee KS, Ernst A, Trentham DE, et al. Relapsing polychondritis: prevalence of expiratory CT airway abnormalities. Radiology 2006;240(2):565–73.

43. Prakash UB, Golbin JM, Edell ES, et al. Airway involvement in Wegener's granulomatosis. Rheum Dis Clin North Am 2007;33:755–75.

44. Gilad R, Milillo P, Som PM. Severe diffuse systemic amyloidosis with involvement of the pharynx, larynx,

and trachea. CT and MR findings. AJNR Am J Neuroradiol 2007;28:1557–8.

45. Poovaneswaran S, Abdul Razak AR, Lockman H, et al. Tracheobronchial amyloidosis: utilization of radiotherapy as a treatment modality. Medscape J Med 2008;10(2):42.

46. Brandstetter RD, Messina MS, Sprince NL, et al. Tracheal stenosis due to sarcoidosis. Chest 1981; 80:656.

47. Restrepo S, Pandit M, Villamil MA, et al. Tracheobronchopathia osteochondroplastica—helical CT findings in 4 cases. J Thorac Imaging 2004;19(2):112–6.

48. Jabbardarjani HR, Radpey B, Kharabian S, et al. Tracheobronchopathia osteochondroplastica: presentation of ten cases and review of literature. Lung 2008; 186:293–7.

49. Devaraj A, Griffin N, Nicholson AG, et al. Computed tomography findings in fibrosing mediastinitis. Clin Radiol 2007;62:781–6.

50. Rossi SE, McAdams HP, Rosado-de-Christenson ML, et al. From the archives of the AFIP- fibrosing mediastinitis. Radiographics 2001;21:737–57.

51. Wilcox P, Miller R, Miller G, et al. Airway involvement in ulcerative colitis. Chest 1987;92(1):18–22.

Bronchiectasis

Cylen Javidan-Nejad, MD*, Sanjeev Bhalla, MD

KEYWORDS

- Airway • Bronchiectasis • HRCT
- High-resolution CT • Cystic fibrosis • Ciliary dyskinesia

Bronchiectasis is defined as the irreversible dilatation of the cartilage-containing airways or bronchi. Enlargement of the bronchi in acute illness, as can be seen in the setting of infectious pneumonia, is usually reversible and would, therefore, not qualify as bronchiectasis (**Fig. 1**). Care must be taken to distinguish this large airway dilatation from dilatation of the small airways (bronchioles) that do not contain cartilage.[1]

MECHANISMS OF DEVELOPMENT

Bronchiectasis may result from one of three main mechanisms: bronchial wall injury, bronchial lumen obstruction, and traction from adjacent fibrosis.[2] The latter two mechanisms are usually apparent on imaging, and are suggested by an endobronchial filling defect or adjacent interstitial lung disease. It is when the first group is encountered that the radiologist is faced with a differential diagnosis and a potential diagnostic conondrum. In this article, we aim to cover the CT appearance of bronchiectasis, potential pitfalls, and a diagnostic approach to help narrow the diverse spectrum of conditions that may cause bronchiectasis.

Many conditions may lead to bronchial wall injury and subsequent bronchiectasis. These include infection and recurrent infections, impaired host defense leading to infection, exaggerated immune response, congenital structural defects of the bronchial wall, and extrinsic insults damaging the airway wall (**Table 1**). These conditions share the common denominator of mucus plugging and superimposed bacterial colonization. The mucus plugging is either a result of abnormal mucus constituency or abnormal mucus clearance. The toxins released by the bacteria and the cytokines and enzymes released by the surrounding inflammatory cells create a vicious cycle of progressive wall damage, mucus plugging, and increased bacterial proliferation.[3,4] Once bronchiectasis begins, therefore, it is sure to progress.

Airway obstruction is most commonly caused by an intraluminal lesion such as carcinoid tumor, inflammatory myofibroblastic tumor, or a fibrous stricture usually from prior granulomatous infection such as histoplasmosis or tuberculosis. The presence of bronchiectasis can be useful in the differential diagnosis of an endoluminal mass, as its presence usually implies a chronic component. Although it may be seen with squamous cell carcinomas arising from papillomas, the presence of bronchiectasis is more suggestive of a slowly growing less malignant lesion, such as a carcinoid tumor (**Fig. 2**). Distal atelectasis and/or postobstructive pneumonitis are common in these conditions.[2] In the post lobectomy or post–lung transplant patient, granulation tissue at the suture line can occasionally result in an intraluminal occlusion and distal bronchiectasis. In these patients, immediate postoperative detection may allow for bronchoscopic removal of granulation tissue and avoid irreversible damage.

When bronchiectasis is from bronchial wall damage or bronchial obstruction, the bronchial wall becomes thickened because of infiltration by mononuclear cells and fibrosis. In cystic fibrosis (CF), an additional neutrophilic infiltration of the walls and airway lumen can be seen. This mural inflammatory process progressively destroys the elastin, muscle, and cartilage. This leads to airway dilatation.

The dilatation can be classified by its gross appearance as tubular (cylindric), varicose, or cystic (saccular). In the former, the bronchiectasis

This article originally appeared in *Radiologic Clinics of North America*, Volume 47, Issue 2, March 2009.
Section of Cardiothoracic Imaging, Mallinckrodt Institute of Radiology, Washington University School of Medicine, 510 South Kingshighway, St Louis, MO, USA
* Corresponding author.
E-mail address: javidanc@mir.wustl.edu (C. Javidan-Nejad).

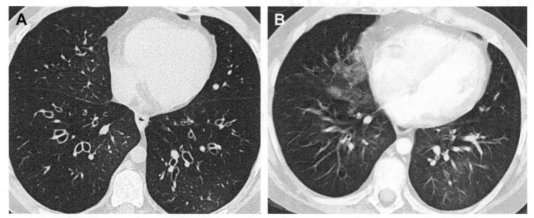

Fig. 1. Reversible lower lobe bronchial dilatation due to pneumonia. Initial CT (*A*) in this 12-year-old girl with hypogammaglobulinemia and pneumonia showed bilateral dilated lower lobe bronchi. Subsequent CT (*B*) performed 6 months later showed resolution of the bronchial dilatation, although it revealed a right middle lobe pneumonia. Because this dilatation is reversible, it would not qualify as bronchiectasis.

is manifest as parallel bronchial walls with failure of normal tapering and squared-off ends of the bronchus. As the process worsens, the bronchi become serpentine with a beaded appearance. This varicose bronchiectasis serves as an intermediate step before the development of grossly dilated, cystic airways. As the airway dilatation increases, there may be progressive collapse and fibrosis of the distal lung parenchyma.[2]

Traction bronchiectasis, as its name implies, is caused by retraction of mature fibrosis of the parenchyma around the bronchi. Such bronchiectasis follows the distribution of the underlying fibrosis. The traction bronchiectasis has an upper lobe distribution in cases of radiation fibrosis, sarcoidosis, and sequela of tuberculosis (**Table 2**) (**Fig. 3**). In cases of usual interstitial pneumonitis (UIP) (idiopathic pulmonary fibrosis) and fibrosing nonspecific interstitial pneumonitis (NSIP), the traction bronchiectasis tends to be mostly in the periphery and the lung bases (**Fig. 4**).[5]

CLINICAL PRESENTATION AND DIAGNOSIS

Symptoms can be very nonspecific. Mild disease may manifest with a mild cough or minimal

Table 1
Bronchiectasis caused by airway wall damage

Mechanism	Disease
Congenital structural defect	Mounier-Kuhn syndrome William-Campbell syndrome
Infection	Pertussis (whooping cough) Tuberculosis Atypical mycobacterium
Impaired immune response	
Abnormal mucociliary clearance	Cystic fibrosis Primary ciliary dyskinesia
Decreased systemic immunity	Hypogammaglobulinemia Lung and bone transplantation
Exaggerated immune response	Allergic bronchopulmonary aspergillosis Inflammatory bowel disease c-ANCA-positive vasculitis Rheumatoid arthritis
Inhalational injury	Smoke and gaseous toxins Chronic gastroesophageal reflux and aspiration

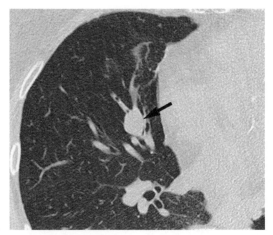

Fig. 2. Bronchiectasis due to obstructing carcinoid tumor. CT through the right middle lobe shows partially mucus-filled bronchiectasis and an endobronchial mass (*arrow*).

dyskinesia, Kartagener syndrome, cystic fibrosis, and diffuse panbronchiolitis.[6]

Hemoptysis, sometimes life-threatening, is caused by chronic airway inflammation and hypoxemia, which leads to bronchial arterial neovascularization.[7,8] These enlarged bronchial arteries are quite fragile and may rupture with even minimal trauma. Pulmonary hypertension can ensue because of underlying hypoxemic vasoconstriction and obstructive endarteritis.[9] The bronchial arteries anastamose with pulmonary arterioles, leading to left-to-right shunting, and if severe enough, can contribute to the pulmonary hypertension.[9]

The severity of airflow limitation is related to the extent and severity of the bronchiectasis. This can be seen in ventilation-perfusion mismatches and retained washout on the ventilation images of ventilation-perfusion scintigraphy. Decreased FEV1 (forced expiratory volume in 1 second) on spirometry can also be seen in the setting of bronchiectasis. Although useful in quantifying the ventilation impairment, spirometry has proven insensitive in detecting early structural damage.

Because of the insensitivity of the other techniques and the high-spatial resolution of CT, high-resolution computed tomography (HRCT) has become the favored diagnostic tool for detection of bronchiectasis.[10,11] Rapid disease progression has a poorer prognosis and has been shown

dyspnea. As it becomes more severe, patients may present with chronic cough, regular and copious sputum production, progressive dyspnea, and repeated pulmonary infections.[3] Digital clubbing, anemia, and weight loss can develop because of chronic hypoxemia and hypercarbia in more severe disease. Severe sinusitis can be seen if the bronchiectasis is due to primary cilia

Table 2
Bronchiectasis based on distribution

Location	Disease
Focal	Congenital bronchial atresia Foreign body Broncholithiasis Endobronchial neoplasm
Diffuse	
Upper lung	Cystic fibrosis Sarcoidosis Progressive massive fibrosis of pneumoconiosis Radiation fibrosis
Central lung	Allergic bronchopulmonary aspergillosis End-stage hypersensitivity pneumonitis (also upper lobes) Mounier-Kuhn (also lower lobes if repeated infections)
Lower lung	Usual interstitial pneumonia (IPF) Nonspecific interstitial pneumonitis Hypogammaglobulinemia Lung and bone transplantation Chronic aspiration Idiopathic
Right middle lobe and lingula	Atypical mycobacterial infection Immotile cilia syndrome (PCD) (also lower lobes)

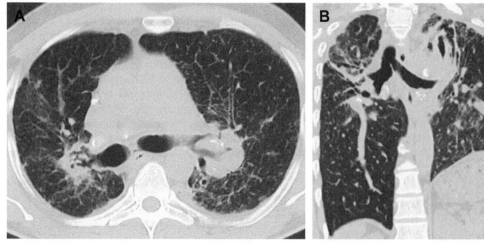

Fig. 3. Upper lobe traction bronchiectasis from end-stage sarcoid. Transaxial image at the level of the carina (*A*) demonstrates tortuous, shortened bronchi amidst upper lobe fibrosis and volume loss. Upper lobe predominance of the bronchiectasis is better appreciated on coronal reconstruction (*B*).

to be associated with increased wall thickening, colonization by *Pseudomonas aeruginosa*, and high concentrations of proinflammatory markers in sputum or serum, such as neutrophilic elastase.[4,12]

Diagnosis is usually suspected by history and confirmed by spirometry and HRCT. Depending on the associated symptoms and age of presentation, the diagnostic workup may include a sweat electrolyte test, serum immunoglobulin levels, or serum *Aspergillus* antibody and precipitin, or even genetic testing. Occasionally electron microscopy of the ciliated cells may be used.[6]

Bronchoscopy is diagnostic and sometimes therapeutic. In localized bronchiectasis caused by a foreign body, an endobronchial neoplasm, bronchiolithiasis, and fibrotic stenosis, bronchoscopy may be used to remove the obstructing lesion. Although the bronchiectasis itself will not revert, the clearance of the airway will improve any postobstructive pneumonia and may prevent progression of the airway damage.[13] Bronchoscopy and lavage is helpful in patients with more diffuse bronchiectasis who present with acute exacerbation or sudden worsening of underlying symptoms. This is usually a sign of acute airway

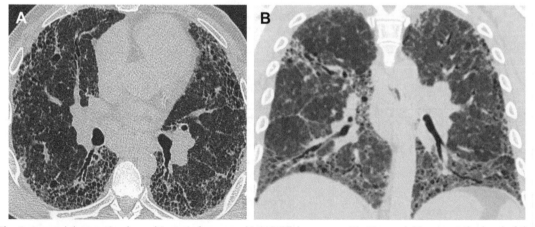

Fig. 4. Lower lobe traction bronchiectasis from usual interstitial pneumonitis. Transaxial image at the level of the superior segmental bronchi (*A*) demonstrates traction bronchiectasis, within peripheral-dominant honeycombing in this 52-year-old man with idiopathic pulmonary fibrosis. Coronal reformatted image (*B*) shows that the basilar and peripheral bronchiectasis follows the distribution of the fibrosis.

infection, commonly by *Pseudomonas* and *Staphylococcus*, and in such patients bronchoscopy is helpful in obtaining samples for culture and determining antibiotic sensitivity, when usual measures of sputum sampling are unsuccessful.[6]

HIGH-RESOLUTION CT IMAGING TECHNIQUE

Because of the nonspecific nature of symptoms associated with bronchiectasis, an accurate way of diagnosis is needed. HRCT provides the most accurate, least invasive technique. It enables the assessment of bronchial abnormalities to the level of the secondary pulmonary lobule level. Conventional HRCT is performed by acquiring 1.0- to 1.5-mm thick images, every 10 mm, reconstructed using a high spatial frequency algorithm. Images can be obtained in a spiral or sequential mode. Using conventional technique, visualization of bronchi 1 to 2 mm in diameter and vessels 0.1 to 0.2 mm in diameter may be achieved.[1] The lungs are scanned twice, during suspended end- inhalation and suspended end-exhalation. The latter phase is performed to reveal subtle air trapping.

Multidetector computed tomography (MDCT) scanners allow fast, volumetric data acquisition, creating contiguous thin sections through the lungs with excellent z-axis spatial resolution. Similar scanning technique is used for all multidetector scanners that have 16 detector rows or higher, where a collimation of 0.50 to 1.25 mm is selected. The scans are performed in inspiration and reconstructed as contiguous 1-mm images or 1-mm-thick images with 10-mm reconstruction interval. Additional advantages are improved anatomic matching of airways with regions of air trapping during inspiration and expiration and providing the ability for postprocessing the axial images to create 3-dimensional (3D) assessment of the airways.[14,15] These postprocessed multiplanar images have become known as volumetric HRCT.[16]

In our center, we use a 16- or 64-row multidetector scanner and image the thorax without use of intravenous contrast during end-inspiration and end-exhalation. Inspiration images are acquired helically and reconstructed as 5×5-mm images and 1×10-mm images; 1×1-mm images are also created in case any mutiplanar or 3D imaging is needed. Exhalation images are also obtained helically and reconstructed as 1×10 mm.

When radiation dose is a consideration (especially in younger patients), a low-dose technique of 30 mAs is used in the expiratory phase. A growing number of authors have advocated the use of low-dose techniques for HRCT, but we have not routinely relied on these.[17]

IMAGING FINDINGS

The imaging findings on conventional radiography are based on visualizing the bronchial wall thickening. This results in ill-defined perihilar linear densities associated with indistinctness of the margins of the central pulmonary arteries. This appearance simulates interstitial pulmonary edema, but lacks the peripheral Kerley B lines. When the bronchus is seen on end, ill-defined ring shadows can be identified because of bronchial wall thickening. The presence of tram lines or parallel lines along the expected courses of the bronchi indicates more severe bronchiectasis, where the dilated bronchial lumen becomes visible on conventional radiography. Tram lines are best identified in the lower lobes, right middle lobe, and lingula (**Fig. 5**). Oftentimes, an abnormality is detected but the specific diagnosis of bronchiectasis is not.

Mucus plugging may appear as elongated opacities, which may be sometimes calcified. These tubular opacities can be confused for pulmonary vascular enlargement. In cystic bronchiectasis, air-fluid levels in thick-walled cysts are seen, associated with variable degrees of surrounding consolidations and atelectasis. Based on the cause and extent of bronchiectasis, the overall lung volume may be increased (**Fig. 6**).[1,2,6]

CT, especially HRCT, is quite reliable in diagnosing bronchiectasis. On CT a diagnosis of bronchiectasis is made when the internal luminal diameter of one or more bronchi exceeds the diameter of the adjacent artery. Other diagnostic criteria of bronchiectasis are the lack of normal tapering of a bronchus, a visible bronchus abutting the mediastinal pleura, or a visible bronchus within 1 cm of the pleura. Signs of bronchiectasis on CT include the signet ring sign, denoted by the artery simulating a jewel abutting the ring, the thick-walled dilated bronchus on a transaxial view, and the tram-track sign, from parallel, thickened walls of a dilated bronchus (**Fig. 7**).

In cylindric bronchiectasis the luminal dilatation is uniform and the wall thickening is smooth. Varicose bronchiectasis denotes a more severe form of disease, where the luminal dilatation is characterized by alternating areas of luminal dilatation and constriction, creating a beaded appearance, and the wall thickening is irregular. In cystic bronchiectasis, the most severe form of bronchiectasis, a dilated, thick-walled bronchus terminates in a thick-walled cyst.[18] Oftentimes, more than

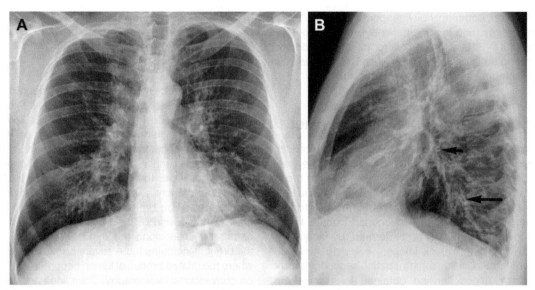

Fig. 5. Diffuse bronchiectasis on conventional radiography. Diffuse bronchiectasis can obscure the perihilar vascular markings, similar to early interstitial pulmonary edema on a pulmonary artery (PA) radiograph (*A*). Identifying dilated bronchi on end (*short arrow*) and tram lines (*long arrow*) leads to the correct diagnosis of bronchiectasis. In this case of cystic fibrosis in a 42-year-old man, the findings are best seen on the lateral radiograph (*B*).

one type of bronchiectasis can be seen in the same patient (**Fig. 8**).

Smooth bronchial wall thickening is seen in all cases of bronchiectasis, except those caused by congenital cartilage deficiency (William-Campbell syndrome, Mounier-Kuhn syndrome) or in allergic bronchopulmonary aspergillosis (ABPA). Bronchial wall thickening alone is a nonspecific finding, as it is also seen in asthma and chronic bronchitis.[6]

A potential pitfall in the diagnosis of bronchiectasis is the double image of a vessel created by cardiac or respiratory motion artifact simulating a dilated bronchus. This is most common in the lingula and left lower lobe where the effect of cardiac motion is most prominent (**Fig. 9**). Caution should be made when diagnosis of bronchial wall thickening is made on HRCT images that have been reconstructed with a very high frequency algorithm.

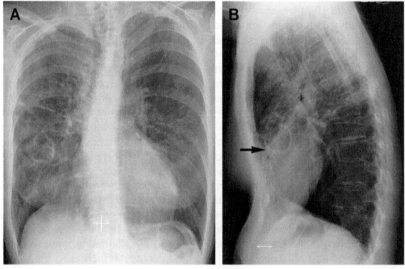

Fig. 6. Cystic bronchiectasis on conventional radiography. Cystic changes are seen in both mid and lower lungs (*arrows*) on the PA chest radiograph (*A*) in this 61-year-old woman with chronic *Mycobacterium avium* intracellulare/complex (MAC) infection. The lateral (*B*) radiograph demonstrates an air-fluid level in cystic bronchiectasis of the right middle lobe (*arrow*).

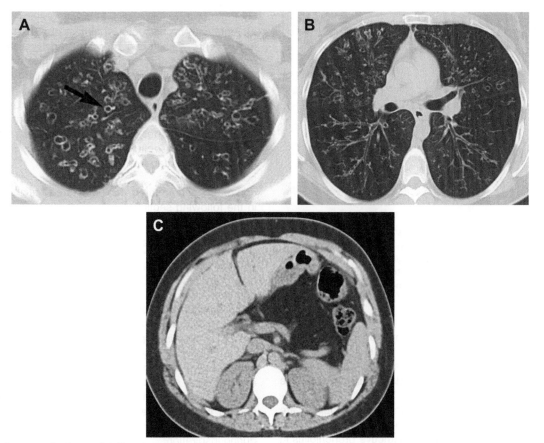

Fig. 7. CT findings of diffuse bronchiectasis in a 27-year-old woman with cystic fibrosis. Transaxial images show the dilated bronchus and adjacent arteriole, seen along their short axis, creating the signet ring sign (*arrow*) (*A*). When the bronchi are visualized along their course, the lack of normal tapering and smooth bronchial wall thickening can be appreciated (*B*). In cystic fibrosis the fatty attenuation of the pancreas is indicative of the pancreatic insufficiency (*C*).

Such algorithm causes the interstitium to appear very thickened and the prominence of the bronchial walls results in a "pseudo-bronchiectasis" appearance (**Fig. 10**).

Mucus plugging of the dilated bronchi and bronchioles appear as branching dense tubular structures, coursing parallel to, but thicker in diameter, than the adjacent artery and arteriole. These

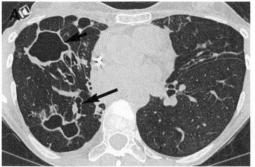
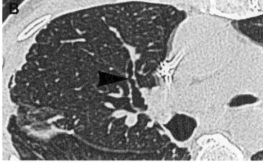

Fig. 8. CT findings of varicose and cystic bronchiectasis. CT images from the same patient as in **Fig. 6** show a more severe form of bronchiectasis, where both varicose (*long arrow*) and cystic (*short arrow*) bronchiectasis is present (*A*). In varicose bronchiectasis, the bronchial lumen has a beaded appearance and nodular wall thickening is seen (*arrowhead*) (*B*).

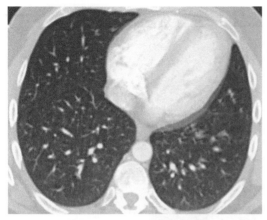

Fig. 9. Pseudo-bronchiectasis due to cardiac motion. The cardiac motion creates a double image, simulating bronchiectasis, usually seen in the left lower lobe and lingula. The artifactual nature of this observation is confirmed by the motion artifact along the posterior wall of the heart.

plugged bronchi are accompanied by adjacent aggregates of nodules, in a "tree-in-bud" pattern, consistent with mucus-filled bronchiolectasis in the center of the secondary pulmonary lobule (**Fig. 11**).

Mosaic attenuation and air trapping are common associated findings. This is felt to be because of coexisting constrictive bronchiolitis in patients with bronchiectasis. The air trapping may be more pronounced when the bronchiectatic airway has a component of bronchomalacia (**Fig. 12**).

BRONCHIECTASIS BASED ON ETIOLOGY

A majority of bronchiectasis encountered in clinical practice will be postinfectious in origin. In fact, in two retrospective studies evaluating the

etiology of bronchiectasis in large cohorts of patients with bronchiectasis, almost one third of the patients were found to have bronchiectasis from prior infection. Idiopathic bronchiectasis, where despite extensive workup the cause was not found, and bronchiectasis related to abnormal mucociliary clearance (cystic fibrosis and primary ciliary dyskinesia) each accounted for almost a quarter of the cases. ABPA and systemic immunodeficiency, due to congenital and acquired causes, were the next most common causes.[3,19] Some of the more commonly encountered etiologies are presented in the following sections.

Traction Bronchiectasis

Traction bronchiectasis is common in UIP, NSIP, and sarcoid and end-stage hypersensitivity pneumonitis.[20,21]

The mechanism of bronchiectasis in fibrotic lung is based on both physiology and mechanical forces involved in inspiration. Patients with widespread fibrosis require increased inspiratory work, leading to a more negative pleural pressure and therefore a greater transpulmonary pressure during inspiration. On the other hand, pulmonary fibrosis increases the elastic recoil of the lung, creating even further expansion of the bronchi during inspiration.

In our practice, we find it helpful to compare bronchiectasis to the adjacent fibrosis. When the bronchiectasis is out of proportion with the adjacent fibrosis, then NSIP secondary to collagen vascular disease may be considered. The explanation may stem from bronchial wall injury caused by collagen vascular disease–related inflammation or secondary to the high incidence of chronic aspiration in this subgroup of patients (**Fig. 13**).

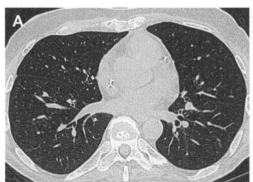
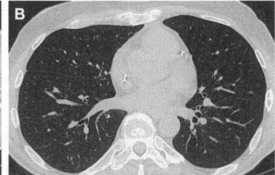

Fig. 10. Imaging pitfall. A very sharp reconstruction algorithm (B80f) of the CT image may result in increased noise, creating the illusion of bronchial wall thickening (*A*). When the same image is reconstructed with a less sharp algorithm (B60f), it becomes clear that the bronchiectasis is not real (*B*).

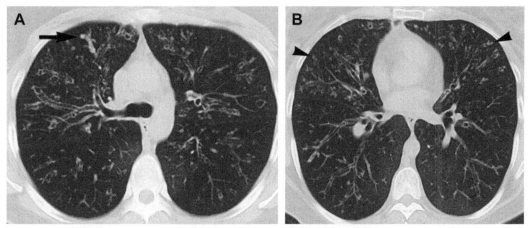

Fig. 11. Mucus plugging on CT. On transaxial images, the filling of bronchiectasis by mucus appears as tubular and branching opacities, with club-like, rounded ends (*arrow*) (*A*). The mucus-filled smaller branching bronchi and bronchioles appear as tree-in-bud opacities (*arrowheads*) (*B*). The mosaic attenuation of the surrounding lung is due to air trapping. In this case, the bronchiectasis was from cystic fibrosis.

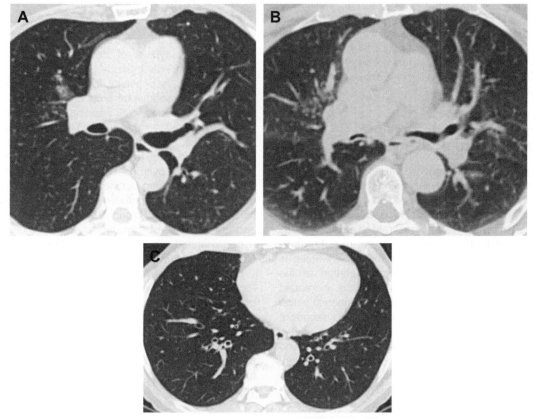

Fig. 12. Bronchomalacia and bronchiectasis: a 68-year-old man with a reported history of asthma nonresponsive to steroid therapy. CT images show a normal caliber of the central bronchi (*A*), and marked collapse of their lumina when imaged during forced exhalation (*B*), consistent with bronchomalacia. The distal bronchi are diffusely dilated and have smooth wall thickening, consistent with mild bronchiectasis (*C*).

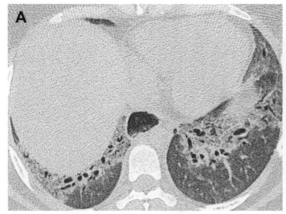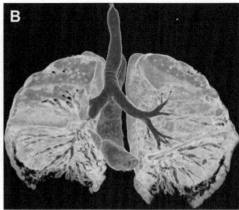

Fig. 13. Bronchiectasis out of proportion of surrounding fibrosis. Transaxial CT of the chest of a 34-year-old woman with scleroderma shows a dilated esophagus, basilar pulmonary fibrosis, and significant bronchiectasis without evidence of honeycombing (*A*). The volume-rendered image demonstrates the extent of the bronchiectasis (*B*) and the markedly dilated esophagus.

Congenital Airway Wall Abnormality

Congenital defects of the cartilage, collagen, or other components of the bronchial wall lead to abnormal physiologic clearing of mucoid excretions, predisposing the bronchial epithelium to repeated infections and a vicious cycle of progressive bronchial dilatation. Structural wall defect is the common feature of Mounier-Kuhn disease or tracheobronchomegaly, William-Campbell syndrome, and congenital bronchial atresia.

TRACHEOBRONCHOMEGALY (MOUNIER-KUHN DISEASE)

Tracheobronchomegaly is an uncommon disease that presents mostly in men, in the fourth and fifth decades. Although believed to be congenital, it may be associated with Ehlers-Danlos syndrome, Marfan syndrome, and generalized elastosis (cutis laxa). Pathological thinning of the muscle, cartilage, and elastic tissue of the airway walls is seen. This results in uniform dilatation of the tracheal and bronchial lumina and increased distensibility of the tracheal and bronchial walls. This tracheobronchomalacia leads to recurrent infections in the dependent lungs.[6]

The disease involves the entire trachea and bronchi of first to fourth order. On imaging, a tracheal diameter exceeding 3 cm in both coronal and sagittal planes and central bronchiectasis is seen without associated airway wall thickening. More distal bronchiectasis, bronchial wall thickening, occasionally fibrosis, and cystic changes in the lower lobes are common because of sequela of repeated pneumonia.[22,23] The net

effect is a progression of the bronchiectasis and lung disease, which, in turn, may result in increased tracheobronchomegaly (**Fig. 14**).

CONGENITAL BRONCHIAL ATRESIA OR MUCOCELE

A focal area of bronchiectasis surrounded by lucent lung is typical of congenital bronchial atresia or congenital mucocele. This condition is characterized by congenital focal obliteration of the lumen of a segmental bronchus, resulting in focal bronchiectasis and air trapping more distally. The dilated airway is commonly filled by inspissated mucus, which may occasionally calcify. Congenital bronchial atresia is usually focal, and is commonly discovered incidentally, as an ovoid, tubular, or branching density on a chest radiograph. It may be confused with a pulmonary nodule. CT reveals its bronchial, branching nature, and the presence of surrounding and more distal hyperexpanded and hyperlucent lung parenchyma, due to the associated air trapping (**Fig. 15**).

Conversely, acquired mucocele is caused by focal scarring of a segmental bronchus because of prior granulomatous infection or from an endobronchial lesion. It should be differentiated from congenital bronchial atresia by the absence of air trapping of the distal lung parenchyma.[24,25] The presence of an acquired mucocele should prompt further interrogation to exclude the possibility of an endobronchial neoplasm (**Fig. 16**).

WILLIAMS-CAMPBELL SYNDROME

Williams-Campbell syndrome is a rare disease in which the cartilage of the fourth-, fifth-, and

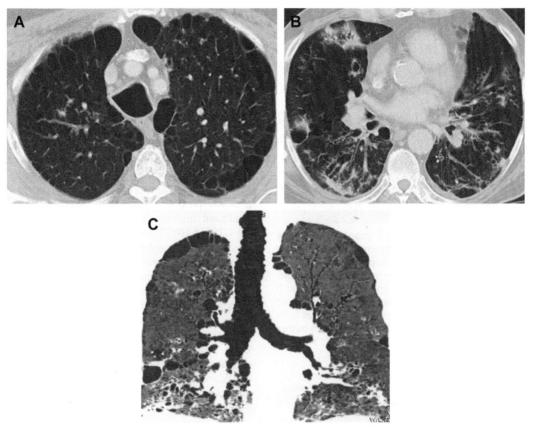

Fig. 14. Mounier-Kuhn Syndrome. Transaxial CT images show tracheomegaly (*A*), and basilar-predominant varicose and cystic bronchiectasis (*B*) seen in Mounier-Kuhn syndrome. The coronal reconstructed image demonstrates the typical corrugated appearance of the tracheal wall (*C*).

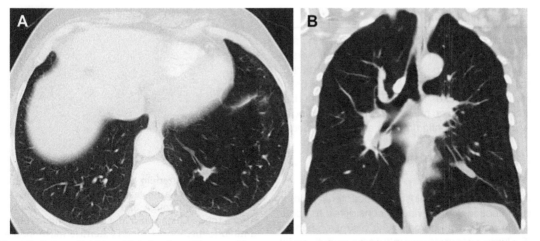

Fig. 15. Congenital bronchial atresia: a 60-year-old woman with pleuritic chest pain. CT with contrast (*A*) shows a nodular density in the left lower lobe with surrounding hyperlucency of the lung parenchyma, due to focal air trapping. Coronal reconstruction (*B*) better demonstrates the tubular nature of that structure, which connects to a dilated bronchus. These features (mucocele with surrounding air trapping) are diagnostic for this condition.

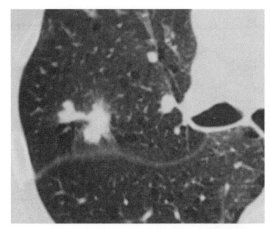

Fig. 16. Acquired mucocele. CT image through the right upper lobe in this 68-year-old man reveals a branching tubular structure representing a mucus-filled dilated subsegmental bronchus or mucocele. The lack of surrounding air trapping suggests that it is not congenital and likely because of an acquired obstruction of the bronchus. In this case, it was from a small squamous cell cancer that was not seen before surgery.

sixth-generation bronchi is defective. The disease may involve the lung focally or diffusely.[26] The congenital form presents in childhood and is commonly associated with congenital heart disease, polysplenia, bronchial isomerism, and situs inversus. The acquired form is likely a sequela of prior adenovirus (measles and pertussis) infections.[27] CT imaging shows cystic bronchiectasis distal to the third-generation bronchi, and inspiratory-expiratory CT imaging reveals ballooning on inspiration and collapse on exhalation.[1]

Acquired Wall Abnormalities

Chronic or past infections, inhalational injury, and cellular infiltration in the setting of graft versus host disease lead to inflammation of the bronchial wall, resulting in structural damage of the bronchial wall. This leads to irreversible bronchial dilatation and increased mucus production, leading to a vicious cycle of inflammation and wall damage.

ATYPICAL OR NONTUBERCULOSIS MYCOBACTERIA

Atypical or nontuberculosis mycobacterial pulmonary infection was previously considered to occur only in adults with chronic lung disease, such as CF, lung cancer, or emphysema; adults with impaired immunity, especially acquired immunodeficiency syndrome (AIDS), or those with thoracic skeletal abnormalities. These organisms, however,

especially mycobacterium avium intracellulare-complex (MAC), are increasingly being recognized as the cause of chronic lung infection in adults with normal immunity and no underlying lung disease, especially older women. In immunocompetent people, MAC has three different forms: a fibrocavitary form, a nodular bronchiectatic form, and hypersensitivity pneumonitis.

The fibrocavitary form, similar to postprimary tuberculosis, involves the apices and upper lobes and causes traction bronchiectasis in the affected lung. It occurs mostly in older men with emphysema. The nodular bronchiectasis form represents a slowly progressive disease, often resistant to treatment and more common in older women. On CT and HRCT imaging it appears as multiple clusters of centrilobular micronodules, in a branching or tree-in-bud pattern, aggregating around air- or mucus-filled cylindric bronchiectasis and bronchiolectasis. Multifocal consolidations and cavities can occur. There is associated mosaic attenuation and air trapping. The disease has a predilection for the right middle lobe, upper lobes, and lingula, but involvement of other lobes may also be seen (**Fig. 17**).[28–30] Scarring and traction bronchiectasis of the right middle lobe and lingula are indicative of long-standing disease (**Fig. 18**).

Mucociliary Clearance Abnormalities

The ciliary ladder is responsible for effective clearing of mucoid excretions of the airway

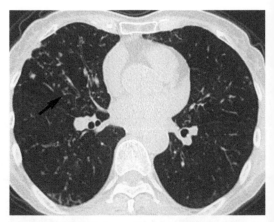

Fig. 17. Mycobacterium avium intracellulare/complex (MAC) infection: a 68-year-old Chinese woman who developed mild cough and intermittent hemoptysis after a trip to China, which did not respond to routine antibiotic therapy. CT shows extensive micronodules, mostly in the right middle lobe, right lower lobe, and lingula, which aggregate in a tree-in-bud pattern around the mildly dilated subsegmental bronchi (*arrow*). Sputum specimen was positive for MAC.

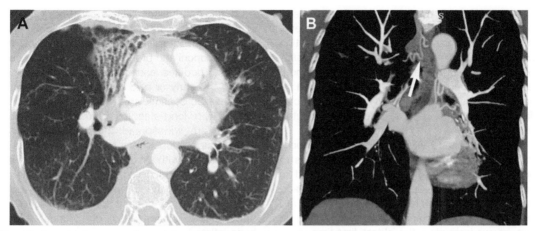

Fig. 18. Bronchial artery collateral formation in bronchiectasis: a 76-year-old woman with chronic productive cough has new-onset of severe, recurrent hemoptysis. CT of chest with intravenous contrast shows severe bronchiectasis and scarring of the right middle lobe (*A*). The dilated bronchial arteries (*white arrow*) providing collateral flow to the lungs are better demonstrated on the coronal thin-MIP (6 mm) reformatted image (*B*).

epithelium. Abnormalities in the consistency of mucus in cystic fibrosis, and abnormalities of the structure and function of the cilia of the airway epithelium, as seen in primary ciliary dyskinesia or immotile ciliary syndrome, leads to ineffective mucus clearance and secondary colonization of the airway lumina by bacteria. This chronic infection and repeated bouts of pneumonia lead to bronchiectasis. The bronchiectasis of cystic fibrosis is typically worse in the upper lobes, as opposed to primary and acquired ciliary dyskinesia, such as Young syndrome where bronchiectasis is associated with azospermia, where the

bronchiectasis is worse in the dependant or lower lungs.

CYSTIC FIBROSIS

CF is an autosomal recessive trait and occurs in approximately 1 in 3000 live births in the United States and Europe. It is caused by a mutation in the CF transmembrane conductance regulator (CFTR). This results in failed secretion of chloride through the CFTR and associated ion channels, leading to dehydration of the endobronchial secretions. This thickened mucus cannot be

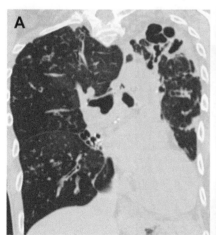
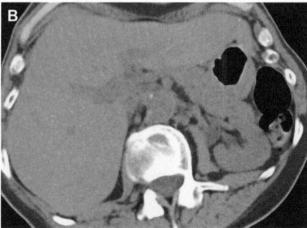

Fig. 19. Initial diagnosis of cystic fibrosis late in life. A 68-year-old woman had undergone left lower lobectomy more than 35 years ago because of recurrent pneumonia of the left lower lobe. Recent dyspnea on exertion and wheezing prompted further workup, which revealed a sweat chloride = 81 mmol/L (normal <40 mmol/L). Coronal reformatted image of HRCT of chest (*A*) shows severe bronchiectasis of the left upper lobe, and relatively mild bronchiectasis throughout the right lung. Transaxial nonenhanced CT of abdomen does not show fatty pancreatic parenchyma (*B*).

efficiently cleared by the mucociliary system, leading to obstructed airways and bacterial infection.[4] Colonization and recurrent infection with *Staphylococcus aureus, Haemophilus influenza,* and *Pseudomonas aeruginosa* is common, leading to progression of airway destruction. A poor prognosis is made when atypical mycobacteria or *Burkholderia cepacia* colonize the dilated airways.[6]

Although CF is usually diagnosed in childhood, the heterogeneity of severity of disease leads to patients with milder disease, first diagnosed in adulthood. As genetic testing improves and awareness of CF increases, milder forms are increasingly being detected later in adulthood. In fact, at our institution, the oldest first-time diagnosis of CF was in a 72-year-old woman with mild bronchiectasis. Sweat chloride test greater than 40 mmol/L indicates the presence of disease.

CT findings include diffuse cylindric, varicose, or even cystic bronchiectasis, bronchial wall thickening. Extensive mucus plugging of the dilated bronchi and bronchioles manifests as centrilobular nodules and branching densities (see **Fig. 7**).[1] In early or mild forms of CF, these findings may be confined to the right upper lobe.[6] In adults with long-standing diffuse disease, the findings are widespread throughout the lungs and the upper lobes may be completely scarred and collapsed with associated traction bronchiectasis. This lobar scarring is due to chronicity of disease where the bronchiectasis has been most severe and present longest. Despite the upper lobe volume loss, the lungs remain hyperinflated.

Typically patients with CF have pancreatic insufficiency and on CT the pancreas has a homogenous fat attenuation. However, in cases of

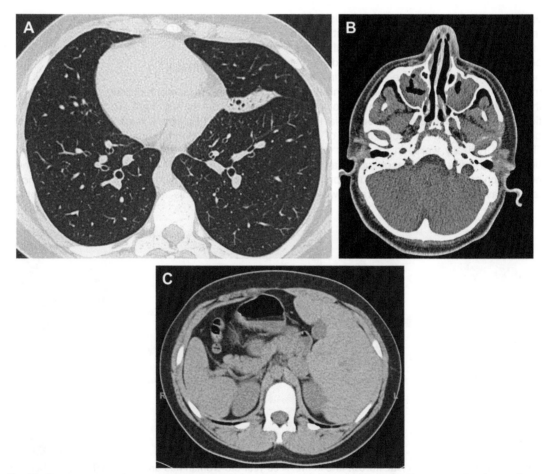

Fig. 20. Kartagener syndrome. Transaxial CT of chest (*A*) in a 12-year-old boy with Kartagener Syndrome shows dextrocardia and bronchiectasis of the lower lobes and scarring of the left middle lobe caused by more severe bronchiectasis and repeated pneumonia. Nonenhanced CT of the paranasal sinuses (*B*) show marked mucosal thickening and opacification of the maxillary sinuses. The transaxial nonenhanced CT image of the upper abdomen (*C*) demonstrates the situs inversus associated with this syndrome.

a milder mutation, which leads to an initial diagnosis later in life, the pancreatic insufficiency is commonly absent (**Fig. 19**).[31]

PRIMARY CILIARY DYSKINESIA

Primary ciliary dyskinesia (PCD) or immotile ciliary syndrome is caused by a defect in structure and function of the airway cilia. This leads to impaired mucociliary clearance.[32] It is a genetically heterogeneous, autosomal recessive trait with a prevalence of approximately 1 in 15,000 to 1 in 30,000 of live births. Patients present with recurrent infections of the lungs, sinuses, and middle ear. Similar to CF, PCD causes progressive bronchiectasis. Thoracoabdominal asymmetry occurs in approximately 50% of patients. Kartagener syndrome or triad is present in half of the PCD patients. This triad consists of situs inversus, bronchiectasis, and sinusitis (**Fig. 20**).[33,34]

PCD tends to be diagnosed relatively late, because of its nonspecific presenting symptoms in children. Clinical suspicion based on a focused history leads to diagnosis. The current diagnostic test of choice is electron microscopic analysis of respiratory cilia in samples of nasal or airway mucosa. This reveals defects in the outer or inner dynein arms of the cilia.[33]

The CT findings of PCD are bronchiectasis of variable severity, associated with tree-in-bud nodules and branching densities because of mucus plugging, and lobar scarring and air trapping (**Fig. 21**). Bronchiectasis in PCD is predominantly in the lingual and middle and lower lobes of the lung. Isolated upper lobe involvement and isolated peripheral bronchiectasis is very rare.

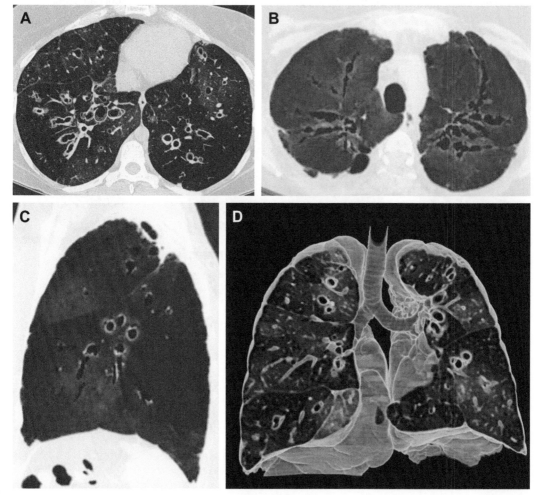

Fig. 21. Primary ciliary dyskinesia: a 37-year-old woman with primary ciliary dyskinesia and chronic pseudomonas aeruginosa infection being evaluated for bilateral lung transplantation. HRCT of chest (*A*) shows mixed tubular, varicose, and cystic bronchiectasis. Minimal intensity reformatted images in axial (*B*) and sagittal (*C*) planes and volume-rendered image (*D*) demonstrate the extent of bronchiectasis and the associated mosaic attenuation.

Hyper-Immune Response

Inflammatory bowel disease, rheumatoid arthritis, Sjogren disease, antineutrophilic cytoplasmic antibody (c-ANCA)–positive vasculitis (Wegener disease), and allergic bronchopulmonary aspergillosis all can lead to bronchiectasis, possibly because of inflammation of the airway wall in the setting of a hyperimmune response to internal or external antigens. The chronic inflammation damages the bronchial walls, leading to bronchiectasis.

ALLERGIC BRONCHOPULMONARY ASPERGILLOSIS

Allergic brochopulmonary aspergillosis (ABPA) is due to a hypersensitivity reaction to *Aspergillus fumigatis* antigens, leading to development of bronchocentric granulomata in the bronchi and bronchioles, associated with mucus impaction.[35]

It is most commonly seen in patients with atopic rhinitis, asthma, or CF.[36] Patients present with wheezing, fever, and pleuritic chest pain and may cough up brown mucus plugs. Clinical diagnosis could be made by detecting an elevated serum IgE level, eosinophilia on peripheral blood smears, or positive skin reaction to *Aspergillus* antigen. Mycelia can occasionally be identified in the exporated mucus plugs.

Chest radiographs and CT show migratory pneumonitis early in the disease. This usually involves the upper lobes. Central and upper lobe bronchiectasis, varicose or cystic subtypes, is best detected by CT, which also helps monitor progression and response to treatment. In more chronic disease, inspissated mucus in the dilated central bronchi created the appearance of the classic finger-in-glove appearance on the chest radiographs (**Fig. 22**). Atelectasis or hyperinflation of the lung distal to the impacted bronchi can occur.[18,35]

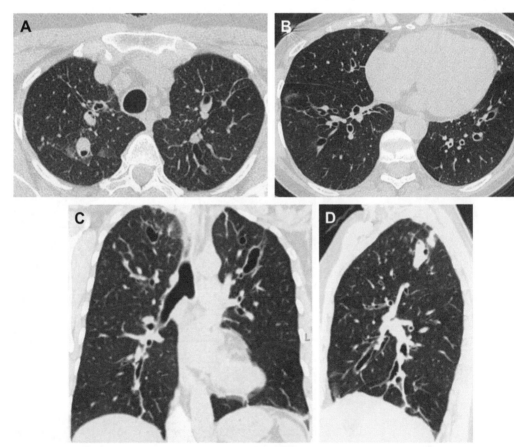

Fig. 22. Allergic bronchopulmonary aspergillosis (ABPA). HRCT of the chest in a 55-year-old woman with history of reactive airway disease at the level of the apices (*A*) and lung bases (*B*) show dilated, thick-walled bronchi. The bronchiectasis is worse in the apices where mucus plugging is seen. Coronal (*C*) and sagittal (*D*) reformatted images better demonstrate the distribution of the bronchiectasis.

SUMMARY

Bronchiectasis, or the irreversible dilatation of bronchi, can present with a host of nonspecific clinical symptoms, including hemoptysis, cough, and hypoxia. The radiologist, then, can play an important role in its detection and characterization. Bronchiectasis must be differentiated from motion artifact and transient bronchial dilatation in acute lung disease. When diagnosed, a logical approach may allow for proper triage of the patient to prevent progression of disease.

The radiologic approach usually begins with CT, which is fast and accurate. The diagnostic approach should be based on the mechanisms of development of bronchiectasis (bronchial wall damage, endobronchial obstruction, and traction) and the location. Once an endobronchial lesion or adjacent fibrosis is excluded, location of the abnormality can be used to help narrow the differential diagnosis. When the bronchiectasis is upper lobe predominant, CF should first be considered but occasionally MAC infection may present with this finding. When the bronchiectasis is mid-upper lobe, then ABPA or chronic hypersensitivity pneumonitis might lead the list of diagnoses. Lower lobe bronchiectasis is usually the sequela of recurrent infection and conditions that predispose to recurrent infections, including Mounier-Kuhn, hypogammaglobulinemia, PCD, and recurrent infections. By using this approach, the radiologist can remain an integral part of the pulmonary team.

REFERENCES

1. Hartman TE, Primack SL, Lee KS, et al. CT of bronchial and bronchiolar diseases. Radiographics 1994;14:991–1003.

2. Shoemark A, Ozerovitch L, Wilson R. Aetiology in adult patients with bronchiectasis. Respir Med 2007;191:1163–70.

3. Muller NL, Fraser RS, Lee KS, et al. Diseases of the lung—radiologic and pathologic correlations. 1st edition. Philadelphia: Lippincott Williams and Wilkins; 2003. p. 280–1. Chapter 15.

4. Lynch DA, Newell JD, Lee JS. Imaging of diffuse lung disease. 1st edition. Hamilton (ON): B.C.Decker Inc; 2000. p. 175–86. Chapter 6.

5. Westcott JL, Cole SR. Traction bronchiectasis in end-stage pulmonary fibrosis. Radiology 1986;161: 665–9.

6. Hirshberg B, Biran I, Glazer M, et al. Hemoptysis: etiology, evaluation, and outcome in a tertiary referral hospital. Chest 1997;112:440–4.

7. Bruzzi JF, Remy-Jardin M, Delhaye D, et al. Multidetector row CT of hemoptysis. Radiographics 2006; 26:3–22.

8. Alzeer AH, Al-Mobeirek AF, Al-Otair HAK, et al. Right and left ventricular function and pulmonary artery pressure in patients with bronchiectasis. Chest 2008;133:468–73.

9. Chang AB, Masel JP, Boyce MC, et al. Non-CF bronchiectasis: clinical and HRCT evaluation. Pediatr Pulmonol 2003;35:477–83.

10. Eshed I, Minski I, Katz R, et al. Bronchiectasis: correlation of high-resolution CT findings with health-related quality of life. Clin Radiol 2007;62: 152–9.

11. Martınez-Garcıa MA, Soler-Cataluna JJ, Perpina-Tordera M, et al. Factors associated with lung function decline in adult patients with stable non-cystic fibrosis bronchiectasis. Chest 2007;132:1565–72.

12. Camacho JR, Prakash UB. 46 year old man with chronic hemoptysis. Mayo Clin Proc 1995;70:83–6.

13. Kwong JS, Muller NL, Miller RR. Diseases of the trachea and main-stem bronchi: correlation of CT with pathologic findings. Radiographics 1992;12: 645–57.

14. Di Scioscio V, Zompatori M, Mistura I, et al. The role of spiral multidetector dynamic CT in the study of Williams-Campbell syndrome. Acta Radiol 2006; 47(8):798–800.

15. Carden KA, Boiselle PM, Waltz DA, et al. Tracheomalacia and tracheobronchomalacia in children and adults: an in-depth review. Chest 2005;127: 984–1005.

16. Nishino M, Hatabu H. Volumetric expiratory HRCT imaging with MSCT. J Thorac Imaging 2005;20(3): 176–85.

17. de Jong PA, Nakano Y, Lequin MH, et al. Dose reduction for CT in children with cystic fibrosis: is it feasible to reduce the number of images per scan? Pediatr Radiol 2006;36(1):50–3.

18. Elizur A, Cannon CL, Ferkol TW. Airway inflammation in cystic fibrosis. Chest 2008;133:489–95.

19. Robinson TE. Computed tomography scanning techniques for the evaluation of cystic fibrosis lung disease. Proc Am Thorac Soc 2007;4:310–5.

20. Kennedy MP, Noone PG, Leigh MW, et al. High-resolution CT of patients with primary ciliary dyskinesia. AJR Am J Roentgenol 2007;188:1232–8.

21. Pasteur MC, Helliwell SM, Houghton SJ, et al. An investigation into causative factors in patients with bronchiectasis. Am J Respir Crit Care Med 2000; 162:1277–84.

22. Misumi S, Lynch DA. Idiopathic pulmonary fibrosis/ usual interstitial pneumonia: imaging diagnosis, spectrum of abnormalities, and temporal progression. Proc Am Thorac Soc 2006;3(4):307–14.

23. Silva CI, Muller NL, Lynch DA, et al. Chronic hypersensitivity pneumonitis: differentiation from idiopathic pulmonary fibrosis and nonspecific interstitial pneumonia by using thin-section CT. Radiology 2008; 246(1):288–97.

24. McAdams HP, Erasmus J. Chest case of the day: Williams-Campbell syndrome. Am J Roentgenol 1995;165:190.

25. Kinsella D, Sissons G, Williams MP. The radiological imaging of bronchial atresia. Br J Radiol 1992;65:681.

26. Jederlinic PJ, Sicilian LS, Baigelman W, et al. Congenital bronchial atresia: a report of 4 cases and review of literature. Medicine 1986;66:73–83.

27. Glassroth J. Pulmonary disease due to nontuberculous mycobacteria. Chest 2008;133:243–51.

28. Kuroishi S, Nakamura Y, Hayakawa H, et al. Mycobacterium avium complex disease: prognostic implication of high-resolution computed tomography findings. Eur Respir J 2008;32:147–52.

29. Kim JS, Tanaka N, Newell JD, et al. Nontuberculous mycobacterial infection—CT scan findings, genotype, and treatment responsiveness. Chest 2005; 128:3863–9.

30. Hansell DM. Bronchiectasis. Radiol Clin North Am 1998;36(1):107–28.

31. Loch C, Cuppens H, Rainisio M, et al. European epidemiologic registry of cystic fibrosis (ERCF): comparison of major disease manifestations between patients with different classes of mutations. Pediatr Pulmonol 2001;31:1–12.

32. Vikgren J, Johnsson AA, Flinck A, et al. High-resolution computed tomography with 16-row MDCT: a comparison regarding visibility and motion artifacts of dose-modulated thin slices and "step and shoot" images. Acta Radiol 2008;23:1–6.

33. Martinez S, Heyneman LE, McAdams HP, et al. Mucoid impactions: finger-in-glove sign and other CT and radiographic features. Radiographics 2008; 28:1369–82.

34. Brown DE, Pittman JE, Leigh MW, et al. Early lung disease in young children with primary ciliary dyskinesia. Pediatr Pulmonol 2008;43:514–6.

35. Bush A, Chodhari R, Collins N, et al. Primary ciliary dyskinesia: current state of the art. Arch Dis Child 2007;92:1136–40.

36. Morozov A, Applegate KE, Brown S, et al. High-attenuation mucus plugs on MDCT in a child with cystic fibrosis: potential cause and differential diagnosis. Pediatr Radiol 2007;37(6):592–5.

Imaging–Bronchoscopic Correlations for Interventional Pulmonology

Tshering Amdo, MD[a], Myrna C.B. Godoy, MD[b],
David Ost, MD, MPH[c], David P. Naidich, MD, FACCP[b],*

KEYWORDS
- Interventional pulmonology • CT • Virtual bronchoscopy
- Endobronchial ultrasound (EBUS)
- Transbronchial needle aspiration (TBNA)

The development and rapid advancement of both bronchoscopic, CT and ultrasound imaging technology has had considerable impact on the management of a wide variety of pulmonary diseases. The synergy between these newer imaging modalities and advanced interventional endoscopic procedures has led to a revolution in diagnostic and therapeutic options in patients with both central and peripheral airway disease. Given the broad clinical implications of these technological advances, only the most important areas of interventional pulmonology in which imaging has had a major impact will be selectively reviewed to highlight fundamental principles.

Whereas interventional pulmonology is often conceptually organized around different technologies and instruments such as stents, lasers, and electrocautery, among others, it is important to emphasize applications of the same technology may vary widely in terms of their methods, risks, and benefits depending on the nature of the indication. For example, while the method in which a stent is placed may not alter, indications and complications are significantly different between patients with benign and malignant disease.[1] As a consequence, particular emphasis will be placed first on evaluation of CT-bronchoscopic correlations in the evaluation and treatment of central airway disease, followed by CT- bronchoscopic correlations in the evaluation of peripheral lung disease, in particular, pulmonary nodules. Following this, the rapidly evolving topic of interventional bronchoscopic approaches to the treatment of emphysema will be reviewed.

Although attention will be primarily be placed on CT bronchoscopic correlations (including CT-fluoroscopy and virtual bronchoscopy), emphasis will also be placed on newer imaging technologies including endobronchial ultrasound (EBUS), electromagnetic navigation and guidance, and Doppler ultrasound site selection for bronchoscopic treatment of emphysema.

BRONCHCOSCOPIC IMAGING CORRELATIONS IN THE EVALUATION OF CENTRAL AIRWAY DISEASE
CT Imaging Technique

Key to the recent ability of imaging to serve as a guide for interventional bronchoscopic procedures has been the introduction and now widespread availability of multidetector CT scanners capable of acquiring contiguous and/or overlapping high-resolution images throughout the entire

This article originally appeared in *Radiologic Clinics of North America*, Volume 47, Issue 2, March 2009.
[a] Division of Pulmonary and Critical Care Medicine, New York University–Langone Medical Center, Tisch Hospital, 560 First Avenue, New York, NY 10016, USA
[b] Department of Radiology, New York University–Langone Medical Center, Tisch Hospital 560 First Avenue, New York, NY 10016, USA
[c] Division of Pulmonary Medicine, MD Anderson Cancer Center, Houston, TX 77030, USA
* Corresponding author.
E-mail address: david.naidich@nyumc.org (D.P. Naidich).

thorax in a single breathhold. This has led to a near revolution in the variety of methods by which the airways and lung can be visualized and evaluated, including the use of quantitative CT techniques.[2,3] Although a truly detailed discussion of this topic is beyond the scope of the present review, the following general points regarding CT technique for evaluating the airways are emphasized.

Optimal evaluation of both the central and peripheral airways requires at a minimum contiguous high-resolution images throughout the entire chest (**Fig. 1**). While contiguous 1- to 1.5-mm sections are sufficient for evaluating both the central and peripheral airways, in our experience, optimal visualization of the peripheral airways is best obtained with use of submillimeter overlapping sections whenever possible (typically 0.75 mm every 0.5 mm) especially in those cases for which three-dimensional (3D) segmentation or virtual bronchoscopic evaluation of the peripheral (sixth to ninth order) airways is deemed clinically important.[4] Although the use of low-dose technique (50 to 80 mAs) is more than sufficient to evaluate the central airways and in most cases the peripheral airways as well, in those cases for which 3D and/or virtual endoscopic views are intended, best results necessitate the use of routine standard CT exposure factors. Additional considerations include acquisition of select expiratory high-resolution images in cases in which tracheal and bronchial dynamics are of concern, or to confirm the presence of obstructive small airway disease.

Axial CT images are sufficient for evaluating most airway abnormalities;[3,5] however, there are inherent limitations of these for assessing the central airways, including (1) limited ability to detect subtle airway stenosis; (2) underestimation of the craniocaudad extent of disease; (3) difficulty displaying the complex 3D relationships of the airway to adjacent mediastinal structures; (4) inadequate representation of airways oriented obliquely to the axial plane; and (5) difficulty assessing the interfaces and surfaces of airways that lie parallel to the axial plane. Another relative limitation of axial CT scanning is the generation of a large number of images for review, especially with multidetector scanners, which may generate data sets containing hundreds of images. As a consequence, use of retrospectively reconstructed 2D and 3D images should be considered routine for bronchoscopic correlation to overcome these limitations.

Virtual bronchoscopy (VB) in particular may facilitate central airway evaluation by allowing the user to "bypass" an obstructing lesion, accurately measure its length and cross-sectional area, and to look backward from distal to proximal, "retroflexing" the virtual bronchoscope, which is not possible with the conventional bronchoscope.[6] Virtual bronchoscopy is especially complementary to bronchoscopy in the assessment of patients with high-grade airway stenoses, particularly for assessing the patency of the airways beyond the site of a stenosis. In one study[7] comparing virtual and conventional bronchoscopy in 20 patients with malignant airway stenoses, while high-grade stenoses were viewed equally well with both techniques, virtual bronchoscopy offered the advantage of viewing the airway beyond the site of

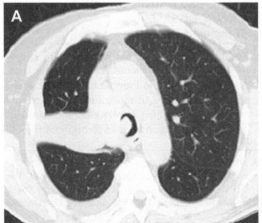 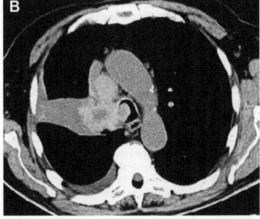

Fig. 1. Central airway lesions. (*A*) Section through the lower trachea imaged with lung windows shows a well-defined obstructing lesion. (*B*) Identical image as in *A* imaged with mediastinal window clearly demonstrates the true extent of tumor which appears denser then adjacent peripheral atelectasis. The ability to demonstrate the extent of tumor is critical to deciding the optimal method for interventional bronchoscopic therapy.

stenosis in 5 (25%) of 20 patients in whom the bronchoscope could not pass the lesion. However, lack of sensitivity for mucosal detail is an important limitation especially when attempting to assess the extent of airway wall involvement in patients in whom a distinction between intrinsic and extrinsic tumor is of clinical consequence.[6,8]

Finally, it is worth emphasizing that in those case in which there are central lesions accompanied by peripheral volume loss, administration of a bolus of intravenous contrast medium may prove indispensable by allowing precise delineation of the true extent of tumor versus atelectatic lung, findings often indispensable for selecting optimal therapeutic interventions.

Transbronchial Needle Aspiration and Biopsy

CT-bronchoscopic correlations

Transbronchial needle aspiration and biopsy (TBNA) is a minimally invasive procedure done via flexible fiber-optic bronchoscopy (FB) that allows sampling of tissue through the tracheal or bronchial wall not directly visualized bronchoscopically. TBNA was first introduced by Schieppati[9] in 1958 for use with the rigid bronchoscope and was later adapted for flexible bronchoscopy (FB) by Wang and colleagues in 1983.[10] This technique has been successfully used since then as a nonsurgical means most often to sample mediastinal nodes or less commonly hilar nodes, endobronchial lesions, and peripheral lesions for the diagnosis of both benign and neoplastic conditions.

The ability of TBNA to sample mediastinal and hilar nodes can reduce the need for invasive mediastinoscopy for assessing paratracheal lymph nodes and the need for open thoracotomy for posterior, subcarinal, and hilar lymph nodes, respectively.[11,12] Importantly, TBNA may provide the only bronchoscopic specimen diagnostic for lung cancer in up to 18% of patients in one reported series.[13] However, TBNA is often a "blind" procedure, especially when limited to sampling peribronchial lesions in the absence of endobronchial abnormalities. As a consequence, use of TBNA has been limited with an overall sensitivity for diagnosing malignant mediastinal adenopathy of 78% with values ranging from 14% to 100%.[14]

Although the sensitivity and specificity of TBNA largely depends on operator technique, the yield of TBNA has been shown to be markedly enhanced by using CT scans to plan optimal biopsy sites before bronchoscopy.[12,15] It should be emphasized, however, that merely identifying an enlarged node adjacent to a central airway on CT may not lead to successful TBNA, as not all endoscopic sites are equally amenable to transbronchial biopsy. As a consequence, optimal endoscopic anatomic landmarks for 14 hilar, intrapulmonary, and mediastinal lymph node stations have been proposed.[11] This classification provides for consistent, reproducible, lymph node mapping that is compatible with the international staging system for lung cancer[16] and is applicable for clinical and surgical-pathologic staging.

Whereas TBNA is most often performed to diagnose and stage NSCLC, it has also been used successfully to diagnose benign diseases as well, including, in particular, sarcoidosis[17] and more recently tuberculous lymphadenopathy in patients with HIV+/AIDS.[18] Especially in the setting of HIV+/AIDS, active tuberculous nodes may appear as rim-enhancing low-density lesions following intravenous contrast administration. In one series, using CT as a guide, mycobacterial infection was diagnosed by TBNA in 21 of 23 cases of documented mycobacterial infection, with TBNA providing the only diagnostic specimen in 13 (57%).[18]

CT fluoroscopic guidance

In 1998, Rong and Cui[19] demonstrated an increase in the yield by performing TBNA under CT guidance. Using conventional CT scanners to provide cross-sectional views of the relevant anatomy during the procedure, the tip of the needle was located and then adjusted until it was documented to be inside targeted mediastinal lymph nodes. Slow CT reconstruction times and significant radiation exposure, however, limit the practical value of this approach.

With the introduction of CT fluoroscopy, real-time imaging during the procedure became feasible enabling continuous image acquisition, permitting precise, real-time localization of the bronchoscopic tip and needle (**Fig. 2**). CT fluoroscopy is less cumbersome than conventional CT guidance, as it is controlled via a foot pedal with the imaging screen mounted next to the bronchoscopist obviating reliance on the technologist's workstation to check the position of the catheter tip. To date, several case series[20,21,22,23] have demonstrated the safety and ease of performing TBNA under CT fluoroscopic guidance with an increase in yield of diagnosis in patients previously undergoing nondiagnostic conventional TBNA.[20,21,23] White and colleagues[23] performed TBNA with CT fluoroscopic assistance on 27 patients, of whom 15 had mediastinal nodes and 12 had lung nodules or focal infiltrates. Mean lesion size was 1.7 cm in the mediastinum and 2.2 cm in the lung. A correct diagnosis was established in 10

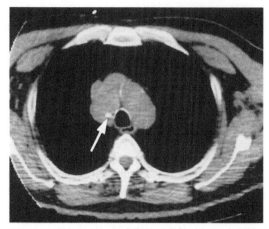

Fig. 2. CT fluoroscopy-guided bronchoscopy. Axial CT section through the distal trachea shows the tip of a TBNA needle in an enlarged right paratracheal lymph node (*arrow*), which on cytology proved to be due to metastatic non–small cell lung cancer. As demonstrated in this case, TBNA not only allows diagnosis, often the sole means for acquiring histologic diagnosis, but may also provide precise tumor staging—in this case Stage IIIA disease, obviating more invasive procedures including mediastinoscopy and/or surgery.

of 12 mediastinal lesions (83%) for which follow-up was available (three patients were lost to follow-up) and in eight lung lesions (67%).[23] These investigators concluded that CT fluoroscopy can provide effective, real-time guidance for TBNA and might be particularly valuable in patients with small or less accessible mediastinal nodes.[23]

Despite these results, a recent randomized trial failed to demonstrate a significant difference between CT fluoroscopic-guided bronchoscopy and conventional approaches, although this may reflect the small sample size of this study as there was a trend toward higher diagnostic yield with CT guidance on a per lymph node versus a per patient basis.[24] Finally, it should be noted that some have advocated the use of virtual bronchoscopic guidance as a means for enhancing the yield of TBNA (**Fig. 3**). Vining and colleagues[6] compared VB images with videotaped bronchoscopy results in 20 patients who had undergone both helical chest CT and FB during clinical evaluation of central airway abnormalities and observed that virtual bronchoscopy simulations accurately represented major endobronchial anatomic findings. As an extension of these findings, McAdams and colleagues[25] assessed the role of virtual bronchoscopy in guiding TBNA in 17 patients and found that it improved the diagnostic yield of this procedure, with an overall sensitivity of 88% on a per-node basis, and reduced both the amount of pre-procedure preparation and the actual procedural time. To date, while suggestive, an actual role for routine VB-guided TBNA remains to be established.

Transbronchial Needle Aspiration–Endobronchial Ultrasound

As discussed above, the yield of TBNA is clearly enhanced by pre-procedural review of CT findings: further advantages accrue from performing TBNA with fluoroscopic guidance. Despite these advantages, the overall yield of TBNA remains suboptimal.[14] As a consequence, and not surprisingly, attention has increasingly focused on developing newer methods for performing image-guided TBNA, most importantly endobronchial ultrasound.

Endobronchial ultrasound (EBUS)-TBNA is a relatively new technique in which a convex ultrasound probe is inserted through the working channel of the bronchoscope allowing real-time ultrasound-guided TBNA. After imaging the target lymph node, a specially designed TBNA needle is passed through the ultrasound catheter into the desired location under real-time ultrasound guidance (**Fig. 4**). EBUS-TBNA can be used to sample all except anterior, prevascular, and aorticopulmonary lymph nodes. This includes the highest mediastinal, upper and lower paratracheal, and subcarinal as well as hilar lymph nodes.[26,27,28] Compared with conventional TBNA, EBUS guidance significantly increases the yield of TBNA in all mediastinal lymph node locations except for subcarinal nodes.[29]

Of particular interest, EBUS has been shown to diagnose malignant mediastinal and hilar nodes in patients in whom both CT and positron emission tomography (PET) scans have proved negative.[30]

Similar findings have been reported by others. Yasufuku and colleagues,[31] for example, in a prospective comparison of EBUS-TBNA with PET and thoracic CT for detection of mediastinal and hilar lymph node metastasis in patients with lung cancer using surgical nodal sampling as a gold standard, showed that the sensitivities of CT, PET, and EBUS-TBNA for mediastinal and hilar lymph node staging were 76.9%, 80.0%, and 92.3%, respectively, with corresponding specificities of 55.3%, 70.1%, and 100%, and diagnostic accuracies of 60.8%, 72.5%, and 98.0%. Other investigators, however, have demonstrated that although EBUS may be useful in this situation, the frequency of occult mediastinal disease may be too low to make routine EBUS worthwhile. Cerfolio and colleagues[32] conducted a prospective trial on patients with NSCLC who were clinically staged N2 negative by both dedicated CT scanning and/or integrated

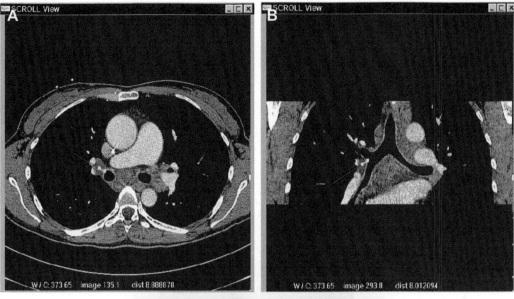

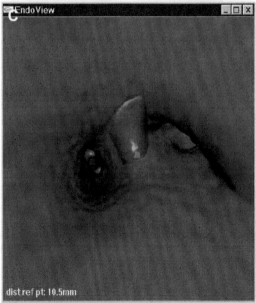

Fig. 3. TBNA: virtual bronchoscopic guidance. Axial (*A*) and coronal (*B*) CT sections imaged with narrow windows at the level of the bronchus intermedius show enlarged bilateral hilar and subcarinal nodes. In this case, right hilar nodes have been semiautomatically outlined and appear in color. Note that the optimal angle for accessing these nodes is also presented (*yellow lines*). (*C*) Virtual bronchoscopic image looking inferiorly from the distal bronchus intermedius showing the bifurcation of the right upper lobe bronchus and bronchus intermedius. The exact location of the right hilar nodes outlined in *A* and *B* are now superimposed on the virtual bronchoscopic image. In this case, virtual bronchoscopy serves as a road map assisting TBNA in accessing nodes in locations less frequently biopsied. Cytologically proven metastatic non–small cell carcinoma. (*From* Naidich DP, Webb WR, Grenier PA, et al. Imaging the airways. Philadelphia: Lippincott Williams and Wilkins; 2005. p. 49; with permission.)

PET/CT. All underwent mediastinoscopy and endoscopic ultrasonography (EUS) esophageal endoscopic ultrasound-guided fine-needle aspiration (FNA). Those with negative N2 nodes underwent thoracotomy with thoracic lymphadenectomy to confirm the findings. Only 2.9% of patients clinically staged as N0 after integrated PET/CT and/or CT had positive mediastinoscopy results and only 3.7% had positive EUS-guided FNA results. Based on these findings, these authors concluded that

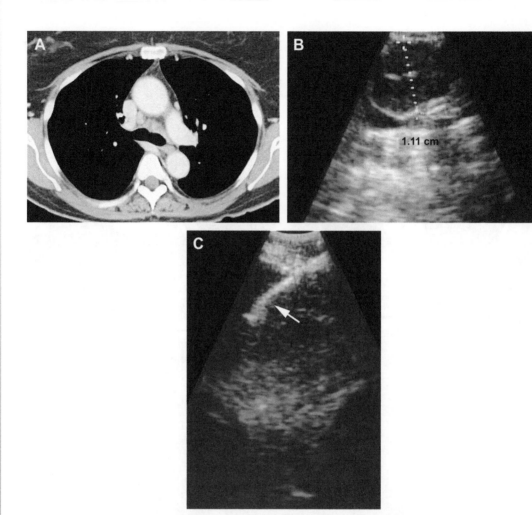

Fig. 4. EBUS-TBNA. (*A*) Contrast-enhanced axial CT image at the level of the carina shows slightly enlarged pre-carinal nodes. (*B*) Endobronchial ultrasound image shows these same nodes adjacent to the airway wall noted at the top of the image, measured at a depth of 1.1 cm. Nodes are especially easy to identify with EBUS separable from adjacent airways and vessels. (*C*) Endoscopic image confirming in real time that the TBNA needle tip is within the center of these nodes (*arrow*). Cytologically proven non–small cell lung cancer. (*Case courtesy of Michael Zervos, MD, New York University–Langone Medical Center, New York, NY.*)

there was no indication for the use of routine EUS-guided FNA in patients with radiographic N0 disease. However, as patients with clinical N1–hilar adenopathy by PET/CT had a relatively higher prevalence of unsuspected N2 disease (a total of 17.6% after mediastinoscopy and 23.5% after EUS-guided FNA) these investigators did conclude that patients with N1 disease be considered for routine EUS-FNA. Despite these findings, the need for preoperative EBUS-TBNA of otherwise normal-appearing mediastinal nodes remains to be determined.

Therapeutic Interventional Bronchoscopy: Imaging Correlations

The past decade has seen the development of a number of interventional bronchoscopic alternatives to routine therapeutic modalities for treating central airway disease. To date, these procedures are most often performed either as complementary to and/or alternatives to surgery, radiation, and/or chemotherapy in the palliative treatment of patients with malignant airway disease. Approximately 30% of lung cancer patients present with lesions obstructing either the trachea or main bronchi resulting in dyspnea, cough, hemoptysis, or symptoms secondary to obstructive pneumonia, especially when the degree of obstruction exceeds 50%.[33,34] Importantly, the ability to recanalize obstructed airways has proved of clinical benefit by alleviating symptoms and, in select cases, prolonging survival.

Currently available ablational procedures include Nd:YAG laser bronchoscopy, photodynamic therapy, argon plasma coagulation, endobronchial stents, brachytherapy, and cryosurgery.[35] Although a detailed description of these various procedures, including their mechanisms of action, is outside the intended scope of the present review, a few basic principles regarding their use warrant emphasis. Airway obstruction may result either from intrinsic tumor, extrinsic disease (typically from adjacent adenopathy, but also including other mediastinal malignancies) or a combination of these causes. In one study of 143 patients in whom stents were placed to alleviate obstruction, of 67% with malignant disease, 42% were because of extrinsic compression whereas 27% had intraluminal tumors.[36] Differentiation between these causes is of significance: stents and brachytherapy, for example, are best suited for extrinsic compression or in cases in which there is extensive submucosal disease (**Fig. 5**).[33] In distinction, in patients with intrinsic airway lesions, options preferentially include tumor debulking with the rigid bronchoscope, laser, cryotherapy, argon plasma coagulation, and photodynamic therapy (**Fig. 6**).[33] Among these latter, cryotherapy, photodynamic therapy, and brachytherapy are generally reserved for smaller endobronchial tumors where distal bronchial segments can be visualized[37] Although choice among these various approaches is individual depending on availability and technical expertise, in all cases CT may prove indispensable by delineating the true extent of disease, both intrinsic and extrinsic, as well as allowing visualization of airways peripheral to points of obstruction otherwise invisible to the bronchoscopist.[3,38]

To date, CT has proved especially useful in the pre- and post-procedural assessment of airway stents. For airway stenting, routine 2D multiplanar reconstructions (MPRs) have proved of greatest utility clinically.[39] Easily obtained, MPRs can be displayed in routine coronal and sagittal planes, orthogonal to a point of reference, or in a curved fashion along the axis of the airway. The 2D reformatted images performed along the axis of the airway offer the advantage of quickly displaying the regional extent of a stenosis on a single image, although more difficult and time consuming to reconstruct.

As an aid, pre-procedural CT planning may prove invaluable by precisely delineating the anatomy, pathology, and severity of airway obstruction.[39] Information provided by CT can help to determine whether the airway obstruction is caused by extrinsic compression, intraluminal disease, or intrinsic airway disease, as occurs in patients with tracheobronchomalacia, for example.[40] CT also provides important complementary information regarding the relationship of the central airways to adjacent structures that are not visible at bronchoscopy.[39] By determining the cause, location, length, and extent of the airway obstruction, CT can help stratify patients into those who are amenable to surgical resection and those who are candidates for palliative

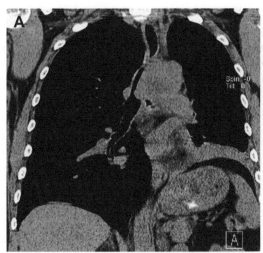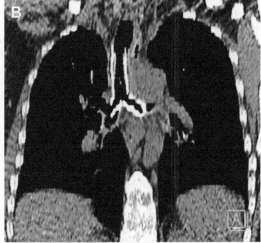

Fig. 5. Airway compression caused by extrinsic disease. (*A*) Non–contrast-enhanced multiplanar coronal reconstruction through the distal trachea and carina shows marked narrowing of these airways with apparent complete obstruction of the left mainstem bronchus resulting in marked volume loss in the left lung. (*B*) Coronal image at the same level as *A* showing the placement of a Y-shaped dynamic silicone stent in the distal trachea and proximal mainstem bronchi resulting in improved aeration of the left lung. Multiplanar reconstructions, in particular, facilitate identification of appropriate candidates for stenting as well as facilitating more precise measurement of airway diameter, lesion length, and airway visualization beyond the reach of the bronchoscope because of obstruction.

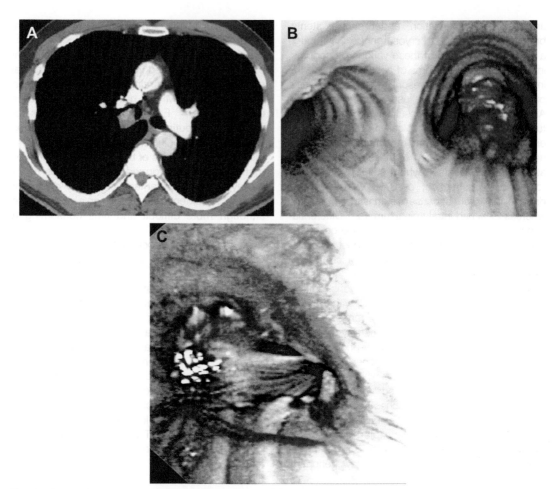

Fig. 6. Airway obstruction caused by intrinsic tumor. (*A*) Contrast-enhanced axial image just below the carina shows near complete obstruction of the right mainstem bronchus by a well-defined soft tissue mass. (*B*) Endoscopic view showing bulky tumor mass appearing to completely occlude the airway lumen. (*C*) Endoscopic view following photodynamic therapy documenting marked decrease in the size of this lesion, which proved to be a mucoepidermoid carcinoma. CT may play an invaluable role by demonstrating the true extent of disease allowing optimal choice of interventional technique.

treatment (see **Fig. 5**). In patients deemed appropriate for airway stenting, CT findings can help to determine the type, size, and length of stent needed. For cases in which the initial bronchoscopic evaluation fails to visualize the airways beyond the site of obstruction, CT serves as an important adjunct study by providing detailed anatomic information of the distal airways.[39]

Less common, although as important, indications for interventional bronchoscopic procedures include the treatment of benign tumors or a number of benign conditions, most often postintubation tracheal strictures. Gluecker and colleagues,[41] for example, compared 2D and 3D CT imaging in the pre- and postoperative evaluation of complex benign laryngeo-tracheal airway stenoses with rigid bronchoscopy, considered as the gold standard. Two-dimensional images and 3D VB of tracheal stenoses proved to be efficient and complementary to rigid bronchoscopy, permitting a reliable endoluminal 3D view and evaluation of the surrounding anatomic structures.

In addition to assisting in pre-procedural planning, CT is also being increasingly used as a first-line study for stent surveillance.[39,42] Because nearly all stents, including metallic stents, cause minimal artifact on multislice CT, the location, shape, and patency of the stents and adjacent airways can be clearly visualized on CT. CT is highly accurate at detecting stent complications, including malpositioning, migration, fracture, incongruence between the stent and airway diameters, external compression with continued stenosis, and local recurrence of malignancy (**Fig. 7**). When compared with fiberoptic bronchoscopy, both MPRs and 3D renderings have been shown to be 88% to 100% sensitive and 100% specific in detecting stent complications.[42,43] In a recent study by Dialani and colleagues,[42] for example, CT accurately detected 15 (100%) of 15 stent complications in a group of patients undergoing surveillance with both CT and bronchoscopy leading these investigators to suggest that CT may be able to replace bronchoscopy for routine surveillance of stents.

Bronchoscopic Imaging Correlations for Peripheral Lesions

It has long been noted that the likely yield of transbronchial needle aspiration or biopsy (TBBx) of peripheral lung nodules or masses is affected by the size and location of lesions. Peripheral lesions (defined as those not visible bronchoscopically beyond the segmental bronchial level) in particular are problematic with sensitivities of 34% for peripheral lesions smaller than 2 cm in diameter versus 63% for lesions with a diameter larger than 2 reported in one recent study including 30 patients with peripheral lung lesions.[44] Additional factors include the type of lesion (solid vs ground-glass), the type of procedure performed (bronchoalveolar lavage vs bronchial brushing vs TBBx), or whether the procedure is performed under fluoroscopic control.

The CT Bronchus Sign/CT Fluoroscopy

It has been shown that the likely yield of TBNA for peripheral lesions is significantly improved in those cases in which a bronchus can be identified leading to or traversing a nodule, a so-called "positive bronchus sign."[45,46] It has also been suggested that improved results from attempted transbronchial biopsy may result when CT fluoroscopy has been used to aid in the diagnosis of peripheral lesions (**Fig. 8**). To date, while there have been several small promising case series reported,[19,20,22,23,47] there has been only one small randomized controlled trial[24] comparing CT fluoroscopy–guided bronchoscopy with conventional bronchoscopy for the diagnosis of peripheral lesions. In this study, there was no significant difference between CT fluoroscopy–guided bronchoscopy and conventional bronchoscopy;[24] however, when CT confirmed entry of the biopsy forceps or needle into peripheral lesions, the diagnostic yield did prove considerably higher. This result suggests that the overall yield of CT-guided bronchoscopy could be considerably enhanced if combined with improved methods of steering, not only using conventional but ultrathin bronchoscopes as well.

In this regard, VB has recently been applied to aid in the diagnosis of peripheral lesions. Asano and colleagues[48] used VB and ultrathin bronchoscopy for peripheral pulmonary lesions. The

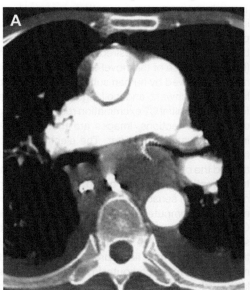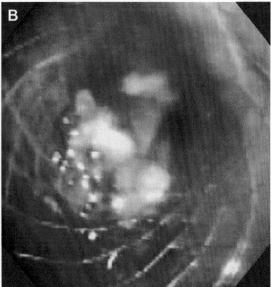

Fig. 7. Stent surveillance. (*A*) Enlargement of a contrast-enhanced axial CT image below the carina shows extensive mediastinal tumor associated with bilateral pleural effusions. Note that there is a stent seen in the left main stem bronchus within which soft tissue density is clearly identifiable, in this case because of tumor invasion of the stent. CT is an effective means for monitoring stents following placement. (*B*) Endoscopic view confirming tumor infiltrating the lumen through the stent.

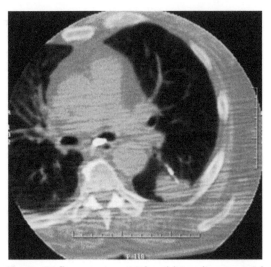

Fig. 8. CT fluoroscopy: peripheral lung disease. Axial non–contrast-enhanced image obtained during fluoroscopic-guided transbronchial biopsy. Note that images obtained during CT fluoroscopy suffer from some degree of motion artifact and increased image noise. In this case it is possible to identify the tip of the biopsy needle within the center of a lesion in the superior segment of the left lower lobe. Cytologically proven non–small cell lung cancer.

diagnosis rate of this procedure was 81.6% for the 38 lesions examined by ultrathin bronchoscopy: 80.8% for 26 lesions 2 cm in size, and 83.3% for 12 lesions larger than 2 cm. Merritt and colleagues[49] and Shinagawa and colleagues[50] have also demonstrated that combining VB and ultrathin bronchoscopy was superior to conventional bronchoscopy for diagnosing peripheral lung lesions. Asahina and colleagues[51] successfully performed transbronchial biopsy (TBB) using EBUS and VB navigation for small peripheral pulmonary lesions smaller than 3 cm in diameter.

Despite these findings, it should be noted that currently available biopsy forceps for use in ultrathin bronchoscopes present an important barrier to the use of this approach, as only minimal tissue can generally be obtained, severely limiting diagnostic efficacy. More promising is the potential use of VB-guided bronchoscopy to precisely direct a pediatric bronchoscope into the lung periphery to sample specific regions in patients with otherwise "diffuse" lung diseases identified on high-resolution CT (HRCT).[4]

Endobronchial ultrasound with radial probe

EBUS using a radial ultrasonic probe has also been used to locate peripheral parenchymal lesions.[52] For this purpose a thin ultrasonic probe is inserted through a guide sheath that is passed

through the working channel of a flexible bronchoscope (FB). Under fluoroscopic guidance, the whole unit is maneuvered to the region of interest. Although the radial probe provides cross-sectional images of the tracheobronchial wall and adjacent mediastinal structures and produces a 360-degree image relative to the long axis of the FB, a major limitation has been the necessity to withdraw the US probe before inserting a biopsy instrument, eliminating the possibility of real-time positioning.

Paone and colleagues[53] conducted a study to compare the diagnostic yield of two bronchoscopic procedures: EBUS transbronchial biopsy (EBUS-TBB) and conventional transbronchial biopsy (TBB) for diagnosing peripheral pulmonary lesions and reported a sensitivity of 79% in the EBUS group versus 55% in the TBB group for establishing malignant diagnoses. In patients with lesions smaller than 3 cm, they found a considerable decline in TBB sensitivity and accuracy (31% and 50%), whereas EBUS-TBB maintained its diagnostic yield (75% and 83%). A similar difference in sensitivity was observed when lesions smaller than 2 cm (23% vs 71%) were compared. Based on these data it may be concluded that in select cases EBUS using a radial probe represents an important option in the diagnosis of peripheral lung cancer, especially in small lesions and/or patients considered ineligible for surgery.

Electromagnetic navigation

The electromagnetic navigation system is an image-guided localization device that assists in placing endobronchial accessories (forceps, brush, or needle) to desired regions of the lung (**Fig. 9**). The use of this novel technology in animal models followed by human subjects was first published by Schwarz and colleagues.[54,55] In brief, following an initial CT examination requiring contiguous 1-mm sections, images are then uploaded into a navigating computer. The electromagnetic navigation system creates an electromagnetic field around the chest by placing the subject on an electromagnetic localization board. An electromagnetic position sensor is then attached to the same navigating computer already loaded with the initial CT scan data, now displayed in virtual bronchoscopic format. As the sensor is positioned within the electromagnetic field, precise spatial coordinates are fed to the computer in real time and correlated with the virtual bronchoscopic CT data by a process of registration. This involves selecting predetermined targets on the virtual bronchoscopic image and then touching the corresponding identical endoscopic targets in real time using the bronchoscopic probe. Targets chosen are points

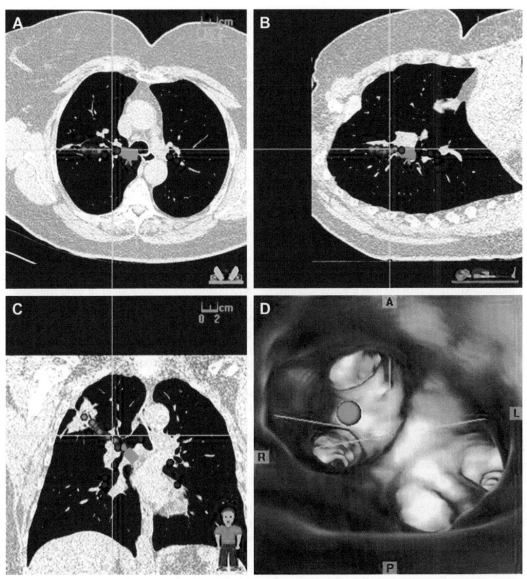

Fig. 9. Electromagnetic registration and guidance: peripheral lung lesions. Screen shot from a commercially available electromagnetic navigation system (SuperDimension, Inc) shows typical interface with axial, sagittal, and coronal CT images, respectively, coupled with virtual bronchoscopic images. Following an initial CT study, data are loaded into the navigating computer. Using virtual bronchoscopy (*lower right image*), anatomic landmarks are chosen as registration points. Typically these are the main carina, right upper lobe carina, middle lobe carina, right lower lobe carina, left upper lobe carina, and left lower lobe carina displayed in this image as purple dots. During actual bronchoscopy, the electromagnetic sensor is touched to each of these points enabling electronic registration of these locations by the computer. A separate path to the target lesion of interest (*green dots*) is also reconstructed. Once the registration process is complete, the bronchoscopist pilots from green dot to green dot until the target lesion is reached.

of airway bifurcation and include the main carina and most proximal lobar bifurcations. Once five to six of these anatomic locations have been so co-registered with the corresponding VB images, the computer can then map the rest of the CT data to real-life coordinates (see **Fig. 9**). Divergence, a measure of the error between the projected

coordinates using these registration points and the actual points, is usually in the range of 3 to 7 mm.

Importantly, the electromagnetic navigation system includes two critical features. The electromagnetic position sensor, which is the size of a bronchoscopy forceps, first is steerable and second may be passed through an extended working channel, which is simply a hollow catheter. Consequently, once the probe reaches its intended target, it can be removed while keeping the extended working channel in place. Biopsy instruments such as forceps and brushes can then be passed back down the extended working channel to the same location.

Schwarz and colleagues[54,55] successfully demonstrated, initially in animal models and subsequently in a human study, safe use of electromagnetic navigation technology coupled with preoperative CT scanning in precisely localizing peripheral lung lesions with a variety of endobronchial accessories. They also demonstrated safety and efficacy in navigating to peripheral lung lesions located beyond the range of a standard FB.[54,55] Subsequent larger studies in human subjects[56,57,58,59] have been conducted with reproducible results, proving that electromagnetic navigation bronchoscopy is a safe method for sampling peripheral and mediastinal lesions with high diagnostic yield independent of lesion size and location. Nonetheless, despite the potential of widespread clinical applicability, it should be emphasized that, to date, no randomized trials demonstrating its superiority to conventional methods for diagnosing peripheral lung lesions has been reported.

Electromagnetic navigation plus endobronchial ultrasound

Although both EBUS using radial probes and electromagnetic navigation bronchoscopy have been used individually to try to improve bronchoscopic diagnosis of peripheral lung lesions, a recent study by Eberhardt and colleagues[60] evaluated whether or not the combination of radial EBUS plus electromagnetic navigation might be superior to either system alone. Focusing on the diagnosis of peripheral lung lesions, this study included three arms: EBUS only, an electromagnetic navigation system only, and a combined procedure using both technologies together. In the combined group, following initial electromagnetic navigation, an ultrasound probe was passed through the extended working channel to enable direct visualization of lesions. Biopsies were taken if ultrasound visualization confirmed that the extended working channel was within the target with retargeting of lesions performed as necessary. For the purpose of this study, primary outcome was defined as diagnostic yield with the reference standard surgical biopsy if bronchoscopic biopsy proved nondiagnostic. The diagnostic yield of the combined procedure (88%) was greater than EBUS (69%) or electromagnetic navigation (59%)

alone, and proved independent of lesion size or lobar distribution. Based on this initial study, it was concluded that combining EBUS and electromagnetic navigation can improve the sensitivity of flexible bronchoscopy when compared with either EBUS or electromagnetic navigation individually for diagnosing peripheral lung lesions without compromising safety.[60] Similarly improved results using a combined approach have also been reported.[61]

Emphysema: CT-Interventional Bronchoscopic Correlations

Bronchoscopic lung volume reduction in severe emphysema

Current treatment of severe emphysema is limited to palliative measures that include supplemental oxygen, bronchodilators, anti-inflammatory drugs, and pulmonary rehabilitation or lung transplantation. Various surgical procedures have been used to treat severe emphysema, including thoracoplasty, excision of bullae, costochondrectomy, phrenic nerve division, autonomic denervation, and lung transplantation. Until the completion of the National Emphysema Treatment Trial (NETT),[62] none of these techniques were accepted as beneficial except for resection of giant bullae and lung transplantation, each indicated in only a small percentage of emphysema patients. The NETT trial established that Lung Volume Reduction Surgery (LVRS) is associated with improvement in health status, dyspnea, and exercise capacity and lung function, when compared with medical treatment in select populations.[62,63] In this regard, the extent and severity of disease as identified by CT has proved one of the most important predictors of a successful outcome, with patients with predominant upper lobe centrilobular disease most likely to respond successfully (**Fig. 10**), while those with more diffuse disease are noncandidates. However, because LVRS is associated with significant morbidity, mortality, and cost, nonsurgical alternatives for achieving volume reduction are being developed.

To date, three bronchoscopic lung volume reduction strategies have shown promise and are currently entering into clinical trials. All are designed to reduce hyperinflation within emphsyematous portions of the lung and thus achieve lung volume reduction without the significant mortality and morbidity associated with surgical LVRS.[64,65,66,67] These include (1) placement of endobronchial one-way valves designed to promote atelectasis by blocking inspiratory flow; (2) formation of airway bypass tracts using drug eluting stents designed to facilitate emptying of

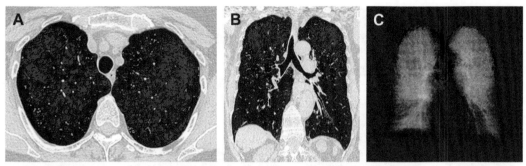

Cluster	Left				Right			
	Total	Upper	Middle	Lower	Total	Upper	Middle	Lower
Class 1 [%]	0.6	0.7	1.1	0.1	0.6	0.7	0.9	0.2
Class 2 [%]	0.6	0.7	1.1	0.0	0.7	1.0	0.9	0.1
Class 3 [%]	0.1	0.2	0.2	0.0	0.1	0.1	0.2	0.0
Class 4 [%]	9.1	23.8	3.3	0.0	6.6	6.6	1.8	0.1
3D BI []	4.6	4.7	4.3	0.0	4.6	4.6	2.6	0.2

Fig. 10. Emphysema: quantitative CT evaluation. Axial (*A, upper left image*), coronal (*B, middle image*), and volumetric rendered coronal sections (*C, upper right image*) show typical appearance of severe centrilobular emphysema almost exclusively restricted to the upper lobes. In this case, contiguous 1-mm images were acquired with quantitative analysis using −950 HU as a cut-off to demonstrate emphysematous foci, visually color-coded. The table below the images shows quantitative assessment of the extent of emphysema as measured by the so-called "cluster" analysis. This allows evaluation of the relative size of low-density foci providing a "bulla index" (3d BI) in which voxels are subdivided as in this example into four arbitrary classes, each separately color coded, with class 1 (*blue*) = all low-density foci ≤ 2 mm; class 2 (*green*) = 2 to 8 mm; class 3 (*yellow*) = 8 to 12 mm; and class 4 (*pink*) = 12 mm, respectively. Note that in this case the majority of low-density foci fall into the class 4 category and are clearly upper lobe in distribution without evidence of discrete subpleural bullae noted—findings ideal for both LVRS and/or bronchoscopic lung volume reduction.

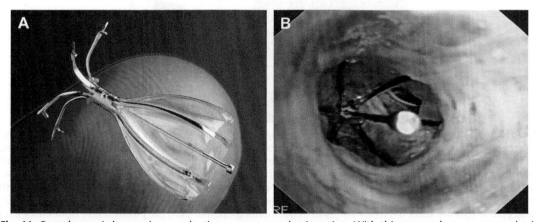

Fig. 11. Bronchoscopic lung volume reduction—one-way valve insertion. With this approach, a one-way valve is inserted under endoscopic guidance in an upper lobe bronchus to block air from entering the emphysematous portion of on inspiration while allowing gas to exit during expiration. (*A*) The appearance of the valve before insertion against the background of a person's finger. (*B*) The appearance of the valve 1 month following deployment within the right upper lobe bronchus, follow-up 9 months later showed marked narrowing of the right upper lobe bronchus consistent with marked volume loss in the right upper lobe.

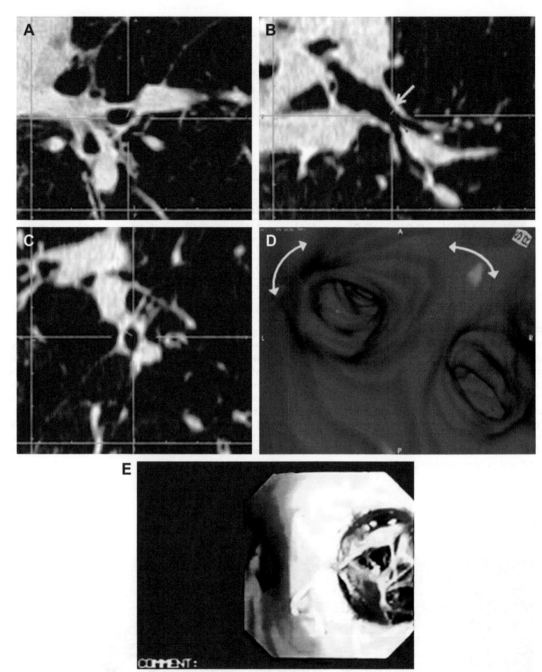

Fig. 12. Airway bypass procedure—drug-eluting airway stents. (*A–D, label from left to right, top to bottom*) Select coned down views of the proximal left lower lobe basilar bronchi in a patient with diffuse emphysema. CT scans are used not only to assess the severity and distribution of emphysema but also to identify blood vessels that need to be avoided during stent placement. With this approach, all lobes except the middle lobe are potential targets for intervention. Drug-eluting airway stents are placed in segmental airways leading to regions with the highest residual volume with the expectation that these will facilitate the escape of trapped air. Virtual bronchoscopic images are also used to further assist in determining optimal stent placement (*lower right image*). (*E*) Endoscopic view showing the appearance of the airway following stent placement. Note that the stent leads directly from a segmental airway to more distal respiratory bronchioles and alveoli.

"damaged" regions of the lung defined by long expiratory times; and (3) instillation of biological adhesives designed to collapse and remodel hyperinflated lung.[64,65,66,67]

For any of these techniques to work, careful delineation of the extent and type and severity of emphysema is essential.[68] Imaging therefore plays a pivotal role in bronchoscopic treatment of emphysema, because it facilitates measurement of the extent and distribution of emphysema as well as identifying concomitant conditions that either require additional evaluation (such as presence of associated severe bronchial disease, concomitant interstitial fibrosis, or potentially malignant lung nodules) that may represent contraindications to routine LVRS. Finally, delineation of airway anatomy relative to adjacent foci of emphysema may aid in the bronchoscopic procedure itself.

Currently, two endobronchial one-way valve systems are currently under evaluation.[64,65,66,67] Both are intended primarily for treatment of heterogeneous upper lobe emphysema again initially identified preferentially using quantitative CT scan data (**Fig. 11**). They are designed to block air from entering the target area during inspiration while allowing gas to exit during expiration with the intention of causing partial or preferably complete lobar collapse resulting in deflation of previously hyperinflated areas of the damaged lung. This allows improved ventilation because of expansion of the less extensively or uninvolved middle and especially lower lobes.

In airway bypass systems,[64,65,66,67] CT images are scored pre-procedure with the extent and severity of emphysema quantified using a variety of software programs currently available in a manner consistent with definitions established in the NETT trial.[62,68] Each lobe of the lung, except the middle lobe, is assessed independently and assigned a grade of 0, 1, 2, 3, or 4 based on the percentage of lung destruction within the lobe. After careful assessment of the pre-procedure CT data and airway anatomy by FB (**Fig. 12**), drug-eluting airway bypass stents are then placed in segmental airways leading to regions with the highest residual volume. This allows escape of excessive trapped gas by the creation of extra-anatomic passages.

SUMMARY

The improvements to patient care that can be achieved by combining advanced imaging techniques and bronchoscopy are considerable. In this regard, CT imaging often plays an indispensable role in both the selection of appropriate candidates for therapy as well as the choice of optimal interventional techniques. However, it is apparent that alternate methods for evaluating the airways and lung including ultrasound and electromagnetic navigation will likely play an increasingly important diagnostic role, necessitating a thorough understanding of their advantages and limitations. Disease-specific applications for which imaging technologies, including CT and VB, are either currently routinely used or show the greatest promise are for suspected or diagnosed lung cancers, central and peripheral, and emphysema. It may be anticipated that with growing experience, the potential for additional indications of these remarkable technologies are likely to increase in the near future.

REFERENCES

1. Chin CS, Litle VR, Yun J, et al. Airway stents. Review. Ann Thorac Surg 2008;85:S792–6.
2. Naidich DP, Gruden JF, McGuinness G, et al. Volumetric (helical/spiral) CT (VCT) of the airways. J Thorac Imaging 1997;12:11–28.
3. Grenier PA, BeigelmanAubry C, Fetita C, et al. Multidetector-row CT of the airways. Semin Roentgenol 2003;38:146–57.
4. Godoy MC, Ost D, Geiger B, et al. Utility of virtual bronchoscopy-guided transbronchial biopsy for the diagnosis of pulmonary sarcoidosis: report of two cases. Chest 2008;134:630–6.
5. Naidich DP, Lee JJ, Garay SM, et al. Comparison of CT and fiberoptic bronchoscopy in the evaluation of bronchial disease. AJR Am J Roentgenol 1987;148:1–7.
6. Vining DJ, Liu K, Choplin RH, et al. Virtual bronchoscopy: relationships of virtual reality endobronchial simulations to actual bronchoscopic findings. Chest 1996;109:549–53.
7. Fleiter T, Merkle EM, Aschoff AJ, et al. Comparison of real-time virtual and fiberoptic bronchoscopy in patients with bronchial carcinoma: opportunities and limitations. Am J Roentgenol 1997;169:1591–5.
8. Finkelstein SE, Schrump DS, Nguyen DM, et al. Comparative evaluation of super high-resolution CT scan and virtual bronchoscopy for the detection of tracheobronchial malignancies. Chest 2003;124:1834–40.
9. Schieppati E. Mediastinal lymph node puncture through tracheal carina. Surg Gynecol Obstet 1958;10(7):243–6.
10. Wang KP, Brower R, Haponik EF, et al. Flexible transbronchial needle aspiration for staging of bronchogenic carcinoma. Chest 1983;84:571–6.
11. Harkin TJ, Wang KP. Bronchoscopic needle aspiration of mediastinal and hilar lymph nodes. J Bronchology 1997;4:238–49.

12. Wang KP. Staging of bronchogenic carcinoma by bronchoscopy. Chest 1994;106:588–93.

13. Harrow EM, Abi-Saleh W, Blum J, et al. The utility of transbronchial needle aspiration in the staging of bronchogenic carcinoma. Am J Respir Crit Care Med 2000;161:601–7.

14. Detterbeck F, Janakiev D, Wallace M, et al. Invasive mediastinal staging of lung cancer: ACCP evidence-based clinical practice guidelines. (2nd edition). Chest 2007;132:202S–20S.

15. Silvestri GA, Gould MK, Margolis M, et al. Noninvasive staging of non-small cell lung cancer: ACCP evidence-based clinical practice guidelines. (2nd edition). Chest 2007;132:S178–201.

16. Mountain CF, Dresler CM. Regional lymph node classification for lung cancer staging. Chest 1997; 111:1718–23.

17. Morales CF, Patefield AJ, Strollo PJ, et al. Flexible transbronchial needle aspiration in the diagnosis of sarcoidosis. Chest 1994;106:709–11.

18. Harkin TJ, Ciotoli C, Addrizzo-Harris DJ, et al. Transbronchial needle aspiration (TBNA) in patients infected with HIV. Am J Respir Crit Care Med 1998; 157:1913–8.

19. Rong F, Cui B. CT scan directed transbronchial needle aspiration biopsy for mediastinal nodes. Chest 1998;114:36–9.

20. Garpestad E, Goldberg SN, Herth F, et al. CT fluoroscopy guidance for transbronchial needle aspiration an experience in 35 patients. Chest 2001;119: 329–32.

21. Goldberg SN, Raptopoulos V, Boiselle PM, et al. Mediastinal lymphadenopathy: diagnostic yield of transbronchial meidastinal lymph node biopsy with CT fluoroscopic guidance. Initial experience. Chest 2000;216:764–7.

22. White CS, Templeton PA, Hasday JD, et al. CT-assisted transbronchial needle aspiration: usefulness of CT fluoroscopy. AJR Am J Roentgenol 1997;169: 393–4.

23. White CS, Weiner EA, Patel P, et al. Transbronchial needle aspiration—guidance with CT fluoroscopy. Chest 2000;118:1630–8.

24. Ost D, Shah R, Anasco E, et al. A randomized trial of CT fluoroscopic-guided bronchoscopy vs conventional bronchoscopy in patients with suspected lung cancer. Chest 2008;135:507–13.

25. McAdams HP, Goodman PC, Kussin P, et al. Virtual bronchoscopy for directing transbronchial needle aspiration of hilar and mediastinal lymph nodes: a pilot study. AJR Am J Roentgenol 1998;170:1361–4.

26. Yasufuku K, Chiyo M, Koh E, et al. Endobronchial ultrasound guided transbronchial needle aspiration for staging of lung cancer. Lung Cancer 2005;50: 347–54.

27. Eloubeidi MA. Endoscopic ultrasound-guided fine-needle aspiration in the staging and diagnosis of patients with lung cancer. Semin Thorac Cardiovasc Surg 2007;19:206–11.

28. Eloubeidi MA, Cerfolio RJ, Chen VK, et al. Endoscopic ultrasound-guided fine needle aspiration of mediastinal lymph node in patients with suspected lung cancer after positron emission tomography and computed tomography scans. Ann Thorac Surg 2005;79:263–8.

29. Herth F, Beck R, Ernst A, et al. Conventional vs endobronchial ultrasound-guided transbronchial needle aspiration: a randomized trial. Chest 2004;125: 322–5.

30. Herth FJF, Eberhardt R, Becker HD, et al. Endobronchial ultrasound-guided transbronchial lung biopsy in fluoroscopically invisible solitary pulmonary nodules. A prospective trial. Chest 2006;129:147–50.

31. Yasufuku K, Nakajima T, Motoori K, et al. Comparison of endobronchial ultrasound, positron emission tomography, and CT for lymph node staging of lung cancer. Chest 2006;130:710–8.

32. Cerfolio RJ, Bryant AS, Eloubeidi MA, et al. Routine mediastinoscopy and esophageal ultrasound fine-needle aspiration in patients with non-small cell lung cancer who are clinically N2 negative: a prospective study. Chest 2006;130:1791–5.

33. Beamis JF. Interventional pulmonology techniques for treating malignant large airway obstruction: an update. Curr Opin Pulm Med 2005;11:292–5.

34. Asimakopoulos G, Beeson J, Evans J, et al. Cryosurgery for malignant endobronchial tumors: analysis of outcome. Chest 2005;127:2007–14.

35. Chan AL, Yoneda KY, Allen RP, et al. Advances in the management of endobronchial lung malignancies. Curr Opin Pulm Med 2003;9:301–8.

36. Wood DE, Liu YH, Vallieres E, et al. Airway stenting for malignant and benign tracheobronchial stenosis. Ann Thorac Surg 2003;76:167–72.

37. Lee P, Kupeli E, Mehta AC, et al. Therapeutic bronchoscopy in lung cancer—laser therapy, electrocautery, brachytherapy stents, and photodynamic therapy. Clin Chest Med 2002;23:241.

38. Boiselle PM, Ernst A. State-of-the-art imaging of the central airways. Respiration 2003;70:383–94.

39. Lee KS, Lunn W, Feller-Kopman D, et al. Multislice CT evaluation of airway stents. J Thorac Imaging 2005;20:81–8.

40. Boiselle PM, FellerKopman D, Ashiku S, et al. Tracheobronchomalacia: evolving role of dynamic multislice helical CT. Radiol Clin North Am 2003; 41:627.

41. Gluecker T, Lang F, Bessler S, et al. 2D and 3D CT imaging correlated to rigid endoscopy in complex laryngo-tracheal stenosis. Eur Radiol 2001;11:50–4.

42. Dialani V, Ernst A, Sun M, et al. MDCT detection of airway stent complications: comparison with bronchoscopy. AJR 2008;191:1576–80.

43. Ferretti GR, Kocier M, Calaque O, et al. Follow-up after stent insertion in the tracheobronchial tree: role of helical computed tomography in comparison with fiberoptic bronchoscopy. Eur Radiol 2003;13:1172–8.

44. Schreiber G, McCrory DC. Performance characteristics of different modalities for diagnosis of suspected lung cancer—summary of published evidence. Chest 2003;123:115S–28S.

45. Gaeta M, Pandolfo I, Volta S, et al. Bronchus sign on CT in peripheral carcinoma of the lung: value in predicting results of transbronchial biopsy. AJR Am J Roentgenol 1991;157:1181–5.

46. Naidich DP, Sussman R, Kutcher WL, et al. Solitary pulmonary nodules: CT-bronchoscopic correlation. Chest 1988;93:595–8.

47. Goldberg SN, Raptopoulos V, Boiselle PM, et al. Mediastinal lymph node biopsy: diagnostic yield of transbronchial mediastinal lymph node biopsy with CT fluoroscopic guidance—initial experience. Radiology 2000;216:764–7.

48. Asano F, Matsuno Y, Shinagawa N, et al. A virtual bronchoscopic navigation system for pulmonary peripheral lesions. Chest 2006;130:559–66.

49. Merritt SA, Gibbs JD, Yu K, et al. Image-guided bronchoscopy for peripheral lung lesions: a phantom study. Chest 2008; 134:1017–26.

50. Shinagawa N, Yamazaki K, Onodera Y, et al. CT-guided transbronchial biopsy using an ultrathin bronchoscope with virtual bronchoscopic navigation. Chest 2004;125:1138–43.

51. Asahina H, Yamazaki K, Onodera Y, et al. Transbronchial biopsy using endobronchial ultrasonography with a guide sheath and virtual bronchoscopic navigation. Chest 2005;128:1761–4.

52. Sheski FD, Mathur PN. Endobronchial ultrasound. Chest 2008;133:264–70.

53. Paone G, Nicastri E, Lucantoni G, et al. Endobronchial ultrasound-driven biopsy in the diagnosis of peripheral lung lesions. Chest 2005;128:3551–7.

54. Schwarz Y, Grief J, Becker HD, et al. Real-time electromagnetic navigation bronchoscopy to peripheral lung lesions using overlaid CT images: the first human study. Chest 2006;129:988–94.

55. Schwarz Y, Mehta AC, Ernst A, et al. Electromagnetic navigation during flexible bronchoscopy. Respiration 2003;70:516–22.

56. Becker H, Herth F, Ernst A, et al. Bronchoscopic biopsy of peripheral lung lesion under electromagnetic guidance: a pilot study. J Bronchology 2005; 12:9–13.

57. Eberhardt R, Anantham D, Herth F, et al. Electromagnetic navigation diagnostic bronchoscopy in peripheral lung lesions. Chest 2007;131:1800–5.

58. Gildea T, Mazzone P, Karnak D, et al. Electromagnetic navigation diagnostic bronchoscopy: a prospective study. Am J Respir Crit Care Med 2006;174:9982–9.

59. Makris D, Scherpereel A, Lerory S, et al. Electromagnetic navigation diagnostic bronchoscopy for small peripheral lung lesions. Eur Respir J 2007; 29:1187–92.

60. Eberhardt R, Anantham D, Ernst A, et al. Multimodality bronchoscopic diagnosis of peripheral lung lesions. Am J Respir Crit Care Med 2007;176:36–41.

61. McLemore TL, Bedekar AR. Accurate diagnosis of peripheral lung lesions in a private community hospital employing electromagnetic guidance bronchoscopy (EMB) coupled with radial endobronchial ultrasound (REBUS). Chest 2007;132:452S.

62. Fishman A, Maartinez F, Naunheim K, et al. National Emphysema Treatment Trial research group. A randomized trial comparing lung-volume reduction surgery with medical therapy for severe emphysema. N Engl J Med 2003;348:2059–73.

63. Group. NETTR. Patients at high risk of death after lung-volume reduction surgery. N Engl J Med 2001;345:1075–83.

64. Brenner M, Hanna NM, Mina-Araghi R, et al. Innovative approaches to lung volume reduction for emphysema. Chest 2004;126:238–48.

65. Ingenito EP, Wood DE, Utz JP, et al. Bronchoscopic lung volume reduction in severe emphysema. Proc Am Thorac Soc 2008;5:454–60.

66. Sahi H, Karnak D, Meli YM, et al. Bronchoscopic approach to COPD. A review. COPD 2008;5: 125–31.

67. Wood DE, McKenna RJ Jr, Yusen RD, et al. A multicenter trial of an intrabronchial valve for treatment of emphysema. J Thorac Cardiovasc Surg 2007;133: 65–73.

68. Washko GR, Hoffman EA, Reilly JJ, et al. Radiographic evaluation of the potential lung volume reduction surgery candidate. Proc Am Thorac Soc 2008;5:421–6.

Volumetric Expiratory HRCT of the Lung: Clinical Applications

Mizuki Nishino, MD[a],*, George R. Washko, MD[b,c],
Hiroto Hatabu, MD, PhD[d,e]

KEYWORDS

- Computed tomography (CT) • Lung • High-resolution CT
- Expiratory high-resolution CT • Volumetric

Expiratory high-resolution CT scan (HRCT) of the chest offers a powerful adjunct to inspiratory HRCT in the detection of lung diseases involving the small airways by reflecting the interplay of air in the alveoli, the pulmonary interstitium, and pulmonary blood volume.[1–5] The hallmark of expiratory airflow obstruction has been the radiographic finding of air trapping where lung regions with a lesser degree of increase in expiratory attenuation than normal are thought to be indicative of retained gas in the secondary pulmonary lobule.[1,3] This process can be found in a variety of lung diseases with obstructive physiology, including asthma, bronchiectasis, and emphysema.

A major limitation to acquiring expiratory CT scans on all patients is the associated radiation exposure. Because of this, in 2003, two of the authors (Nishino and Hatabu) and their colleagues[6,7] developed a clinical volumetric expiratory HRCT protocol with the decreased tube current that provides volumetric data sets of the entire thorax at end-inspiration and at end-expiration without increasing radiation dose and examination time. These volumetric data sets of expiratory HRCT images allow for full visualization of the airway and lung parenchyma, with the added value of the three-dimensional and multiplanar capability (**Fig. 1**).[6,7] Volumetric expiratory HRCT has since been used for evaluation of diffuse lung disease with suspected airway abnormalities. More recently, the Chronic Obstructive Pulmonary Disease Gene (COPDGene) Study, a multicenter investigation of the genetic epidemiology of subjects with chronic obstructive pulmonary disease (COPD) supported by National Institute of Health, adopted volumetric inspiratory and expiratory HRCT for its protocol.

COPD

COPD is defined as incompletely reversible expiratory airflow obstruction.[8] It is typically related to tobacco smoke exposure and is the result of remodeling of the small airways with obliteration of their lumen and loss of lung elastic recoil due to emphysematous destruction of the parenchyma.[9] Standard objective measures of both of these processes, airway disease and emphysema have been well established using inspiratory CT scanning.[10] Less well recognized are the potential contributions that expiratory CT scanning can be made to further understanding of these processes

This article originally appeared in *Radiologic Clinics of North America*, Volume 48, Issue 1, January 2010.

[a] Department of Radiology, Dana-Farber Cancer Institute, Harvard Medical School, 44 Binney Street, Boston, MA 02215, USA

[b] Division of Pulmonary and Critical Care Medicine, Brigham and Women's Hospital, 75 Francis Street, Boston, MA 02215, USA

[c] Harvard Medical School, Boston, MA, USA

[d] MRI Program, Center for Pulmonary Functional Imaging, Brigham and Women's Hospital, 75 Francis Street, Boston, MA 02215, USA

[e] Department of Radiology, Center for Pulmonary Functional Imaging, Brigham and Women's Hospital, Harvard Medical School, 75 Francis Street, Boston, MA 02215, USA

* Corresponding author.

E-mail address: Mizuki_Nishino@dfci.harvard.edu (M. Nishino).

Thorac Surg Clin 20 (2010) 121–127
doi:10.1016/j.thorsurg.2009.12.009
1547-4127/10/$ – see front matter

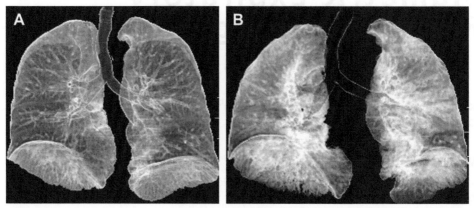

Fig. 1. A 70-year-old woman with a history of bronchial asthma. (*A, B*) The reconstructed images with volume rendering of the posterior two-thirds of the lungs at end-inspiration and end-expiration using an ADW workstation. Volume and attenuation changes after expiration are visually displayed in a 3-dimensional fashion, providing easy recognition of air trapping. There are marked changes in the configuration of the airway conducting to the areas of air trapping. (*From* Nishino M, Boiselle PM, Copeland JF, et al. Value of volumetric data acquisition in expiratory high-resolution CT of the lung. J Comput Assist Tomogr 2004;28:209–14; with permission.) ADW, Advanced Development Workstation.

using quantitative measures of gas trapping and CT attenuation gravitational gradients.

Densitometric assessments of the lung parenchyma have been accepted methods for quantitatively examining CT scan burdens of emphysema since the 1980s.[10] These methods have been benchmarked against histopathologic examination and have been integral to most CT scan-based epidemiologic studies of subjects with COPD.[10–13] With the advent of volumetric expiratory CT scan imaging protocols came the recognition that similar densitometric methods can be applied to these images. Recently, Akira and colleagues[14] found that such objective analysis of the expiratory images of subjects with COPD may offer stronger correlates to lung function than inspiratory scans in subjects with severe disease. Additional studies in larger cohorts will likely support such observations and further argue for the phenotypic information available in expiratory CT scans.

It has been known that CT demonstrates an attenuation gradient in the normal lung, with the greatest density in dependent lung regions and the least density in nondependent lung regions. In 1993, Webb and colleagues[2] reported that the anteroposterior attenuation gradient is discontinuous at the major fissure, and that the posterior aspect of the upper lobe has greater attenuation than the anterior aspect of the lower lobe. It was also noted that the anteroposterior intralobar attenuation gradient was accentuated during expiration. Departure from these gradients could imply local abnormalities in lung compliance, distribution

of mechanical stress, or distensibility of vessels.[2,15] However, the significance of the loss of this intralobar attenuation gradient has not been determined in detail.

The authors investigated 21 consecutive patients with emphysema studied with volumetric expiratory HRCT, and 6 patients with normal HRCT. The anterior-posterior intralobar attenuation gradients were quantified on end-inspiratory and end-expiratory sagittal reformations using a lung analysis software program.[16] The quantitative values of the intralobar attenuation gradients were correlated with pulmonary function test results (**Figs. 2** and **3**). The intralobar attenuation gradients in the patients with forced expiratory volume in 1 second (FEV_1), by percent, of less than 70% were significantly smaller compared with those in patients with FEV_1(%) greater than 70% in right lower lobe at end-inspiration, and right and left lower lobes at end-expiration. There was a significant positive correlation between the intralobar attenuation gradient and pulmonary function test results in bilateral lower lobes, when the cutoff values of 70% for FEV_1(%) and 0.002 for attenuation gradient were used. The intralobar attenuation gradients in bilateral lower lobes at end-expiration were significantly correlated with FEV_1 and FEV_1 per forced vital capacity (FVC). These results indicated that the quantitatively measured intralobar attenuation gradients correlate with obstructive changes on pulmonary function tests in patients with emphysema, especially at end-expiration in the lower lobes, suggesting a potential utility of

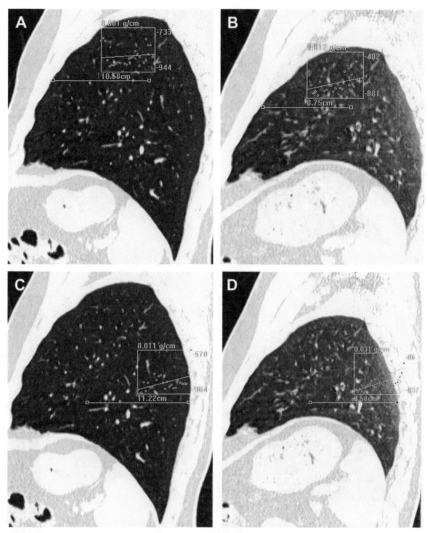

Fig. 2. A 38-year-old man presenting with cough and wheezing, with normal pulmonary function test results of FEV_1 (% predicted): 84, FVC (% predicted): 84, FEV_1/FVC (% predicted): 100. Quantitative measurement of the intralobar anteroposterior attenuation gradient in the left upper lobe shows attenuation gradient of 0.001 g/cm at (*A*) end-inspiration, which increased to 0.012 g/cm at (*B*) end-expiration, demonstrating the presence of normal attenuation gradient accentuated at end-expiration. Quantitative measurement of the intralobar anteroposterior attenuation gradient in the left lower lobe shows attenuation gradient of 0.011 g/cm at (*C*) end-inspiration, which increased to 0.031 g/cm at (*D*) end-expiration, also demonstrating the presence of normal attenuation gradient accentuated at end-expiration. (*From* Nishino M, Roberts DH, Sitek A, et al. Loss of anteroposterior intralobar attenuation gradient of the lung: correlation with pulmonary function. Acad Radiol 2006;13(5):589–97; with permission.)

these gradients as a functional indicator of emphysema.[16]

BRONCHIECTASIS

Bronchiectasis is an airway disease associated with chronic progressive inflammatory changes of the bronchial wall, which leads to irreversible abnormal bronchial dilatation and airflow obstruction.[17,18] The pathophysiologic mechanism is generally considered as multifactorial. Air trapping is often seen in patients with bronchiectasis on expiratory CT scan, and is considered one of the major determinants of airflow obstruction in bronchiectasis.[19,20] In addition to bronchial dilatation, the chronic airway inflammation in bronchiectasis may cause bronchial wall weakness and loss of dynamic integrity, resulting in excessive collapsibility of the airway, namely bronchomalacia. In mid 1960s, Fraser and colleagues[21] reported the prominent collapse of the large airways on expiration in bronchiectasis based on the evaluation

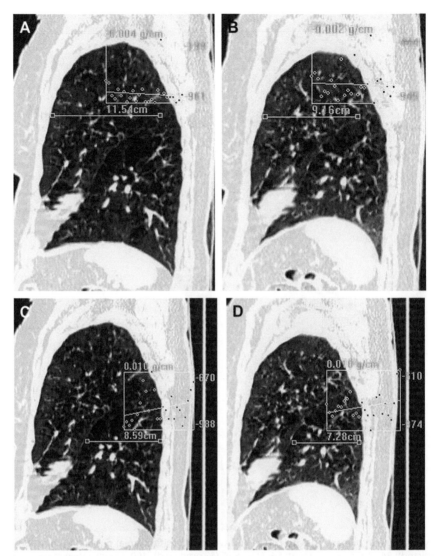

Fig. 3. A 70-year-old woman with emphysema, with obstructive changes on pulmonary function test; FEV_1 (% predicted): 35, FVC (% predicted): 78, FEV_1/FVC (% predicted): 45. Quantitative measurement of the intralobar anteroposterior attenuation gradient in the left upper lobe shows attenuation gradient of −0.004 g/cm at (*A*) end-inspiration, and −0.002 g/cm at (*B*) end-expiration, demonstrating loss of intralobar attenuation gradient on both images. Quantitative measurement of the intralobar anteroposterior attenuation gradient in the left lower lobe shows attenuation gradient of 0.010 g/cm both at (*C*) end-inspiration, and at (*D*) end-expiration, demonstrating loss of normal attenuation gradient. (*From* Nishino M, Roberts DH, Sitek A, et al. Loss of anteroposterior intralobar attenuation gradient of the lung: correlation with pulmonary function. Acad Radiol 2006;13(5):589–97; with permission.)

using cinefluorography evaluation. However, the frequency and severity of bronchomalacia in association with the resultant air trapping remained to be determined in patients with bronchiectasis. The authors studied 46 patients with bronchiectasis evaluated by volumetric expiratory high-resolution CT scan and pulmonary function tests to evaluate the frequency and severity of bronchomalacia in bronchiectasis, to compare the extent

of air trapping in bronchiectasis patients with or without bronchomalacia, and to correlate the severity of bronchomalacia and the extent of air trapping versus pulmonary function. Of 46 patients with bronchiectasis, 32 patients (70%) were noted to have bronchomalacia. Air trapping was observed in 43 patients (93%). The extent of air trapping in patients with bronchomalacia was significantly greater compared with the patients

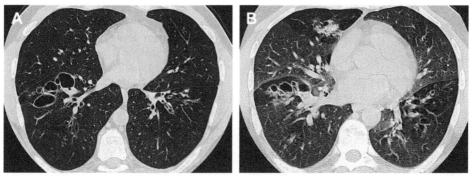

Fig. 4. A 47-year-old woman with bronchiectasis. Pair of (*A*) end-inspiratory and (*B*) end-expiratory scans obtained at the level of inferior pulmonary veins show cystic bronchiectasis in right lower lobe and (*A*) cylindrical bronchiectasis in lower lobes at end-inspiration, which demonstrate excessive collapsibility at end-expiration, indicating bronchomalacia (grade 2). (*B*) Note multiple radiolucent areas compared with adjacent lung at end-expiration in the bilateral lower lobes, indicating air trapping (grade 3). (*From* Nishino M, Siewert B, Roberts DH, et al. Excessive collapsibility of bronchi in bronchiectasis: evaluation on volumetric expiratory high-resolution CT. J Comput Assist Tomogr 2006;30(3):474–8; with permission.)

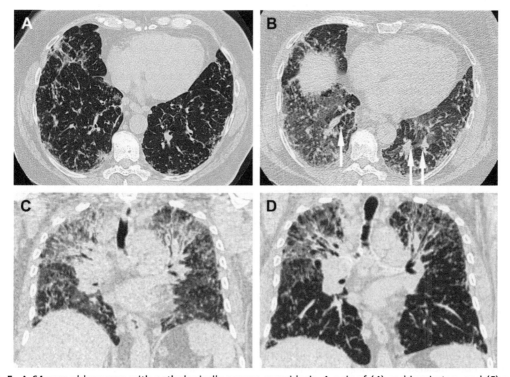

Fig. 5. A 64-year-old woman with pathologically proven sarcoidosis. A pair of (*A*) end-inspiratory and (*B*) end-expiratory scans obtained at the lung base showing nodular thickening of the interlobular septum and fissures. At end-expiration, multiple areas of air trapping in both lower lobes are noted. (*B*) The segmental and subsegmental bronchi conducting to the areas of air trapping are severely collapsed, indicating bronchomalacia (*arrows*). Reformatted coronal images on (*C*) end-inspiration and (*D*) end-expiration at the level of the carina showing marked peribronchovascular interstitial thickening, ground-glass opacities, and small nodules, predominantly in the upper lobes. (*D*) Note the severely narrowed bronchi at end-expiration. (*From* Nishino M, Kuroki M, Roberts DH, et al. Bronchomalacia in sarcoidosis: evaluation on volumetric expiratory high-resolution CT of the lung. Acad Radiol 2005;12(5):596–601; with permission.)

without bronchomalacia ($P = .0308$, chi-squared test) **(Fig. 4)**.[22]

SARCOIDOSIS

Sarcoidosis is a multisystemic disease of unknown cause characterized by the presence of noncaseating granulomatous inflammation that may involve all parts of the lung, including the airways. Characteristic HRCT findings of pulmonary sarcoidosis include nodular thickening of bronchovascular bundles, small nodules, and ground-glass opacities.[23] The presence of air trapping on expiratory CT scan in sarcoidosis was described by Gleeson and colleagues[24] in 1996. Since then, air trapping on expiratory CT scan is considered as evidence of small-airway obstruction and has been reported in sarcoidosis in association with incomplete lung emptying at end-expiration.[25–27]

In the authors' preliminary review of cases of sarcoidosis evaluated with volumetric expiratory HRCT, bronchomalacia was unexpectedly but frequently observed on the end-expiratory images. The authors examined the CT scans of 18 subjects with pathologically proven sarcoidosis who underwent clinical volumetric expiratory high-resolution computed tomography. Bronchomalacia was noted in 11 of 18 patients (61%) with sarcoidosis (mild, n = 6; moderate, n = 4; and severe, n = 1). Air trapping was observed in 17 of 18 patients (94%; grade 1 [1%–25%], n = 8; grade 2 [26%–50%], n = 9) **(Fig. 5)**. The extent of air trapping in patients with bronchomalacia was significantly greater than that in patients without bronchomalacia ($P = .027$, chi-squared test).[28] Given the propensity of sarcoidosis to involve the central and peripheral airways, sarcoidosis may cause increased airway collapsibility resulting in bronchomalacia. These results demonstrated that bronchomalacia may be frequently associated with sarcoidosis. Further investigation is required to determine the clinical sequela of bronchomalacia in this population.

SUMMARY AND FUTURE DIRECTIONS

Volumetric HRCT is useful in the evaluation of a variety of diffuse lung diseases with suspected airway abnormalities, including emphysema, bronchiectasis, and sarcoidosis. It also provides volumetric assessment of the entire thorax at end-inspiration and at end-expiration and allowing for detailed analysis of the airway and parenchyma. Obviously, this field of volumetric expiratory HRCT is work-in-progress. While the HRCT provides a static view of lung morphology, volumetric expiratory HRCT provides complementary dynamic and functional information of the pulmonary airway and parenchyma. Without question, quantified data analysis of volumetric expiratory HRCT is crucial for further use and application of volumetric expiratory HRCT. Standardization of image acquisition and postprocessing in CT examinations will be necessary for the real application of such quantified data derived from volumetric expiratory HRCT to daily clinical medical practice.[29] The authors are confident that more advanced works in this field will be published, and this technique will come into practice in the next 3 to 5 years.

REFERENCES

1. Stern EJ, Webb WR, Warnock ML, et al. Bronchopulmonary sequestration: dynamic, ultrafast, high-resolution CT evidence of air trapping. AJR Am J Roentgenol 1991;157:947–9.
2. Webb WR, Stern EJ, Kanth N, et al. Dynamic pulmonary CT: findings in healthy adult men. Radiology 1993;186:117–24.
3. Stern EJ, Webb WR, Gamsu G. Dynamic quantitative computed tomography. A predictor of pulmonary function in obstructive lung diseases. Invest Radiol 1994;29:564–9.
4. Arakawa H, Webb WR. Air trapping on expiratory high-resolution CT scans in the absence of inspiratory scan abnormalities: correlation with pulmonary function tests and differential diagnosis. AJR Am J Roentgenol 1998;170:1349–53.
5. Arakawa H, Webb WR, McCowin M, et al. Inhomogeneous lung attenuation at thin-section CT: diagnostic value of expiratory scans. Radiology 1998; 206:89–94.
6. Nishino M, Hatabu H. Volumetric expiratory high-resolution CT of the lung. Eur J Radiol 2004;52:180–4.
7. Nishino M, Boiselle PM, Copeland JF, et al. Value of volumetric data acquisition in expiratory high-resolution CT of the lung. J Comput Assist Tomogr 2004; 28:209–14.
8. Pauwels RA, Buist AS, Calverley PM, et al. GOLD Scientific Committee. Global strategy for the diagnosis, management, and prevention of chronic obstructive pulmonary disease. NHLBI/WHO Global Initiative for Chronic Obstructive Lung Disease (GOLD) Workshop summary. Am J Respir Crit Care Med 2001;163:1256–76.
9. Hogg JC, Macklem PT, Thurlbeck WM. Site and nature of airway obstruction in chronic obstructive lung disease. N Engl J Med 1968;278:1355–60.
10. Müller NL, Staples CA, Miller RR, et al. "Density mask". An objective method to quantitate emphysema using computed tomography. Chest 1988;94:782–7.
11. Gevenois PA, de Maertelaer V, De Vuyst P, et al. Comparison of computed density and macroscopic

morphometry in pulmonary emphysema. Am J Respir Crit Care Med 1995;152:653–7.

12. Gevenois PA, De Vuyst P, de Maertelaer V, et al. Comparison of computed density and microscopic morphometry in pulmonary emphysema. Am J Respir Crit Care Med 1996;154:187–92.

13. Patel BD, Coxson HO, Pillai SG, et al. Airway wall thickening and emphysema show independent familial aggregation in chronic obstructive pulmonary disease. Am J Respir Crit Care Med 2008; 178:500–5.

14. Akira M, Toyokawa K, Inoue Y, et al. Quantitative CT in chronic obstructive pulmonary disease: inspiratory and expiratory assessment. AJR Am J Roentgenol 2009;192:267–72.

15. Millar AB, Denison DM. Vertical gradients of lung density in supine subjects with fibrosing alveolitis or pulmonary emphysema. Thorax 1990;45:602–5.

16. Nishino M, Roberts DH, Sitek A, et al. Loss of anteroposterior intralobar attenuation gradient of the lung: correlation with pulmonary function. Acad Radiol 2006;13(5):589–97.

17. Reid LM. Reduction in bronchial subdivision in bronchiectasis. Thorax 1950;5:233–47.

18. Ip M, Lauder IJ, Wong WY, et al. Multivariate analysis of factors affecting pulmonary function in bronchiectasis. Respiration 1993;60:45–50.

19. Roberts HR, Wells AU, Milne DG, et al. Airways obstruction in bronchiectasis: correlation between computed tomography features and pulmonary function tests. Thorax 2000;55:198–204.

20. Hansell DM, Wells AU, Rubens MB, et al. Bronchiectasis: functional significanceof areas of decreased attenuation at expiratory CT. Radiology 1994;193: 369–74.

21. Fraser RG, Macklem PT, Brown WG. Airway dynamics in bronchiectasis: a combined cinefluorographic-manometric study. AJR Am J Roentgenol 1965;93:821–35.

22. Nishino M, Siewert B, Roberts DH, et al. Excessive collapsibility of bronchi in bronchiectasis: evaluation on volumetric expiratory high-resolution CT. J Comput Assist Tomogr 2006;30(3):474–8.

23. Muller NL, Kullnig P, Miller RR. The CT findings of pulmonary sarcoidosis: analysis of 25 patients. AJR Am J Roentgenol 1989;152:1179–82.

24. Gleeson FV, Traill ZC, Hansell DM. Evidence of expiratory CT scans of small-airway obstruction in sarcoidosis. AJR Am J Roentgenol 1996;166: 1052–4.

25. Hansell DM, Milne DG, Wilsher ML, et al. Pulmonary sarcoidosis: morphologic associations of airflow obstruction at thin-section CT. Radiology 1998;209: 697–704.

26. Davies CW, Tasker AD, Padley SP, et al. Air trapping in sarcoidosis on computed tomography: correlation with lung function. Clin Radiol 2000;55:217–21.

27. Magkanas E, Voloudaki A, Bouros D, et al. Pulmonary sarcoidosis. Correlation of expiratory high-resolution CT findings with inspiratory patterns and pulmonary function tests. Acta Radiol 2001;42: 494–501.

28. Nishino M, Kuroki M, Roberts DH, et al. Bronchomalacia in sarcoidosis: evaluation on volumetric expiratory high-resolution CT of the lung. Acad Radiol 2005;12(5):596–601.

29. Hatabu H. Are we ready? A time for measurement of physiological parameters of the lung using multidetector row CT scans. Acad Radiol 2009;16: 249.

Acute Pulmonary Embolism

Jean Kuriakose, MBBS, MRCP, FRCR[a],
Smita Patel, MBBS, MRCP, FRCR[b],*

KEYWORDS

- CT pulmonary angiography • Pulmonary embolism
- CT venography • Radiation exposure

Imaging plays a crucial role in the diagnosis of pulmonary embolism (PE) and deep venous thrombosis (DVT), a spectrum of the same disease entity. PE is the third most common cause of cardiovascular death in the United States, following ischemic heart disease and stroke, with an annual incidence of 300,000 to 600,000 per year.[1,2] Despite the high prevalence, PE is difficult to diagnose, with only 43 to 53 patients per 100,000 being accurately diagnosed, and up to 70% of clinically unsuspected PE diagnosed at autopsy.[1,3] In the past few decades, the incidence of PE has decreased by 45%, whereas that of DVT is unchanged.[4,5] Death occurs in up to 90% of patients with unrecognized PE, whereas in treated patients PE accounts for less than 10% of deaths.[6,7]

Rapid and timely diagnosis of this life-threatening disease is important to improve patient outcome as the signs and symptoms as well as ancillary tests are nonspecific. The recent rapid growth in CT technology over the past decade has seen the emergence of CT pulmonary angiography (CTPA) as the single first line test in the diagnosis of PE because of its high diagnostic accuracy and ability to provide alternate diagnosis for diseases of the lung parenchyma, pleura, pericardium, aorta, heart, thoracic lymph nodes, and mediastinum.

The widespread availability and use of CTPA has made the diagnosis of PE easier in most cases, but has raised the need for optimal use of this technique in the appropriate patient population, in order to minimize unnecessary medical radiation exposure.

Pretest risk stratification using Wells criteria, clinical probability scores, assessing premorbid conditions, past history, and a thorough clinical examination should precede an appropriate, timely, and accurate diagnostic test.[8,9] In some common scenarios like pregnancy and in critically ill patients, the diagnosis of PE still remains challenging.

DIAGNOSIS OF ACUTE PULMONARY EMBOLISM
Ventilation-Perfusion Scintigraphy

Combined ventilation and perfusion (V/Q) scintigraphy had been the imaging technique of choice for decades. A V/Q scan with normal findings essentially excludes pulmonary embolism with an NPV (Negative Predictive Value) close to 100%, thereby precluding the use of anticoagulation, whereas a high-probability scan is highly specific for the diagnosis of PE, allowing definitive treatment. In the original PIOPED (Prospective Investigation of Pulmonary Embolism Diagnosis) study only 14% of patients had a normal V/Q scan and 13% a high-probability V/Q scan, rendering a definitive diagnosis in only a small group of patients; most (73%) had an indeterminate (nondiagnostic) or low-probability test result.[10] This high degree of uncertainty makes initiation of definitive anticoagulant therapy difficult because

This article originally appeared in *Radiologic Clinics of North America*, Volume 48, Issue 1, January 2010.
a Division of Cardiothoracic Radiology, Department of Radiology, University of Michigan Health System, 1500 East Medical Center Driver, Ann Arbor, MI, USA
b Department of Radiology, University of Michigan Health System, Cardiovascular Center - Room 5338, 1500 East Medical Center Drive, Ann Arbor, MI 48109-5868, USA
* Corresponding author.
E-mail address: smitap@med.umich.edu (S. Patel).

thoracic.theclinics.com

of risk of bleeding and necessitates additional tests to diagnose or exclude pulmonary embolism.

The criteria for reporting V/Q scans have improved significantly.[11] Recent use of V/Q scanning with SPECT allows 3-dimensional visualization of segments previously not identified on planar imaging, such as the medial basal segment of the right lower lobe. The lung segments are more clearly defined and can be viewed in any orthogonal plane, resulting in better detection and characterization of defects.[12] SPECT also improves image contrast, thus decreasing the rate of intermediate scan reports. Large-scale trials are needed to fully assess this modality and compare its performance with CTPA. Currently the definitive primary role of V/Q scanning is in patients where CTPA is contraindicated as in severe renal impairment or history of iodine or contrast allergy.

Catheter Pulmonary Angiography

Catheter pulmonary angiography has been considered as the reference test for the diagnosis of PE since the late 1960s. However, the invasive nature and expense of the study along with a small but definite risk in morbidity has contributed to its underutilization. Two studies, done 12 years apart in 1240 patients, showed that following an inconclusive V/Q scan result, catheter pulmonary angiography was performed in less than 15% of patients.[13,14] Many patients were treated with anticoagulants without a definitive result. Accurate diagnosis is important, as anticoagulants themselves account for significant morbidity (up to 6.5%), that increases with age and with comorbid conditions.[15,16]

With the newer generation of MDCT (multidetector CT) scanners, the role of catheter pulmonary angiography as the gold standard test has been questioned and is considered to be flawed, particularly at the subsegmental level.[17–19] The interobserver agreement at the subsegmental level on the original PIOPED study was reported to be only 66%.[10] In PIOPED II, in the 20 discordant cases, PE was missed at the lobar, segmental, and subsegmental levels in 13 patients; 8 of 13 were at the subsegmental level.[19] The current role of catheter pulmonary angiography is when CTPA is inconclusive, or when the clinical findings are discordant with CTPA results.

CT Pulmonary Angiography

Incidental detection of PE was first documented by Sinner in 1978.[20] The advent of single-detector helical CT in the early 1990s, made it possible to obtain volumetric datasets with good contrast in a single breath-hold, allowing diagnosis predominantly of central and segmental PE. With rapid evolvement of CT technology, the CT diagnosis of PE has been a subject of much research in the past couple of decades, and has resulted in CTPA becoming a first-line imaging test at many centers.[21] CTPA is a relatively safe, accurate, readily available and cost-effective noninvasive test that not only diagnoses PE, but also provides diagnosis of alternative pathologies in the thorax accounting for patient symptoms, particularly in the inpatient and emergency department settings.

Faster multidetector scanners have set the way for a potential new gold standard test. With newer 128 and higher slice scanners, the sensitivity and specificity is likely to increase albeit at a cost of increased radiation.

Advances in MDCT

MDCT has several advantages over SDCT (single detector CT) in the diagnosis of PE, which include improved z-axis resolution, shorter scan times, reduction in volume of contrast, and the ability to do a combined CTPA/CT venography (CTV) exam at the same setting with a single bolus of contrast.

Z-Axis Resolution

Advances in MDCT technology with improved gantry rotation speeds and increased detector width allow rapid acquisition of large volumetric datasets over a greater craniocaudal distance than with SDCT. While reduction in slice collimation with SDCT results in a longer breath hold and a likelihood of increased respiratory motion artifact, with MDCT reduction in slice thickness leads to better visualization of subsegmental pulmonary arteries, with 94% of fifth order and 74% of sixth order pulmonary arteries being visualized.[22–24] Reducing the reconstruction thickness decreases partial volume averaging and also results in better visualization of the obliquely oriented middle lobe and lingular arteries, in which an estimated 20% of emboli occur.[17] Reducing the slice thickness also improves the interobserver agreement for diagnosis of PE.[25]

Shorter Scan Acquisition Time

A shorter breath hold translates into decreased respiratory motion artifact which in turn results in less indeterminate studies and allows better visualization of the subsegmental pulmonary arteries. The scan range for SDCT typically ranges from 15 to 20 cm from the top of the aortic arch to the dome of the diaphragm, with a breath hold of 30 to 40 seconds or longer, whereas the entire chest can be scanned with 16-slice or higher generation

MDCT scanners at a shorter breath hold of 3 to 10 seconds.

Decrease in Contrast Volume

The shorter acquisition time enables a reduction in volume and tighter bolus of contrast for optimal opacification of the pulmonary arteries. With SDCT and early generation MDCT, contrast volumes of 120 mL or higher were commonly used, whereas on the current generation of MDCT scanners, studies can be performed with doses of 80 mL or less. A saline chase can also be used to further reduce the volume of contrast and to decrease beam hardening artifact from the SVC as is done for imaging of the coronary arteries.

CT Pulmonary Angiography Technique

With rapidly advancing MDCT technology, the techniques and protocols are continually evolving. Precise techniques vary between the different generation of scanners and between vendors. **Table 1** suggests parameters for CTPA using different generations of MDCT scanners. The imaging acquisition on the current generation of scanners includes the entire lungs with resolution of 1.25 mm or less. The aim is to perform the study at thinnest slice collimation with a single short breath hold in full suspended respiration. With the 64-slice and higher generation scanners, it is possible to obtain the entire study with a breath hold of less than 5 seconds. In intubated patients, because of the short acquisition time, respiration can be suspended for the duration of the study. With such short breath holds, it does not matter whether the scan is acquired in a caudocranial or craniocaudal direction.

Power injectors are required for rapid contrast delivery to obtain adequate enhancement of the pulmonary arteries. An 18- to 20-gauge intravenous cannula is placed in the antecubital vein. The degree and quality of pulmonary arterial enhancement depends on the amount and concentration of contrast, injection rate, and the scan delay. On the 64-slice scanner we use 70 mL of contrast (Isovue 370, Bracco Diagnostics, New Jersey) for CTPA imaging of the chest alone, and for a combined CTPA/CTV study we use 120 mL of contrast (Isovue 370 Bracco Diagnostics) at 4 mL/s. A greater degree of arterial enhancement can be achieved by increasing the rate of contrast, independent of the concentration of iodine contrast medium.

Timing Bolus/Bolus Tracking

The timing of contrast bolus administration is critical to obtain optimal opacification of the pulmonary arteries. Incorrect timing is a common cause of suboptimal studies. A fixed scan delay of 20 to 25 seconds was used especially for SDCT and early generation of MDCT scanners, which leads to adequate opacification of the pulmonary arteries in at least 85% of patients with normal cardiac function. However, with the current generation of scanners, a timing bolus or bolus tracking method is more commonly used to optimize opacification of pulmonary arteries.

A timing bolus is usually performed by injecting 15 to 20 mL of intravenous contrast material and placing a region of interest in the pulmonary trunk to obtain a time-density curve from which the scan-delay can be calculated. When comparing empirical delay with test bolus, Hartmann and colleagues reported that despite objective improvement in pulmonary artery enhancement, there was no significant difference in image quality.[26] Additionally, 16% of the studies had to be excluded because of uninterpretable time density curves.

Alternatively, bolus tracking method can be used with a cursor in the main pulmonary artery that triggers scanning at a preset threshold. For the 16-slice scanner, the scan is triggered when a threshold of 120 HU is reached and for the 64-slice scanner, at the first sight of contrast in the pulmonary artery. A timing or bolus tracking method should be used in patients with suspected or known cardiac dysfunction because the optimal scan delay time can be 40 seconds or more.

In larger patients, a larger volume of high-density contrast should be injected at a higher flow rate to improve the signal to noise, a higher kVP should be used, and images should be acquired at thicker collimation of 2.0 to 2.5 mm to decrease quantum mottle.

ECG Gating

The benefit of ECG gating in diagnostic PE evaluation is controversial.[27] Only 1% of subsegmental pulmonary arteries are inadequately visualized secondary to cardiac motion artifact using a 4-row scanner at 1-mm collimation.[22] The higher radiation dose secondary to ECG gating is therefore not justified. ECG gating in patients with high or irregular heart rates would lead to considerable artifacts. With MDCT scanners, 16-slice and higher, the addition of ECG gating to the CTPA study can be helpful when there is a need for a double/triple rule-out study to detect or exclude pathology within the pulmonary arteries, aorta, and/or the coronary arteries. Significant stenosis of coronary arteries or nonenhancement of the myocardium in patients with acute myocardial infarction may offer an alternative differential

Table 1
CT pulmonary angiography protocols with evolution of MDCT technology at our institution

Indication	Suspected Thromboembolic Disease			
Scan type	Lightspeed QXi 4-row	Lightspeed Ultra 8-row	Lightspeed 16 16-row thin/ultrathin collimation	VCT 64-row
Detector rows	4-row	8-row	16-row[a]	64-row[a]
Tube setting				
kVp	140	140	120	120
mA	380	380	400	500
Gantry speed (s):	0.8	0.7	0.7	0.6
Table speed (mm/rotation):	7.5	13.5	27.5[a]/13.75[a]	55
Pitch	1.5	1.35:1	1.375:1	1.375:1
Slice collimation (mm):	1.25	1.25	1.25[a]/0.625[a]	1.25/0.625
Breath-hold:	Suspended Respiration			
Anatomic coverage:	Mid diaphragm to lung apices (25 cm)			Entire lungs
Acquisition time (s):	27.6	13.8	7.0[a]/13.5[a]	3–5
Recon kernel:	Standard			
Reconstruction thickness (mm):	1.25	1.25	1.25/0.625	0.625
Effective slice thickness (mm):	2.5	1.6	1.6/0.8	
Reconstruction interval (mm):	0.625	0.625	0.625	0.625

Note that protocols vary depending on types of scanners and with different vendors.
[a] The 16-row and 64-row scanner allows for a choice of rapid acquisition using a 1.25-mm collimation, which is particularly useful in dyspneic patients, or thinner collimation for greater spatial resolution.

diagnosis on these studies. In patients with large central emboli or a large thrombus burden, right ventricular function can be assessed on ECG-gated studies, albeit at increased radiation exposure. Poor right ventricular function has prognostic implications in patients with significant pulmonary embolic disease.[28]

Image Interpretation

Given the large volume datasets and the increased number of images generated for these studies, CTPA is now routinely read off a dedicated work station or PACS system and not on hard copy images. The window level and width are adjusted on the fly while scrolling to optimally visualize the opacified pulmonary arterial lumen. At some institutions, coronal and sagittal reformats are routinely generated to aid fast review of the pulmonary arterial tree. In an interobserver study evaluating the utility of multiplanar reconstructions in CTPA, the authors report that generated sagittal and coronal reformats do not increase diagnostic accuracy, but do increase reader agreement and reader confidence, and may decrease interpretation time (Espinosa et al, presented at Society of Thoracic Radiology Annual Meeting, 2008).

The paddle wheel technique helps delineate the vessel and its branches in continuity as the artery radiates from the hilum, allowing visualization of the extent of thrombus burden on a single image (**Fig. 1**). There is no significant difference between the paddle wheel technique and axial images for detecting central PE.[29,30] However, for the diagnosis of peripheral pulmonary emboli, there is significantly lower sensitivity and specificity for the paddle wheel method alone without the concurrent use of axial images.[29]

CT FINDINGS OF PULMONARY EMBOLISM
Direct Findings

The diagnosis of PE is made on CT by direct visualization of a low attenuation filling defect that partially (**Fig. 2**) or completely occludes a contrast filled artery. A vessel "cut-off" sign is seen when the distal artery is not opacified owing to the presence of occlusive PE (**Fig. 3**). The involved artery could be significantly larger than the well-enhanced corresponding artery on the opposite side, particularly with occluded smaller-sized arteries (**Fig. 4**).[31] When PE partially occludes an artery, the "rim-sign" (**Fig. 2**A, C) is seen on short axis views of the vessel, when the low attenuation embolus is surrounded by a rim of high attenuation contrast, or the "railway-track"/"tram-track" sign, on the long axis view of the vessel (**Fig. 2**B).

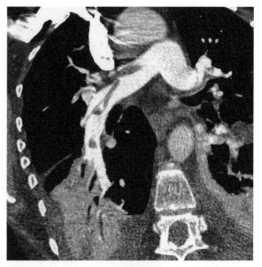

Fig. 1. Contrast-enhanced paddle wheel view depicts pulmonary emboli in the bilateral main pulmonary arteries, with embolus extending into the right lower lobe segmental and subsegmental arteries. Note that the vessels can be followed in a continuous manner from the hilum.

Indirect Findings

Pulmonary hemorrhage can occur as a result of PE and usually resolves within a week. Pulmonary infarction is seen more frequently in the lower lobes as wedge-shaped peripheral areas of consolidation with central low attenuation that do not enhance and represent uninfarcted secondary pulmonary lobules (see **Figs. 4** and **5**).[32] Air bronchograms are typically not seen in the areas of infarcted lung.[33,34] The vascular sign (**Fig. 4**A, B) increases the specificity for infarction and corresponds to acute embolus in a dilated vessel leading to the apex of the consolidation (see **Fig. 4**).[35,36] Other indirect signs of acute PE include areas of linear parenchymal bands, focal oligemia, atelectasis or small pleural effusions.[33] Although mosaic attenuation is more common with chronic PE, it can sometimes be seen with acute PE.

Acute large central pulmonary emboli can lead to right heart strain (**Fig. 6**). The effect of PE on the right heart can be assessed by dilatation of the right ventricle (RV) when the short axis diameter of the RV to left ventricle (LV) ratio is greater than one, straightening or deviation of the interventricular septum toward the LV and compression of the LV (**Fig. 6**) or acute enlargement of the central pulmonary arteries.[28,37,38] Signs of right heart strain need to be promptly communicated to the referring physician so that appropriate

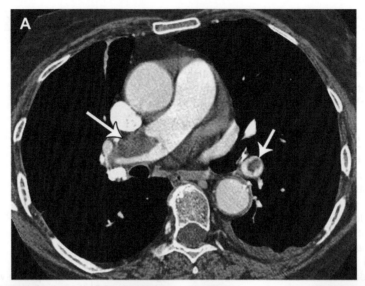

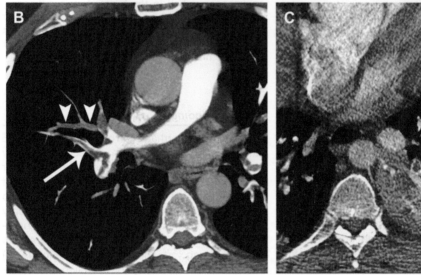
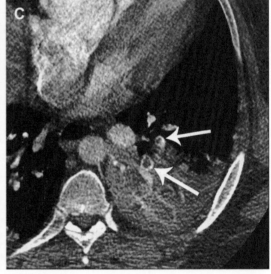

Fig. 2. "Rim-sign" and "railway-track" sign. (*A*) A low attenuation filling defect from nonocclusive embolus is completely surrounded by a rim of contrast on cross-sectional view of the left lower lobe pulmonary artery. Note large central PE in the right upper lobe artery. (*B*) On the long axis view of a segmental pulmonary artery, contrast is seen on either side of the nonocclusive embolus in the lateral segmental artery of the middle lobe. Occlusive thrombus is seen in the middle lobe medial segmental artery and its branches. (*C*) The "rim-sign" (*arrows*) can be identified even in the presence of consolidation in the right lower lobe.

therapy can be implemented immediately to prevent circulatory collapse.

ARTIFACTS
Technical

Respiratory motion artifact is a common cause for an indeterminate study. The use of 16-slice and higher generation scanners result in shorter breath holds. Routine use of oxygen via a nasal cannula and practicing breath holding with the patient before the acquisition can also help to reduce this artifact. Motion artifact can cause doubling of vessels creating a pseudo filling defect (**Fig. 7**).[39]

A common pitfall is poor contrast opacification of the pulmonary arteries. This may be because of poor cardiac function and can be overcome by delaying the trigger point by using bolus tracking or timing bolus. Improper coordination of the total contrast injection dose and injection flow rate may lead to a pseudo filling defect in the pulmonary artery that mimics pulmonary embolism (**Fig. 8**).

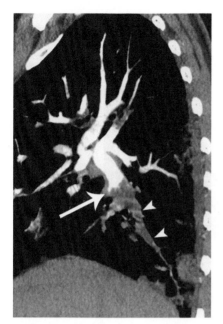

Fig. 3. Vessel cutoff sign of PE. Multiplanar sagittal oblique reformat of the lower lobe an abrupt cutoff (*long arrow*) of the contrast column from embolus that completely occludes the lobar artery in the artery and its distal branches (*short arrows*).

A soft tissue reconstruction algorithm should be used to avoid high attenuation around vessels that mimics PE. Image noise because of large body habitus increases the quantum mottle and makes it difficult to evaluate the subsegmental arteries. Increasing the collimation, volume, concentration, and rate of contrast helps to increase the signal-to-noise ratio.

Streak artifacts from beam hardening can occur from dense contrast material in the superior vena cava or of from a Swan Ganz balloon catheter in the pulmonary artery. This may obscure emboli or may mimic pulmonary embolism. Using a saline push immediately after the intravenous (IV) contrast injection and scanning in the caudal-to-cranial direction reduces the density of the contrast material in the SVC. A Swan-Ganz balloon catheter must ideally be pulled out of the pulmonary artery and placed in the heart or superior vena cava before CTPA acquisition in order to avoid this artifact.

A pulmonary arterial flow artifact called the stripe sign is caused by deep inspiration immediately before scanning that results in an inhomogeneous admixture of contrast material from the superior vena cava and unopacified blood from the inferior vena cava within the right atrium that leads to transient interruption of the contrast column in the pulmonary arteries.[40] This can be reduced by scanning in suspended inspiration.

Anatomical

Lymph nodes in the intersegmental region can be confused for emboli. This is less of a problem with thin collimation and active scrolling on the workstation. Low-density mucus-filled bronchi and pulmonary veins might also mimic filling defects. This can be differentiated from the corresponding artery by tracing the structure proximally to its origin.

Accuracy of CT Pulmonary Angiography

In the first prospective study by Remy-Jardin and colleagues[21] in 1992, single detector CTPA at 5-mm collimation was compared with catheter angiography, in an ideal group of patients with optimal contrast, with reported sensitivity of 100% and specificity of 96%, demonstrating promise for the use of this technique.[41] This study was followed by several studies that compared single-detector CTPA with catheter angiography as the reference test, with sensitivity ranging from 53% to 97% and specificity from 78% to 97%.[42] The wide variability in sensitivity and specificity partly reflects differences in technique and selection bias, as many of these studies were performed on selective patient groups rather than in consecutive patients with suspected PE. In a systematic literature review of accuracy for PE detection by Eng and coworkers, combined sensitivity for PE detection ranged from 66% to 93% and combined specificities from 89% to 97%.[43] Most of these studies were performed on SDCT. With continuously evolving technology, the true accuracy of the technique is difficult to know.

With the advent and evolution of MDCT techniques over the past decade, the higher spatial and temporal resolution of near isotropic data sets, with shorter breath holds at thinner collimation, has increased the sensitivity and specificity of MDCT for PE detection when compared with SDCT, with reported sensitivity ranging from 83% to 100%, and specificity from 89% to 97%.[18,23,44–46] The recently published PIOPED II study, which was mainly performed on four-slice MDCT scanners, that compared CT with a composite reference standard, a sensitivity of 83% and specificity of 96% was reported for CTPA.[18] When CTV was also performed, the sensitivity for the combined CTPA/CTV exam increased to 90%.[18]

Comparison of CT Pulmonary Angiography with Ventilation and Perfusion Scan

In a study of 179 patients by Blachere and colleagues a statistically significant greater accuracy for CTPA was reported (sensitivity, 94.1%;

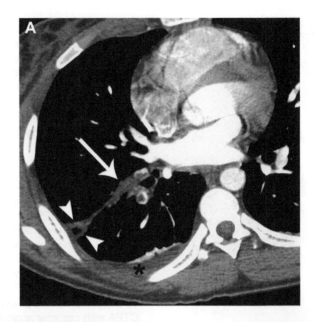

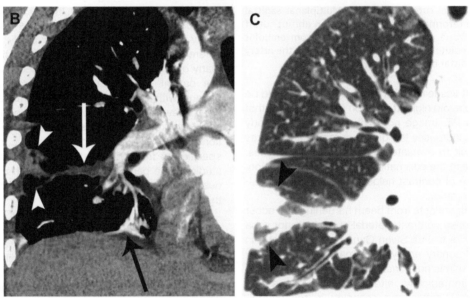

Fig. 4. Pulmonary infarct and the "vascular-sign". (*A*) Axial CT shows an occluded and dilated (*white arrow*) right lower lobe (RLL) pulmonary artery owing to the presence of PE. The vessel is enlarged (vascular sign) courses to the apex of a subpleural nonenhancing triangular opacity, which is an infarct (*arrowheads*). The asterisk indicates a small right pleural effusion. (*B*) Coronal reformatted image along the long axis of the vessel shows embolus (*white arrow*) occluding the RLL segmental pulmonary artery. Note the nonenhancing infarct along the lateral pleura (*arrowheads*), and enhancing atetectasis adjacent to the diaphragm (*black arrow*). (*C*) On lung window images the infarct is triangular in shape and has a broad base with the pleura (*arrowheads*).

specificity, 93.6%; positive predictive value [PPV], 95.5%; NPV, 96.2%) than for planar V/Q scans (sensitivity, 80.8%; specificity, 73.8%; PPV, 95.5%; NPV, 75.9%).[47] Similar results were reported by Grenier: sensitivities, specificities, and kappa values with helical CT and scintigraphy were 87%, 95%, and 0.85 and 65%, 94%, and 0.61, respectively.[48] Many believe these results are sufficient justification for CT pulmonary angiography to replace V/Q scintigraphy in the diagnostic algorithm for suspected acute pulmonary embolism. PIOPED II is the largest and most significant study that has assessed the use of MDCT in the diagnosis of PE in outpatients and inpatients, with reported sensitivity of 83% for CTPA, which is comparable to V/Q scanning.

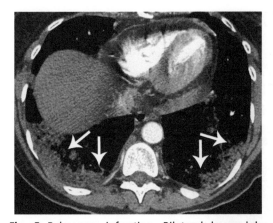

Fig. 5. Pulmonary infarction. Bilateral lower lobe infarction with wedge-shaped areas of peripheral consolidation (*arrows*) showing central lucencies, a reliable finding of infarction in the presence of PE. Air bronchograms are absent. The patient had extensive bilateral central and peripheral PE.

Comparison of CT Pulmonary Angiography and Catheter Angiography

Baile and coworkers[28] evaluated the accuracy of CTPA with catheter pulmonary angiography for the detection of subsegmental PE using postmortem methacrylate casts of the pulmonary arteries in a porcine model. CT and pulmonary angiography were both performed. The sensitivity for 1-mm collimation helical CT of 87% (95% confidence interval [CI] 79%–93%) was the same as catheter angiography, 87% (95% CI 79%–93%) (*P* = .42).[49] Note that catheter angiography

did not show 100% sensitivity, but only 87%. In the PIOPED II study, in the 20 cases with discordant CTPA and catheter angiography results, an expert panel concluded that CTPA was accurate in 14 of 20 cases, with 13 cases false-negative and one false-positive on conventional catheter angiography and CT results were false-negative in 2/20 cases. In the remaining 4/20 cases, the panel thought that the CTPA was initially truly negative, however the subsequent pulmonary angiogram showed the presence of PE.[19] This resulted in the sensitivity for detection of PE of 87% with CT, and 32% with conventional angiography (*P* = 0.007). With better visualization of subsegmental pulmonary arteries on CT and greater interobserver agreement, investigators have questioned whether catheter pulmonary angiography should still be considered the gold standard test by which MDCT is judged.

Interobserver Agreement

For CTPA, interobserver agreement for the detection of acute PE is moderate to almost excellent, with kappa values ranging from 0.59 to 0.94.[39,45,50–54] Remy-Jardin and colleagues[41] report that using thinner collimation of 2 mm versus 3 mm, the kappa values improve, 0.98 versus 0.94 (*P*<.05).[53]

For subsegmental PE, interobserver agreement is significantly better with MDCT (k = 0.56–0.85) than with SDCT (k = 0.21–0.54), with worse agreement in the obliquely oriented arteries of the middle lobe and lingula.[55–57]

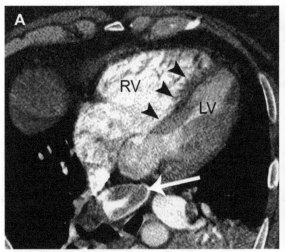
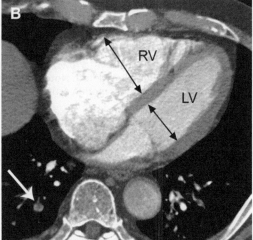

Fig. 6. Right ventricular strain. (*A*) The interventricular septum (*arrowheads*) is bowed toward the left ventricle (LV) and the LV is compressed. Note central PE in the RLL pulmonary artery (*arrow*). (*B*) In another patient with central and peripheral PE (*arrow*), the right atrium and right ventricle are dilated. The short axis diameter of the RV is greater than that of the LV.

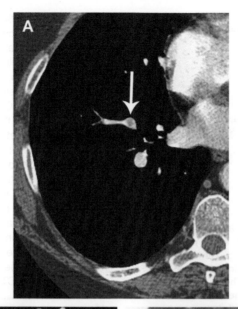

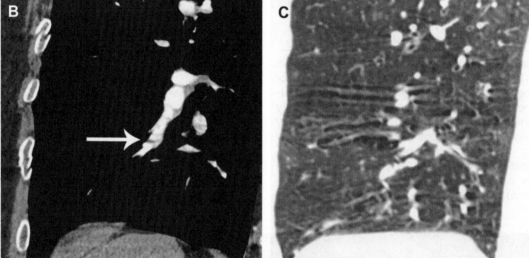

Fig. 7. Technical and interpretative pitfall. (*A*) Axial CT shows a filling defect (*arrow*) in a segmental RLL pulmonary artery suggestive of PE, discordant with clinical findings. (*B*) Coronal reformat at soft tissue window shows a horizontal linear filling defect (*arrows*) in the corresponding pulmonary artery, which was an artifact corresponding to the pseudofilling defect. Note step artifacts in the ribs from respiratory motion. (*C*) Lung window settings also show respiratory motion artifact.

For catheter angiography the interobserver agreement is moderate to poor at the subsegmental level. The interobserver agreement for central arteries is reported as 89%, whereas that for subsegmental pulmonary arteries is only 13% to 66%.[58–60]

Isolated Subsegmental Pulmonary Embolism

Ninety-four percent of segmental and 88% of subsegmental pulmonary arteries are well visualized using 16-MDCT (Patel and colleagues, 2003

Society for Computed Body Tomography and Magnetic Resonance annual meeting). There is not only improved visualization of the subsegmental pulmonary arteries using 1-mm collimation, but also improved interobserver agreement regarding the presence or absence of emboli.[25]

The prevalence of isolated subsegmental PE (ISSPE) varies from 3% to 36% at pulmonary angiography or CT (**Fig. 9**).[10,22,44,59,61,62] With better subsegmental artery visualization at MDCT, and the increased diagnosis of subsegmental PE, the question arises as to clinical significance of these

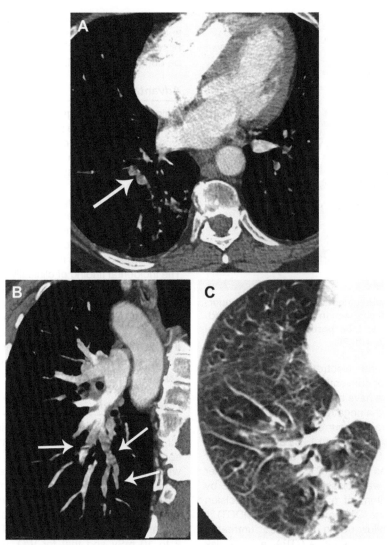

Fig. 8. Technical pitfall because of poor enhancement. (*A*) Axial CT shows low attenuation in the lower lobe pulmonary arteries mimicking PE. (*B*) Sagittal reformats show poor enhancement of the lower lobe pulmonary arteries because of poor bolus. This can be differentiated from vessel cut-off sign by the gradual and not abrupt margin of the contrast column. Respiratory motion artifact is also seen.

small emboli. Should we treat ISSPE? Subsegmental PE are common at autopsy, and when the pulmonary arteries are carefully examined, can be seen in 50% to 90% of patients, suggesting that these small emboli are usually asymptomatic and many resolve naturally.[1,63]

Currently there is no clear recommendation for treatment of ISSPE. Small PE can be clinically important and may benefit from anticoagulant therapy in patients with poor cardiopulmonary reserve, in those with coexistent DVT or a prothrombotic stage, in those with chronic pulmonary hypertension, and in cases of ISSPE with right ventricular dilatation, as the risk of death is increased in these patients.[21,38,64,65] When

treatment is withheld because of risks associated with anticoagulation, a lower extremity study is warranted to exclude a DVT.

EVIDENCE FOR MDCT IN THE DIAGNOSIS OF ACUTE PULMONARY EMBOLISM

A meta-analysis published in 2005 by Quiroz and colleagues found the overall negative likelihood ratio after a negative CTPA for PE was 0.07 (95% CI, 0.05–0.11); and the NPV was 99.1% (95% CI, 98.7%–99.5%).[66] The clinical validity of using a CT scan to rule out PE is similar to that reported for conventional pulmonary angiography, namely 1.0% to 2.8% for CT (including single-section,

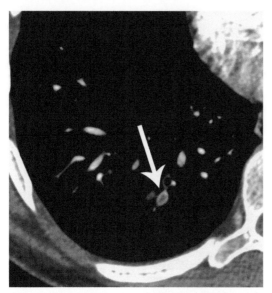

Fig. 9. Isolated subsegmental PE. An isolated nonocclusive filling defect is seen in a subsegmental branch of the right lower lobe posterior basal segmental artery compatible with PE.

multidetector, and electron-beam CT) versus 1.1% to 2.9% for conventional pulmonary angiography.[67,68] There have been a number of outcome studies following a negative CTPA with SDCT that report an average recurrence of VTE (venous thromboembolic disease) in 1.3% and that of fatal PE in 0.3%. Similar results are reported for outcome studies with MDCT. In the Christopher study, patients were classified as having a PE by using an algorithm of a dichotomized decision rule, D-dimer and CT (both SDCT and MDCT).[69] At 3-month follow-up in the 1505 untreated patients following a negative CTPA, a 1.1% risk of thromboembolic disease was reported. In a prospective management study in 756 ED (emergency department) patients with suspected PE, all patients with high clinical probability or non-high clinical probability and positive D-dimer, underwent both CTPA with MDCT and lower limb ultrasonography. Proximal DVT was found in only 3 of 318 patients (0.9%).[70] Righini and colleagues compared two diagnostic strategies that did or did not include lower extremity ultrasound along with D-dimer and MDCT. In the arm that did not use lower extremity ultrasound, the untreated patients with negative D-dimer and MDCT had a 3-month risk of VTE of only 0.3%.[71] These studies demonstrate that a negative MDCT in patients without a high clinical probability is adequate to exclude PE. Therefore, in most patients with suspected acute PE and no symptoms of DVT, especially in an outpatient setting, anticoagulation therapy can be safely withheld

after negative CTPA. The PIOPED II study suggests that in patients with high clinical probability and negative CTPA, further testing should be considered to exclude PE.[18]

Advantages

A significant advantage of CTPA is that it identifies additional findings like pneumothorax, pneumonia, lung cancer, pleural effusions, aortic dissection, pericardial effusion, mediastinitis, and so forth to account for patient symptoms. Alternative diagnosis rates can be seen in 25% to 67% of cases.[72,73] Of the negative CTPA studies in the emergency department, 7% had an alternative diagnosis that required specific and immediate action.[74] Aortic dissection and undiagnosed lung cancer were detected in about 7% of these cases. The incidental finding of clinically relevant disease is a powerful benefit of this modality.[75] There is improved visualization of the segmental and subsegmental pulmonary arteries using MDCT in patients with underlying pulmonary disease (**Fig. 2**C).[76] Cost analysis of different imaging algorithms show that per life saved, CT is the least expensive imaging modality.[77]

Disadvantages

CTPA is commonly used as a first-line imaging test for suspected acute PE. An increasing number of scans are performed especially in the ED setting, with a lower yield of positive PE test results. The high radiation dose is of concern particularly in the younger female patients, as it results in significant radiation dose to the female breast. The average whole-body doses for CTPA range from 2 to 10 mSv and that for V/Q, 0.6 to 1.5 mSv. CTPA causes significant breast radiation of at least 20 mGy (range 10 mGy–70 mGy).[78,79] This is equivalent to 10 to 25 two view mammograms or 100 to 400 chest radiographs. The Biological Effects of Ionizing Radiation, seventh report (BEIR VII) estimates that the lifetime attributable risk for breast cancer from a dose of 20 mGy is approximately 1 in 1200 for a woman aged 20, 1 in 2000 for a woman age 30, and 1 in 3500 for a woman aged 40. That is, if a woman aged 30 has a CTPA with a breast dose of 20 mGy, there would be an additional 1/2000 chance of her developing breast cancer.[78] Studies using bismuth breast shields have shown radiation dose reductions of 34% to 57% to the breast, without significant decrease in image quality or diagnostic accuracy.[80]

Other dose-reduction strategies include increasing pitch, dose modulation of tube current, and lowering tube current–time product (milliampere–second) as well as using a lower kVP of 80 to 100 mSV.[81–83]

CT VENOGRAPHY

Most PE originate as thrombi in the lower extremity veins. These thrombi break off and propagate cranially to lodge in the pulmonary arteries. Sonography is the gold standard test for evaluating lower extremity DVT. Loud and colleagues first demonstrated the potential use for indirect CTV in combination with CTPA as a single exam.[84] Multiple studies followed that compared indirect CTV to sonography, with reported sensitivity and specificity greater than 95% in symptomatic patients. The development of indirect CTV has enabled a rapid and accurate combined evaluation for both DVT and PE with one exam.

A variety of techniques ranging from incremental to helical acquisition from the tibial plateaux to the iliac crests have been used, with similar accuracy results. Controversy remains between the use of helical versus incremental images with short skip intervals of 2 to 4 cm.[85] Helical scans minimize the likelihood of missing small DVT, but result in a higher radiation dose. Agreement with incremental discontinuous imaging is good but not perfect; however, the radiation dose is significantly reduced.

CT Venography Technique

CT venography is performed after a 2.5- to 4.0-minute delay following start of injection bolus for CTPA.[86] Eighty-five percent of patients are within 10% of their peak enhancement around this time, whereas in patients with peripheral vascular disease or poor cardiac output, the delays could vary from 145 to 210 seconds.[87,88] Scans are obtained from the tibial plateaus to the iliac crests at 5- to 10-mm collimation.

DVT is seen as a low attenuation filling defect partially or completely occluding the vein, with or without vessel dilatation. Additional findings include dense rim enhancement owing to contrast straining of the vasa vasorum (**Fig. 10**), perivenous soft tissue edema, and presence of collateral vessels.

Technical Pitfalls

Venous return depends on cardiac function, arterial inflow, and venous integrity. Flow artifacts owing to suboptimal contrast opacification and early scanning, can lead to streaming of contrast in the periphery of the vessel, mimicking DVT.[89] In patients with severe atherosclerotic disease, there are arterial inflow problems with delayed venous return, and poor opacification of veins. Streak artifacts from orthopedic hardware,

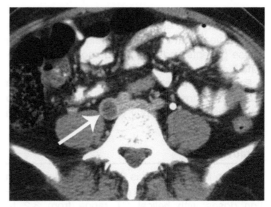

Fig. 10. Indirect CTV with deep venous thrombosis. A low-attenuation filling defect completely occludes the right common iliac vein (*arrow*).

vascular calcification, and contrast pooling in the urinary bladder can obscure portions of adjacent vein.[89]

Evidence for CT Venography

Multiple studies comparing indirect CTV to lower extremity ultrasound, the gold standard test, report sensitivities of 71% to 100%, specificity 97% to 100%, PPV 67% to 100%, and NPV 97% to 100%. In a large retrospective study by Loud and colleagues in 308 patients, the reported sensitivity was 97% and specificity 100%.[90] There were only two false negative and no false positive results. Among other prospective studies, the sensitivity ranges from 93% to 100% and specificity, 97% to 100%.[91–93] The interobserver agreement is also moderate to excellent kappa (0.59–0.88).[18,51,92]

The question arises whether the addition of CTV to the CTPA exam alters clinical management. In a study by Richman and colleagues in 800 ED patients, CTPA was positive in 5% of patients, combined CTPA/CTV in 4%, and CTV alone in 2%.[94] Several studies report an increased detection rate of 2% to 5% of VTE when CTV is added to the CTPA part of the exam. In PIOPED II, there was 95% concordance between ultrasound and CTV. Fourteen (8%) of 181 subjects had DVT alone and the addition of CTV to CTPA increased the overall sensitivity for VTE to 90% versus 83% for CTPA alone.[18] CT is better for diagnosing pelvic DVT and possibly nonobstructive DVT; however, patients with pelvic DVT often have a thrombus load in the leg veins.

Advantages

CTV can be combined with CTPA without requiring any additional intravenous contrast material and offers a one-stop comprehensive test in about 20 minutes. It is also superior for evaluating the inferior vena cava and iliac veins especially in obese patients and those with anomalous, duplicated, and complex venous anatomy.

Patients with recent surgery and with a cast in the lower extremity who are unable to undergo compression sonography can be assessed with CTV.

Disadvantages

The main disadvantage is the additional radiation incurred to the thighs and pelvis. Calculated radiation doses with helical CT range from 3.2 to 9.1 mSV, whereas with discontinuous axial images, radiation is reduced to 0.6 to 2.3 mSv.[85,95] Radiation dose can be minimized by the use of incremental sections, tube current modulation, and scanning only up to the acetabuli as incidence of DVT is low in the IVC (inferior vena cava) and pelvic veins, reported in only 3% in the PIOPED II study.[18] Given the high radiation doses, combined CTPA/indirect CTV should not be part of a routine test especially in the young female of childbearing years. The Fleischner Society Guidelines recommend the use of the combined test, when the emphasis is placed on a complete vascular exam.[79]

PULMONARY EMBOLISM IN PREGNANCY

Venous thromboembolic disease is challenging to diagnose, and is the second commonest cause of mortality in pregnancy following hemorrhage.[96] Even though the risk of radiation is high, the risk of fetal death is much greater if the mother has untreated PE.[97] The incidence of DVT is increasing and is significantly higher than in the nonpregnant female, whereas the incidence in PE between the two groups is not significantly different.[98] Controversy remains as to which is the best test to diagnose VTE in the pregnant female. Initial evaluation should begin with venous ultrasound of the lower extremities. If this is negative, then the question arises as to the preference for an imaging test that delivers the highest yield of a definitive test result, at the lowest radiation risk to the fetus. In the pregnant female, the likelihood of a normal V/Q is high (74%) and a high probability scan low (2%), with a significantly fewer number of patients (24%) having indeterminate scans compared with the general population with suspected VTE, probably because of young age and fewer comorbidities.[99]

The Fleischner society advocates CT as the first line imaging test in pregnancy following leg ultrasound. The fetal radiation exposure for CTPA varies from 3.3 mGy to 130.0 mGy; the dose increases at each trimester as the fetus enlarges and approaches the imaged area in the thorax.[100] The worst estimated absorbed dose for the fetus in the third trimester with CTPA is 130 mGy. The estimated fetal radiation dose for V/Q scanning is 100 to 370 mGy, ie, the dose may be more than three times greater than for CTPA. Based on the average background radiation to an adult, the equated dose to the fetus in utero for 9 months is about 1000 mGy.[101] So a third trimester CTPA delivers only about seven times less than the natural background radiation. All radiation to the fetus carries a potential risk. The absorbed dose to the fetus (0.2 to 0.3 mSv) is well below the level that would increase the risk of congenital abnormality.

Breast radiation dose from CTPA is an additional consideration. The female breast is extremely radiosensitive and a radiation dose of 100 cGy is associated with an increased risk of breast cancer of 40% in young Western women. Epidemiological studies have not detected a significantly increased risk of breast cancer below a dose of 20 cGy. Female breast radiation exposure during CTPA has been calculated at an effective minimum dose of 20 mGy (2 cGy)[64] and that for ventilation/perfusion scanning 0.28 mGy. These estimates are significantly below the level of 20 cGy, below which no effect on the breast can be demonstrated. This exposure should not be ignored and the use of breast shields may reduce this dose by up to 73%.[102]

Although CTPA is advocated as the initial imaging test after ultrasound of the legs, the quality of the scan may not be optimal in pregnant patients. Two recently published articles report a significantly lower enhancement of pulmonary arteries on CTPA in pregnant women with nondiagnostic rates of 7.5% or 27.5%.[103,104] This is thought to occur as a result of a combination of physiological factors: increased cardiac output, increased plasma volume, increased body weight, hyperdynamic circulation, and increased effects of a Valsalva maneuver. Contrast injection protocols need to be modified to address this problem. In pregnant women, the contrast material arrives early within the pulmonary arteries and the peak enhancement is lower. Therefore, the scan should be performed on the highest generation of scanners by using bolus tracking and increased concentration of the contrast material at higher rates of injection.[105] Scarsbrook and colleagues suggest radiation dose–reducing methods with CTPA such as reduced mAs, reduced kVp, increased pitch, increased detector and beam collimation, reducing z-axis range and field of view, and the use of abdominal shielding.[96]

Another consideration is the effect of contrast on a developing fetus, which has not been fully investigated. It is recommended that the infant has thyroid function testing within a week of birth because of the theoretical risk of contrast-induced hypothyroidism.[106]

Magnetic resonance angiography is another alternative to V/Q scanning and CTPA. MR is advantageous because the fetus is not exposed to ionizing radiation or to intravenous contrast material.

IMAGING ALGORITHM FOR DIAGNOSIS OF PE

Imaging algorithms vary, depending on the clinical probability (**Fig. 11**).

Low Pretest Probability

In the low and intermediate probability population, a cost-effective algorithm would be to perform a D-dimer. The value is in a negative test that effectively rules out significant VTE. If the test is positive, a diagnostic imaging study should be performed depending on local availability, easy access, cost, radiation, and clinician preference.

The chest x-ray (CXR) may be helpful to strategize management. If the CXR is abnormal, the patient should undergo CTPA. If the CXR is normal, either CTPA or V/Q scan can be done. The perfusion portion of the V/Q scan alone can be performed initially if there is radiation concern. The greatest drawback of the V/Q scan is the likelihood of intermediate probability scans which in a setting of a raised D-dimer necessitates another exam such as CTPA thereby increasing cost, radiation, and a delay in diagnosis.

High Pretest Probability

In high-risk cases and with strong pretest probability, D-dimer testing need not be performed because a negative D-dimer result in a patient with a high-probability clinical assessment may not exclude VTE. Depending on local preference, an early CTPA or V/Q scan can be performed if the CXR is normal. If the test is negative, the leg veins should be evaluated with compression sonography. If either CT angiography is positive or DVT is diagnosed, definitive treatment is recommended.

If the CTPA is nondiagnostic, the test can be repeated. If repeat examination is unlikely to alter image quality owing to known patient parameters (poor cardiac output, large patient habitus,

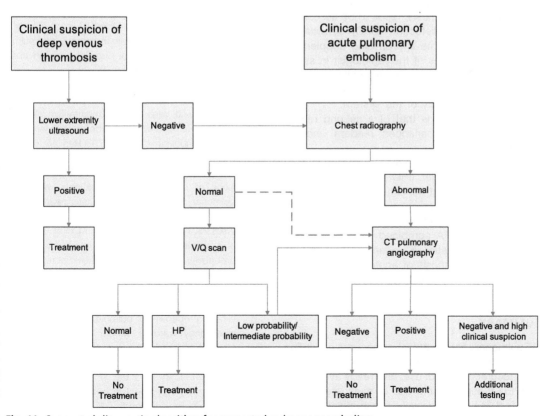

Fig. 11. Suggested diagnostic algorithm for suspected pulmonary embolism.

extensive respiratory motion), then pulmonary angiography can be performed. If both CT angiography and leg vein studies are negative or CTPA/CTV results are negative, options include serial venous ultrasound examinations, pulmonary digital subtraction angiography, and pulmonary scintigraphy.

In the critically ill patient, bedside echocardiogram to assess the right ventricle and for right heart strain and ultrasound examination of the legs can be performed until the patient is stabilized for further imaging tests. CTPA can be a challenging technique to perform in ICU patients because of respiratory motion, suboptimal bolus with poor cardiac reserve, and streak artifact from lines and tubes. However, in one series of 50 consecutive ICU patients with suspected pulmonary embolism, 76% of CT pulmonary angiography examinations were of diagnostic quality in this challenging group of patients.[107]

Future of Pulmonary Imaging

Research is now aimed at ways of radiation dose reduction of CT angiographic data and in computer-aided detection of luminal thrombus and perfusion defects. A large-scale study evaluating MR is under way (PIOPED III). With refinements in SPECT imaging, the role of SPECT V/Q scanning for PE diagnosis needs to be assessed.

Computer-aided detection (CAD) software is anticipated to become a promising supplement to the work and eyes of the radiologist in aiding detection of PE on CTPA. The high false-negative results demand technologic improvement to increase the sensitivity of the system.[108,109] The current role of CAD is that of a second reader particularly for inexperienced readers and for residents.

The Prospective Investigation of Pulmonary Embolism Diagnosis III (PIOPED III) that just completed enrollment will estimate the diagnostic accuracy of gadolinium-enhanced magnetic resonance angiography of the pulmonary arteries (Gd-MRA) and Gd-MRA combined with gadolinium-enhanced magnetic resonance venography (MRV) for the diagnosis of acute PE. If it proves to have high accuracy for diagnosis of PE, it would avoid radiation, which is a big problem with CT.

SUMMARY

CT pulmonary angiography has become a first-line imaging test for evaluation of PE because of its high accuracy, ease of use, and ready availability. PIOPED II supports the use of multidetector CT as a first-line test especially in outpatients. Technological advances continue to evolve, and with refinements in technology, we will continue to optimize imaging for PE detection. Ionizing radiation remains a concern particularly in the young and in pregnant patients, and methods to decrease these are being advocated. SPECT V/Q may play a bigger role in PE diagnosis in the future and the role of MR is yet to be determined in the PIOPED III study, with the potential of solving some of the issues regarding radiation in a select group of patients.

REFERENCES

1. Egermayer P. Follow-up for death or recurrence is not a reliable way of assessing the accuracy of diagnostic tests for thromboembolic disease. Chest 1997;111:1410–3.
2. Goldhaber SZ, Morpurgo M. Diagnosis, treatment, and prevention of pulmonary embolism. Report of the WHO/International Society and Federation of Cardiology Task Force. JAMA 1992;268:1727–33.
3. Stein PD, Beemath A, Olson RE. Trends in the incidence of pulmonary embolism and deep venous thrombosis in hospitalized patients. Am J Cardiol 2005;95:1525–6.
4. Patel S, Kazerooni EA. Helical CT for the evaluation of acute pulmonary embolism. AJR Am J Roentgenol 2005;185:135–49.
5. Silverstein MD, Heit JA, Mohr DN, et al. Trends in the incidence of deep vein thrombosis and pulmonary embolism: a 25-year population-based study. Arch Intern Med 1998;158:585–93.
6. Laporte S, Mismetti P, Decousus H, et al. Clinical predictors for fatal pulmonary embolism in 15,520 patients with venous thromboembolism: findings from the Registro Informatizado de la Enfermedad TromboEmbolica venosa (RIETE) Registry. Circulation 2008;117:1711–6.
7. Nijkeuter M, Hovens MM, Davidson BL, et al. Resolution of thromboemboli in patients with acute pulmonary embolism: a systematic review. Chest 2006;129:192–7.
8. Wells PS, Anderson DR, Rodger M, et al. Derivation of a simple clinical model to categorize patients' probability of pulmonary embolism: increasing the models utility with the SimpliRED D-dimer. Thromb Haemost 2000;83:416–20.
9. Wicki J, Perneger TV, Junod AF, et al. Assessing clinical probability of pulmonary embolism in the emergency ward: a simple score. Arch Intern Med 2001;161:92–7.
10. PIOPED Investigators. The value of the ventilation/perfusion scan in acute pulmonary embolism. Results of the prospective investigation of pulmonary embolism diagnosis (PIOPED). JAMA 1990; 263:2753–9.

11. Freeman LM, Haramati LB. V/Q scintigraphy: alive, well and equal to the challenge of CT angiography. Eur J Nucl Med Mol Imaging 2009;36: 499–504.

12. Miles S, Rogers KM, Thomas P, et al. A comparison of single-photon emission CT lung scintigraphy and CT pulmonary angiography for the diagnosis of pulmonary embolism. Chest 2009;136(6): 1546–53.

13. Schluger N, Henschke C, King T, et al. Diagnosis of pulmonary embolism at a large teaching hospital. J Thorac Imaging 1994;9:180–4.

14. Sostman HD, Gottschalk A. The stripe sign: a new sign for diagnosis of nonembolic defects on pulmonary perfusion scintigraphy. Radiology 1982;142: 737–41.

15. Beyth RJ, Quinn LM, Landefeld CS. Prospective evaluation of an index for predicting the risk of major bleeding in outpatients treated with warfarin. Am J Med 1998;105:91–9.

16. Levine MN, Raskob G, Landefeld S, et al. Hemorrhagic complications of anticoagulant treatment. Chest 1998;114:511S–23S.

17. Ghaye B. Peripheral pulmonary embolism on multidetector CT pulmonary angiography. JBR-BTR 2007;90:100–8.

18. Stein PD, Fowler SE, Goodman LR, et al. Multidetector computed tomography for acute pulmonary embolism. N Engl J Med 2006;354:2317–27.

19. Wittram C, Waltman AC, Shepard JA, et al. Discordance between CT and angiography in the PIOPED II study. Radiology 2007;244:883–9.

20. Sinner WN. Computed tomographic patterns of pulmonary thromboembolism and infarction. J Comput Assist Tomogr 1978;2:395–9.

21. Torbicki A, Perrier A, Konstantinides S, et al. Guidelines on the diagnosis and management of acute pulmonary embolism: the Task Force for the Diagnosis and Management of Acute Pulmonary Embolism of the European Society of Cardiology (ESC). Eur Heart J 2008;29:2276–315.

22. Ghaye B, Szapiro D, Mastora I, et al. Peripheral pulmonary arteries: how far in the lung does multi-detector row spiral CT allow analysis? Radiology 2001;219:629–36.

23. Patel S, Kazerooni EA, Cascade PN. Pulmonary embolism: optimization of small pulmonary artery visualization at multi-detector row CT. Radiology 2003;227:455–60.

24. Remy-Jardin M, Remy J, Artaud D, et al. Peripheral pulmonary arteries: optimization of the spiral CT acquisition protocol [comments]. Radiology 1997; 204:157–63.

25. Schoepf UJ, Holzknecht N, Helmberger TK, et al. Subsegmental pulmonary emboli: improved detection with thin-collimation multi-detector row spiral CT. Radiology 2002;222:483–90.

26. Hartmann IJ, Lo RT, Bakker J, et al. Optimal scan delay in spiral CT for the diagnosis of acute pulmonary embolism. J Comput Assist Tomogr 2002;26:21–5.

27. Marten K, Engelke C, Funke M, et al. ECG-gated multislice spiral CT for diagnosis of acute pulmonary embolism. Clin Radiol 2003;58:862–8.

28. van der Meer RW, Pattynama PM, van Strijen MJ, et al. Right ventricular dysfunction and pulmonary obstruction index at helical CT: prediction of clinical outcome during 3-month follow-up in patients with acute pulmonary embolism. Radiology 2005;235: 798–803.

29. Brader P, Schoellnast H, Deutschmann HA, et al. Acute pulmonary embolism: comparison of standard axial MDCT with paddlewheel technique. Eur J Radiol 2008;66:31–6.

30. Chiang EE, Boiselle PM, Raptopoulos V, et al. Detection of pulmonary embolism: comparison of paddlewheel and coronal CT reformations—initial experience. Radiology 2003;228:577–82.

31. Remy J, Remy-Jardin M, Wattinne L, et al. Pulmonary arteriovenous malformations: evaluation with CT of the chest before and after treatment. Radiology 1992;182:809–16.

32. Revel MP, Triki R, Chatellier G, et al. Is it possible to recognize pulmonary infarction on multisection CT images? Radiology 2007;244:875–82.

33. Coche EE, Müller NL, Kim KI, et al. Acute pulmonary embolism: ancillary findings at spiral CT. Radiology 1998;207:753–8.

34. Shah AA, Davis SD, Gamsu G, et al. Parenchymal and pleural findings in patients with and patients without acute pulmonary embolism detected at spiral CT. Radiology 1999;211:147–53.

35. Balakrishnan J, Meziane MA, Siegelman SS, et al. Pulmonary infarction: CT appearance with pathologic correlation. J Comput Assist Tomogr 1989; 13:941–5.

36. Ren H, Kuhlman JE, Hruban RH, et al. CT of inflation-fixed lungs: wedge-shaped density and vascular sign in the diagnosis of infarction. J Comput Assist Tomogr 1990;14:82–6.

37. Findik S, Erkan L, Light RW, et al. Massive pulmonary emboli and CT pulmonary angiography. Respiration 2008;76:403–12.

38. Ghaye B, Ghuysen A, Willems V, et al. Severe pulmonary embolism:pulmonary artery clot load scores and cardiovascular parameters as predictors of mortality. Radiology 2006;239:884–91.

39. Perrier A, Howarth N, Didier D, et al. Performance of helical computed tomography in unselected outpatients with suspected pulmonary embolism. Ann Intern Med 2001;135:88–97.

40. Gosselin MV, Rassner UA, Thieszen SL, et al. Contrast dynamics during CT pulmonary angiogram: analysis of an inspiration associated artifact. J Thorac Imaging 2004;19:1–7.

41. Remy-Jardin M, Remy J, Wattinne L, et al. Central pulmonary thromboembolism: diagnosis with spiral volumetric CT with the single-breath-hold technique—comparison with pulmonary angiography. Radiology 1992;185:381–7.

42. Safriel Y, Zinn H. CT pulmonary angiography in the detection of pulmonary emboli: a meta-analysis of sensitivities and specificities. Clin Imaging 2002; 26:101–5.

43. Eng J, Krishnan JA, Segal JB, et al. Accuracy of CT in the diagnosis of pulmonary embolism: a systematic literature review. Am J Roentgenol 2004;183. 1819–7.

44. Coche E, Verschuren F, Keyeux A, et al. Diagnosis of acute pulmonary embolism in outpatients: comparison of thin-collimation multi-detector row spiral CT and planar ventilation-perfusion scintigraphy. Radiology 2003;229:757–65.

45. Qanadli SD, Hajjam ME, Mesurolle B, et al. Pulmonary embolism detection: prospective evaluation of dual-section helical CT versus selective pulmonary arteriography in 157 patients. Radiology 2000;217: 447–55.

46. Winer-Muram HT, Rydberg J, Johnson MS, et al. Suspected acute pulmonary embolism: evaluation with multi-detector row CT versus digital subtraction pulmonary arteriography. Radiology 2004; 233:806–15.

47. Blachere H, Latrabe V, Montaudon M, et al. Pulmonary embolism revealed on helical CT angiography: comparison with ventilation-perfusion radionuclide lung scanning. Am J Roentgenol 2000;174:1041–7.

48. Grenier PA, Beigelman C. Spiral computed tomographic scanning and magnetic resonance angiography for the diagnosis of pulmonary embolism. Thorax 1998;53:S25–31.

49. Baile EM, King GG, Muller NL, et al. Spiral computed tomography is comparable to angiography for the diagnosis of pulmonary embolism. Am J Respir Crit Care Med 2000;161:1010–5.

50. Domingo ML, Marti-Bonmati L, Dosda R, et al. Interobserver agreement in the diagnosis of pulmonary embolism with helical CT. Eur J Radiol 2000; 34:136–40.

51. Garg K, Kemp JL, Russ PD, et al. Thromboembolic disease: variability of interobserver agreement in the interpretation of CT venography with CT pulmonary angiography. Am J Roentgenol 2001;176: 1043–7.

52. Mayo JR, Remy-Jardin M, Muller NL, et al. Pulmonary embolism: prospective comparison of spiral CT with ventilation-perfusion scintigraphy. Radiology 1997;205:447–52.

53. Remy-Jardin M, Remy J, Baghaie F, et al. Clinical value of thin collimation in the diagnostic workup of pulmonary embolism. Am J Roentgenol 2000; 175:407–11.

54. van Rossum AB, Treurniet FE, Kieft GJ, et al. Role of spiral volumetric computed tomographic scanning in the assessment of patients with clinical suspicion of pulmonary embolism and an abnormal ventilation/perfusion lung scan [comment]. Thorax 1996;51:23–8.

55. Brunot S, Corneloup O, Latrabe V, et al. Reproducibility of multi-detector spiral computed tomography in detection of sub-segmental acute pulmonary embolism. Eur Radiol 2005;15:2057–63.

56. Patel S, Kazerooni EA, Cascade PN. 16-slice MDCT optimization of small pulmonary artery visualization for pulmonary embolism detection vs 4-slice. MDCT. SCBT/MR Annual Meeting. Rancho Mirage, CA, March, 2003.

57. Ruiz Y, Caballero P, Caniego JL, et al. Prospective comparison of helical CT with angiography in pulmonary embolism: global and selective vascular territory analysis. Interobserver agreement. Eur Radiol 2003;13:823–9.

58. Diffin DC, Leyendecker JR, Johnson SP, et al. Effect of anatomic distribution of pulmonary emboli on interobserver agreement in the interpretation of pulmonary angiography. Am J Roentgenol 1998; 171:1085–9.

59. Quinn MF, Lundell CJ, Klotz TA, et al. Reliability of selective pulmonary arteriography in the diagnosis of pulmonary embolism. Am J Roentgenol 1987; 149:469–71.

60. Stein PD, Henry JW, Gottschalk A. Reassessment of pulmonary angiography for the diagnosis of pulmonary embolism: relation of interpreter agreement to the order of the involved pulmonary arterial branch. Radiology 1999;210:689–91.

61. Eyer BA, Goodman LR, Washington L. Clinicians' response to radiologists' reports of isolated subsegmental pulmonary embolism or inconclusive interpretation of pulmonary embolism using MDCT. Am J Roentgenol 2005;184:623–8.

62. Stein PD, Henry JW. Prevalence of acute pulmonary embolism in central and subsegmental pulmonary arteries and relation to probability interpretation of ventilation/perfusion lung scans [comment]. Chest 1997;111:1246–8.

63. Ryu JH, Olson EJ, Pellikka PA. Clinical recognition of pulmonary embolism: problem of unrecognized and asymptomatic cases. Mayo Clinic Proceedings 1998;73:873–9.

64. Perrier A, Bounameaux H. Accuracy or outcome in suspected pulmonary embolism. N Engl J Med 2006;354:2383–5.

65. Quiroz R, Kucher N, Schoepf UJ, et al. Right ventricular enlargement on chest computed tomography. prognostic role in acute pulmonary embolism. Circulation 2004;109(20):2401–4.

66. Quiroz R, Kucher N, Zou KH, et al. Clinical validity of a negative computed tomography scan in

patients with suspected pulmonary embolism: a systematic review. JAMA 2005;293:2012–7.

67. Henry JW, Relyea B, Stein PD. Continuing risk of thromboemboli among patients with normal pulmonary angiograms. Chest 1995;107:1375–8.

68. Novelline RA, Baltarowich OH, Athanasoulis CA, et al. The clinical course of patients with suspected pulmonary embolism and a negative pulmonary arteriogram. Radiology 1978;126:561–7.

69. van Belle A, Buller HR, Huisman MV, et al. Effectiveness of managing suspected pulmonary embolism using an algorithm combining clinical probability, D-dimer testing, and computed tomography. JAMA 2006;295:172–9.

70. Perrier A, Roy PM, Sanchez O, et al. Multidetector-row computed tomography in suspected pulmonary embolism. N Engl J Med 2005;352:1760–8.

71. Righini M, Le Gal G, Aujesky D, et al. Diagnosis of pulmonary embolism by multidetector CT alone or combined with venous ultrasonography of the leg: a randomised non-inferiority trial. Lancet 2008; 371:1343–52.

72. Cross JJ, Kemp PM, Walsh CG, et al. A randomized trial of spiral CT and ventilation perfusion scintigraphy for the diagnosis of pulmonary embolism [comments]. Clin Radiol 1998;53:177–82.

73. Kim KI, Muller NL, Mayo JR. Clinically suspected pulmonary embolism: utility of spiral CT. Radiology 1999;210:693–7.

74. Richman PB, Courtney DM, Friese J, et al. Prevalence and significance of nonthromboembolic findings on chest computed tomography angiography performed to rule out pulmonary embolism: a multicenter study of 1,025 emergency department patients. Acad Emerg Med 2004;11:642–7.

75. Paul GK, Charles SW. Acute Pulmonary Embolism: Imaging in the Emergency Department. Radiol Clin North Am 2006;44:259–71.

76. Remy-Jardin M, Tillie-Leblond I, Szapiro D, et al. CT angiography of pulmonary embolism in patients with underlying respiratory disease: impact of multislice CT on image quality and negative predictive value. Eur Radiol 2002;12:1971–8.

77. Doyle NM, Ramirez MM, Mastrobattista JM, et al. Diagnosis of pulmonary embolism: a cost-effectiveness analysis. Am J Obstet Gynecol 2004;191: 1019–23.

78. Parker MS, Hui FK, Camacho MA, et al. Female breast radiation exposure during CT pulmonary angiography. Am J Roentgenol 2005;185:1228–33.

79. Remy-Jardin M, Pistolesi M, Goodman LR, et al. Management of suspected acute pulmonary embolism in the era of CT angiography: a statement from the Fleischner Society. Radiology 2007;245: 315–29.

80. Hurwitz LM, Yoshizumi TT, Goodman PC, et al. Radiation dose savings for adult pulmonary embolus 64-MDCT using bismuth breast shields, lower peak kilovoltage, and automatic tube current modulation. Am J Roentgenol 2009;192:244–53.

81. Coche E, Vynckier S, Octave-Prignot M. Pulmonary embolism: radiation dose with multi-detector row CT and digital angiography for diagnosis. Radiology 2006;240:690–7.

82. Heyer CM, Mohr PS, Lemburg SP, et al. Image quality and radiation exposure at pulmonary CT angiography with 100- or 120-kVp protocol: prospective randomized study. Radiology 2007; 245:577–83.

83. Schueller-Weidekamm C, Schaefer-Prokop CM, Weber M, et al. CT angiography of pulmonary arteries to detect pulmonary embolism: improvement of vascular enhancement with low kilovoltage settings. Radiology 2006;241:899–907.

84. Loud PA, Grossman ZD, Klippenstein DL, et al. Combined CT venography and pulmonary angiography: a new diagnostic technique for suspected thromboembolic disease. Am J Roentgenol 1998; 170:951–4.

85. Goodman LR, Stein PD, Beemath A, et al. CT venography for deep venous thrombosis: continuous images versus reformatted discontinuous images using PIOPED II data. Am J Roentgenol 2007;189:409–12.

86. Bruce D, Loud PA, Klippenstein DL, et al. Combined CT venography and pulmonary angiography: how much venous enhancement is routinely obtained? Am J Roentgenol 2001;176:1281–5.

87. Szapiro D, Ghaye B, Willems V, et al. Evaluation of CT time-density curves of lower-limb veins. Invest Radiol 2001;36:164–9.

88. Yankelevitz DF, Gamsu G, Shah A, et al. Optimization of combined CT pulmonary angiography with lower extremity CT venography. Am J Roentgenol 2000;174:67–9.

89. Ghaye B, Szapiro D, Willems V, et al. Pitfalls in CT venography of lower limbs and abdominal veins. Am J Roentgenol 2002;178:1465–71.

90. Loud PA, Katz DS, Bruce DA, et al. Deep venous thrombosis with suspected pulmonary embolism: detection with combined CT venography and pulmonary angiography. Radiology 2001;219:498–502.

91. Begemann PG, Bonacker M, Kemper J, et al. Evaluation of the deep venous system in patients with suspected pulmonary embolism with multi-detector CT: a prospective study in comparison to Doppler sonography. J Comput Assist Tomogr 2003;27: 399–409.

92. Coche EE, Hamoir XL, Hammer FD, et al. Using dual-detector helical CT angiography to detect deep venous thrombosis in patients with suspicion of pulmonary embolism: diagnostic value and additional findings. Am J Roentgenol 2001;176: 1035–9.

93. Loud PA, Katz DS, Klippenstein DL, et al. Combined CT venography and pulmonary angiography in suspected thromboembolic disease: diagnostic accuracy for deep venous evaluation. Am J Roentgenol 2000;174:61–5.

94. Richman PB, Wood J, Kasper DM, et al. Contribution of indirect computed tomography venography to computed tomography angiography of the chest for the diagnosis of thromboembolic disease in two United States emergency departments. J Thromb Haemost 2003;1:652–7.

95. Goodman LR, Sostman HD, Stein PD, et al. CT venography: a necessary adjunct to CT pulmonary angiography or a waste of time, money, and radiation? Radiology 2009;250:327–30.

96. Scarsbrook AF, Evans AL, Owen AR, et al. Diagnosis of suspected venous thromboembolic disease in pregnancy. Clin Radiol 2006;61:1–12.

97. Matthews S. Short communication: imaging pulmonary embolism in pregnancy: what is the most appropriate imaging protocol? Br J Radiol 2006;79:441–4.

98. Stein PD, Hull RD, Kayali F, et al. Venous thromboembolism in pregnancy: 21-year trends. Am J Med 2004;117:121–5.

99. Chan WS, Ray JG, Murray S, et al. Suspected pulmonary embolism in pregnancy: clinical presentation, results of lung scanning, and subsequent maternal and pediatric outcomes. Arch Intern Med 2002;162:1170–5.

100. Winer-Muram HT, Boone JM, Brown HL, et al. Pulmonary embolism in pregnant patients: fetal radiation dose with helical CT. Radiology 2002;224:487–92.

101. Committee to Assess Health Risks from Exposure to Low Levels of Ionizing Radiation, National Research Council. Health risks from exposure to low levels of ionizing radiation: BEIR VII Phase 2, 2006. Available at: http://www.lnapledu./books/030909156X/html. Accessed October 10, 2009.

102. Hurwitz LM, Yoshizumi TT, Goodman PC, et al. Radiation dose savings for adult pulmonary embolus 64-MDCT using bismuth breast shields, lower peak kilovoltage, and automatic tube current modulation. Am J Roentgenol 2009;192:244–53.

103. Andreou AK, Curtin JJ, Wilde S, et al. Does pregnancy affect vascular enhancement in patients undergoing CT pulmonary angiography? Eur Radiol 2008;18:2716–22.

104. Jm UK-I, Freeman SJ, Boylan T, et al. Quality of CT pulmonary angiography for suspected pulmonary embolus in pregnancy. Eur Radiol 2008;18:2709–15.

105. Schaefer-Prokop C, Prokop M. CTPA for the diagnosis of acute pulmonary embolism during pregnancy. Eur Radiol 2008;18:2705–8.

106. Webb JA, Thomsen HS, Morcos SK. The use of iodinated and gadolinium contrast media during pregnancy and lactation. Eur Radiol 2005;15:1234–40.

107. Kelly AM, Patel S, Kazerooni EA. CT pulmonary angiography for acute pulmonary embolism in ICU patients: clinical experience 2002 [abstract]. Radiology 2002:225(P):385.

108. Maizlin ZV, Vos PM, Godoy MB, et al. Computer-aided detection of pulmonary embolism on CT angiography: initial experience. J Thorac Imaging 2007;22:324–9.

109. Walsham AC, Roberts HC, Kashani HM, et al. The use of computer-aided detection for the assessment of pulmonary arterial filling defects at computed tomographic angiography. J Comput Assist Tomogr 2008;32:913–8.

MDCT Evaluation of Acute Aortic Syndrome

Seung Min Yoo, MD, PhD[a], Hwa Yeon Lee, MD, PhD[b], Charles S. White, MD[c],*

KEYWORDS

- Acute aortic syndrome • Aortic dissection
- Intramural hematoma • Penetrating atherosclerotic ulcer
- Multidetector CT (MDCT)

Acute aortic syndrome (AAS) comprises aortic dissection (AD), intramural hematoma (IMH), penetrating atherosclerotic ulcer (PAU), and unstable aortic aneurysm. Because the highest mortality of AAS, particularly AD, occurs during the first 48 hours after onset of symptoms, prompt diagnosis and immediate initiation of appropriate therapy is essential for a favorable outcome.[1] Unfortunately, several studies have reported that a delay in diagnosis of more than 24 hours after admission occurs in up to 39% of patients with AD.[2,3] This is mainly because of a significant overlap of clinical symptoms between AAS and acute coronary syndrome (ACS) or pulmonary embolism (PE). In addition, the annual incidence of AAS, ACS, and PE has been estimated at 0.5 to 3.0, 440.0, and 69.0 per 100,000 in the United States, respectively.[4,5] This relatively rare occurrence of AAS compared with ACS and PE increases the likelihood of delayed diagnosis or misdiagnosis of AAS as ACS or PE. Although radiologists are not directly involved with history taking or physical examination of patients with suspicious AAS, a precise understanding of both the pretest probability and typical clinical symptoms and signs of AAS is valuable for radiologists to get the broadest perspective of AAS.

Current multidetector CT (MDCT) equipped with state-of-the art tube and detector technology, and optimal temporal and spatial resolution has become widely available globally. With appropriately obtained MDCT data in patients who have findings suspicious for AAS, the diagnostic accuracy of MDCT is nearly 100%.

This article provides a summary of AAS, focusing especially on MDCT technique and findings of AAS, as well as recent concepts regarding the subtypes of AAS, consisting of AD, IMH, PAU, and unstable aortic aneurysm.

AORTIC DISSECTION
Pathogenesis of Aortic Dissection

The exact mechanism of AD still remains unclear.[6] AD is characterized by intimal rupture and subsequent formation of a false lumen parallel to the original aortic lumen. An entry tear is likely to be a primary event for development of most AD. In some cases, intramural hemorrhage in the media followed by intimal rupture may also be an initiating event. Most patients with AD have hypertension. The most common sites of entry tear are the right lateral wall of the ascending aorta and the descending aorta just distal to the left subclavian artery, where the shearing stress against the aortic wall generated by hypertensive blood flow is maximal. Once an entry tear is made, propagation of AD ensues along the aortic lumen, either in an

This article originally appeared in *Radiologic Clinics of North America*, Volume 48, Issue 1, January 2010.
[a] Department of Diagnostic Radiology, 351 Yatop-dong Bundang-gu, CHA Medical University Hospital, Bundang 463-712, Korea
[b] Department of Diagnostic Radiology, 65-207 Hangang-ro 3 ga Youngsan-gu, Chung-Ang University College of Medicine, Seoul 140-757, Korea
[c] Department of Diagnostic Radiology, 22 South Greene Street, University of Maryland, Baltimore, MD 21201, USA
* Corresponding author.
E-mail address: cwhite@umm.edu (C.S. White).

Thorac Surg Clin 20 (2010) 149–165
doi:10.1016/j.thorsurg.2009.12.011
1547-4127/10/$ – see front matter © 2010 Elsevier Inc. All rights reserved.

antegrade or retrograde fashion. When an ascending aortic dissection propagates into the aortic arch and descending aorta, the dissection often extends along the greater curvature of the aortic arch, resulting in frequent involvement of aortic arch branches (**Fig. 1**).[7] The term intimal flap is a misnomer. As the dissection flap is composed of intima and the inner two-thirds of media, intimomedial flap is a more appropriate terminology. The thickness of the outer wall of false lumen is only one-third of the intimomedial flap and one-quarter of the original aortic wall. The outer wall of the false lumen is thus vulnerable to aortic rupture.[7,8] Surgeons operating on AD often describe this structure as paper-thin. Most aortic ruptures occur in the vicinity of the entry tear. The presence and location of the high-density hematoma on pre–contrast-enhanced CT suggests the site of aortic rupture. Hemopericardium or right hemothorax indicates rupture of the ascending aorta, whereas hemomediastinum and left hemothorax suggest rupture of the aortic arch and descending aorta, respectively (**Fig. 2**).[7]

Predisposing Factors

Predisposing factors related to AD are hypertension, aortic disease (eg, bicuspid aortic valve, aortic coarctation, and aortic aneurysm),[9] connective tissue diseases of the aorta (eg, Marfan's syndrome and Ehler-Danlos syndrome),[10,11] direct trauma to the aortic wall,[12] cocaine abuse,[13] and pregnancy.[14]

Most AD occurring in young patients is related to Marfan's syndrome.[9] Cocaine use may result in rapid increase of blood pressure, making cocaine users vulnerable to intimal tear. AD occurring in young women is often associated with pregnancy-induced hypertension during the third trimester or labor.[15]

CLINICAL FINDINGS OF AORTIC DISSECTION AND CHOICE OF IMAGING MODALITIES

Typical AD has been associated with severe chest or back pain of sudden onset with a tearing or ripping quality in an older patient (ie, sixth or seventh decade) who has hypertension.[3] However, ripping or tearing chest pain may not be a typical descriptor in patients with AD. According to a study performed by the International Registry of Acute Aortic Dissection (IRAD), the incidence of tearing or ripping pain (51%) was less frequent than that of sharp pain (64%) in patients with AD.[4] The location of pain is related to the site of AD: patients with ascending AD are more likely to have anterior chest pain, whereas those with descending aortic dissection more often complain of posterior chest, back, or abdominal pain. A migratory nature of the pain (16.6%) and radiation of pain (28.3%) to the interscapular region, back, or abdomen are fairly typical of AD.[4]

Focal neurologic signs or symptoms, and a pulse deficit or pressure difference between the two extremities are also characteristic of AD. For example, in a patient with severe chest pain of sudden onset, a nonpalpable unilateral extremity pulse is highly suggestive of AD, regardless of the nature of the pain (**Fig. 3**).

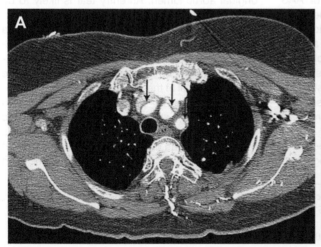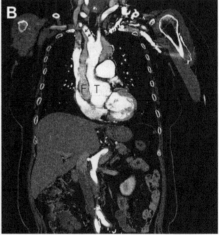

Fig. 1. Extension of intimomedial flap into all of three aortic arch branches in 67-year-old woman with Stanford type A aortic dissection. (*A*) Intimomedial flap (*arrows*) is noted in brachiocephalic, left common carotid, and left subclavian artery on contrast-enhanced axial CT image at the level of left brachiocephalic vein. (*B*) Intimomedial flap (*arrows*) extending into brachiocephalic artery is clearly noted on coronal MPR image. The contrast enhancement of true lumen (T) is higher than that of false lumen (F) owing to slow flow of the false lumen.

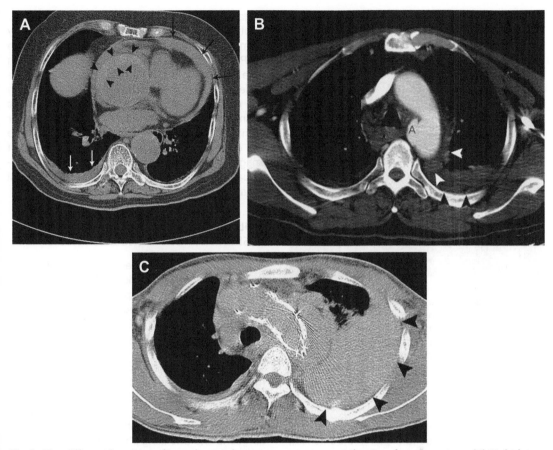

Fig. 2. The different locations of intrathoracic hematoma may suggest the site of aortic rupture. (*A*) Right hemo-thorax (*white arrows*) and hemopericardium (*black arrows*) of high attenuation are seen in a patient with ruptured Stanford type A dissection on pre–contrast-enhanced axial CT image at the level of left atrium. Note the high attenuation of ascending aortic wall (*black arrowheads*) owing to partial thrombosis of false lumen. (*B*) Mediastinal hemorrhage (*white arrowheads*) is demonstrated on contrast-enhanced axial CT image at the level of aortic arch in a patient with traumatic aortic pseudoaneurysm (*A*) at the aortic isthmus. Left pleural effu-sion (*black arrowheads*) is also noted. (*C*) Left hemothorax (*arrowheads*) of high attenuation is noted on pre–contrast-enhanced axial CT image at the level of aortic arch in a patient in whom aortic stent-graft was inserted owing to ruptured Stanford type B dissection.

Acute aortic regurgitation is one of the most deleterious consequences of AD. A new diastolic murmur at the apex may therefore suggest AD.

With respect to imaging, mediastinal widening or displacement of aortic intimal calcifications away from the outer aortic wall on chest radiog-raphy can be an important clue of AD, although these signs are not specific.[4,16]

Von Kodolitsch and colleagues[16] reported a clin-ical prediction model of AD. In their study, there were three independent predictors of AD: chest pain of abrupt onset with a tearing or ripping nature, or both, a pulse or blood pressure differen-tial, and substantial mediastinal widening on chest radiograph. The presence of one of these variables was detected in 96% of patients with AD. The pretest probability of AD was low (7%) in the absence of three variables, intermediate with one of characteristic chest pain or mediastinal widening (31%), and high (>83%) in patients with either pulse or blood pressure differential, or any combination of three variables. Therefore, these variables can provide an important guide for further imaging evaluation.

MDCT has both advantages and disadvantages with respect to other imaging techniques such as ultrasound and MRI for the evaluation of AD. Because of the inability of transthoracic echocar-diography (TTE) to visualize the aorta beyond the root, transesophageal echocardiography (TEE) is mainly used for assessment of AD. A major advan-tage of TEE is its portability, which is useful in unstable patients. The disadvantages of TEE are operator dependency, limited acoustic window,

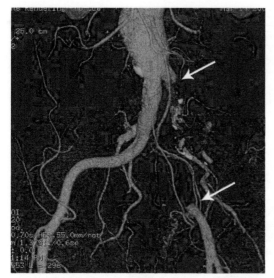

Fig. 3. Total occlusion of left common iliac and external iliac artery owing to false lumen thrombosis in a patient with Stanford type B dissection. Volume rendering (VR) image intuitively shows total occlusion (*arrows*) of left common iliac and external iliac artery. Left common femoral artery is opacified by collateral circulation. This patient had a sudden onset of sharp chest pain and a loss of left femoral pulse.

innate blind spot (ie, the distal ascending aorta and proximal aortic arch due to the air in the trachea), and inability to visualize the entire aorta. By contrast, a major strength of MDCT is the ability to image aortic branch vessels as well as the entire aorta without any limitations encountered on TEE. Another advantage of MDCT over TEE is the ability to make alternative extracardiac diagnoses such as PE. Because of a relatively long examination time and difficulty in monitoring the unstable patients in the magnetic field, the role of MRI in the evaluation of acute AD is limited.[7] MRI is mainly used for follow-up of chronic AD rather than MDCT to avoid radiation exposure and the use of contrast material. Therefore, the choice of imaging modality for evaluating AD should be individualized according to the specific clinical situations.

MULTIDETECTOR CT TECHNIQUE IN THE ASSESSMENT OF AORTIC DISSECTION

The 64-slice MDCT has become widely used and can provide iso-volumetric, 3-dimensional information without loss of spatial resolution during a single breath-hold. Because of a diagnostic accuracy approaching 100%, MDCT has become the first-line imaging study for evaluating patients with suspicious AD.[7]

Various postprocessing techniques such as multiplanar reformation (MPR), maximum intensity projection (MIP), and volume rendering (VR) help to facilitate understanding of complex aortic pathology and to expedite communication with surgeons and attending physicians.[17]

The standard protocol for evaluating AAS should include a pre–contrast-enhanced CT to recognize the presence of IMH and high-density

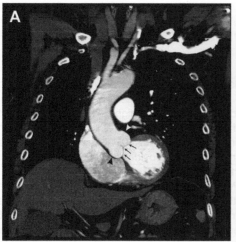
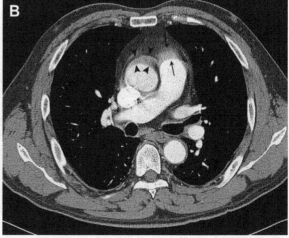

Fig. 4. The advantages of ECG-gated aortic CT and differential point between intimomedial flap and aortic pulsation artifact. (*A*) Artifact-free ascending aortic root (*arrowheads*) and normal coaptation of aortic valves (*arrows*) are noted on coronal MPR image of mid-diastolic phase. (*B*) Aortic (*arrowheads*) and pulmonary arterial motion artifact (*arrows*) are noted on non-ECG gated axial CT image at the level of right main pulmonary artery. Simultaneous visualization of crescent-shaped low attenuation in both ascending aorta and pulmonary artery suggests motion artifact rather than aortic dissection.

blood in the pericardium, pleural space, or mediastinum, indicating aortic rupture. Pre–contrast-enhanced CT with low-dose technique accompanied by thick collimation (collimation, 1.5 mm; slice thickness, 5 mm; reconstruction interval, 5 mm) may be used to reduce total radiation dose.[18,19] In addition, the scan range of pre–contrast-enhanced CT can be restricted from the lung apex to upper abdomen, instead of a full-scan range from the thoracic inlet to femoral head.[20]

The scan range of contrast-enhanced CT is from the thoracic inlet to femoral head in our institution to exclude involvement of major aortic arch branches and both iliac arteries.[21] However, if there is no evidence of AD during scanning of the thorax and upper abdomen (ie, at least at the level of celiac axis), further scanning should be stopped to avoid unnecessary radiation exposure.

There is no standard iodine concentration for a dedicated MDCT protocol of AD. In general, a body weight–adapted iodine concentration accounting for flow rate of 1.0 to 1.6 g per second is sufficient to opacify the entire aorta in most patients.[17,22] For example, in a nonobese patient, an iodine concentration of 3 to 4 mL of 300 mg I/mL per second (ie, 0.9–1.2 g per second) may be adequate, whereas in a patient with higher body mass index, 5 mL of 300 mg I/mL per second (ie, 1.5 g per second) may be necessary to obtain satisfactory opacification of the aorta.

The starting time point for a contrast-enhanced scan can be best achieved using a bolus tracking method.[19] When the CT attenuation value in the ascending aorta reaches 100 Hounsfield Units, scanning starts with a scan delay time of 5 to 7 seconds. A saline chaser technique with a dual-head injector is used to reduce the amount of

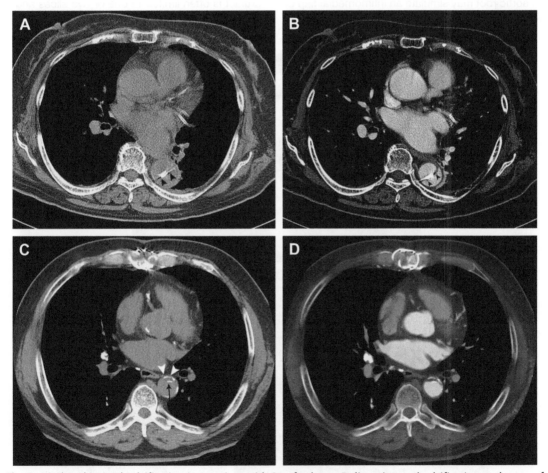

Fig. 5. Displaced intimal calcification in a patient with Stanford type B dissection and calcification at the top of mural thrombus in an asymptomatic patient. Displaced intimal calcification (*arrowheads*) is noted on pre-enhanced (*A*) and contrast-enhanced (*B*) axial CT image at the level of left atrium. Calcifications lying on intima (*arrowheads*) and top of mural thrombus (*arrow*) are noted on preenhanced (*C*) and contrast-enhanced (*D*) axial CT image at the level of left atrium.

contrast material while maintaining the flow rate of contrast material. It is feasible to obtain adequate opacification of the entire aorta if contrast material is administered at least as long as scan time plus the scan delay time. For example, if scan time and scan delay time are 15 and 5 seconds, respectively, a 20-second injection of contrast material followed by a 50-mL saline chase is sufficient. With 64-slice MDCT, it is possible to scan the entire aorta with submillimeter collimation (collimation, 0.625 mm; slice thickness, 0.625 mm; reconstruction interval, 0.3 mm) within a single breath-hold, thus making high-resolution 3-dimensional reconstruction and other postprocessing displays possible.

ECG-GATED MULTIDETECTOR CT FOR AORTIC DISSECTION

Artifacts caused by the pendular or circular motion of aortic root may simulate an intimomedial flap of AD, particularly in the ascending aorta. With an ECG-gated acquisition, the aortic motion artifact can be completely eliminated (**Fig. 4**A), thus increasing diagnostic confidence.[17,23] Other advantages of retrospectively ECG-gated aortic CT include precise evaluation of involvement of coronary arteries by intimomedial flap extension, detection of myocardial perfusion defect as evidence of ischemia, indirect assessment of aortic regurgitation based on lack of coaptation of the aortic valve leaflets, calculation of left ventricular ejection fraction, and evaluation of ventricular wall motion.[17,24] As the entry tear is often perpendicular to the long axis of the aorta, it can be better visualized on an ECG-gated multiplanar reformatted image.[17] These advantages may help in deciding therapeutic strategy and presurgical prognosis.

However, in most cases, aortic motion artifact is not a major diagnostic problem because it can be differentiated from intimomedial flap.[25] Motion artifact is often limited to one or two slices and is accompanied by pulmonary artery motion

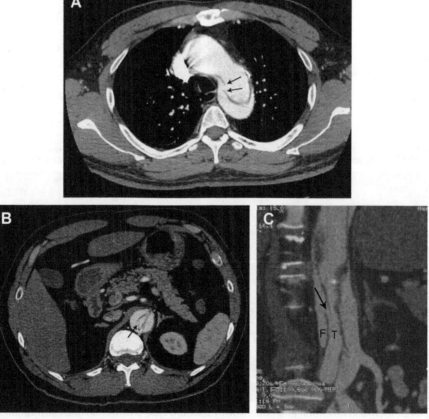

Fig. 6. Entry and reentry tear in a patient with Stanford type B dissection. Entry (*arrows*) and reentry tear (*arrow*) are noted on contrast-enhanced axial CT image at the level of aortic arch (*A*) and upper pole of left kidney (*B*), respectively. (*C*) Curved multiplanar reformatted image (MPR) shows reentry tear (*arrow*) to connect true lumen (T) with false lumen (F) in distal abdominal aorta more intuitively.

(**Fig. 4**B). A study with four-slice MDCT in a tertiary referral hospital indicated no false positive case caused by aortic motion artifact among 373 cases of AD.[26] Therefore, the use of ECG-gated MDCT is controversial. In particular, a major disadvantage of retrospective ECG-gated acquisition is increased radiation exposure. Therefore, it may be advisable to limit use of ECG-gated acquisition to cases in which a non–ECG-gated scan mandates further investigation (eg, equivocal involvement of coronary artery by the intimomedial flap or aortic regurgitation).

MULTIDETECTOR CT FINDINGS OF AORTIC DISSECTION

The following information should be provided when interpreting MDCT in patients with AD: extent of AD (ie, Stanford classification); site of entry tear; side branch involvement such as coronary, carotid, subclavian, celiac, superior mesenteric, inferior mesenteric, renal, and iliac artery; the presence of aortic rupture; differentiation between the true and false lumen; the size of false lumen diameter as a predictor for aortic rupture.

Inwardly displaced intimal calcification can be a sign of AD on precontrast MDCT (**Fig. 5**A, B). However, this finding may be confused with calcified mural thrombus in patients without AD (**Fig. 5**C, D).[21]

An intimomedial flap is the major finding demonstrated on contrast-enhanced MDCT. Identification of the precise location of the entry tear is important because current endovascular stent-graft therapy targets the exclusion of the entry tear. The entry tear is often at the most proximal location of the intimomedial flap and can be identified on contrast-enhanced MDCT in most cases. Conversely, a reentry tear is usually in the descending thoracic or abdominal aorta, or iliac arteries (**Fig. 6**),[17] and is not frequently identified because it typically consists of a minute defect or defects. The Stanford classification is based on the extent of intimomedial flap. By definition, a Stanford type A dissection involves the ascending aorta regardless of involvement of descending aorta, whereas a type B dissection affects only the descending aorta. A Stanford Type B dissection is more frequent in radiological and surgical series of AD, whereas Type A dissection is more prevalent in autopsy series.[8] This discrepancy is because substantial numbers of patients with type A dissection die before reaching the hospital. As a Stanford type A dissection is frequently associated with deadly complications such as pericardial tamponade, acute aortic regurgitation, or the involvement of aortic arch branch,

aortic replacement is the mainstay of therapy. The worst outcome is expected in patients with Stanford type A dissection treated conservatively because of old age or severe comorbidity. Conversely, Stanford type B dissection is usually managed conservatively because emergent operation is associated with a mortality rate of up to 40%. However, operative or interventional treatment is mandatory for the following situations: uncontrollable hypertension and the presence of symptoms or signs such as intractable pain or shock suggesting impending rupture.

Endovascular stent-graft repair is an emerging therapeutic option in patients with complicated Stanford type B dissection. This procedure is aimed at the complete exclusion of the false lumen by sealing up the entry tear site with a stent-graft. Candidates for aortic stent-graft placement include those with a sufficient landing zone without excessive aortic tortuosity (ie, proximal neck of more than 5 mm distal to left subclavian artery) and adequate vascular access (ie, iliac arterial diameter larger than 9 mm). However, in the absence of long-term follow-up data and complications such as retrograde extension of the dissection flap into the ascending aorta or endoleak occurring after insertion of aortic stent-graft (**Fig. 7**), the exact role of aortic stent-graft in patients with acute type B dissection remains to be elucidated.[27–29]

The differentiation between the true and false lumen is extremely important because major side branches originating from the false lumen may be

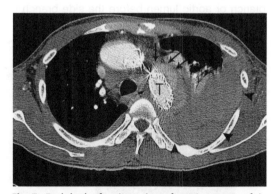

Fig. 7. Endoleak after insertion of aortic stent-graft in a patient with ruptured Stanford type B dissection. Aortic stent-graft was emergently inserted in 40-year-old man because of symptoms and signs of rupture. The presence of contrast material (*arrows*) within false lumen is noted on axial CT image at the level of tracheal carina obtained after interventional procedure, consistent with endoleak. Left hemothorax (*arrowheads*) is also noted. The patient died 2 days after CT as a result of shock. Note aortic stent-graft in true (T) lumen.

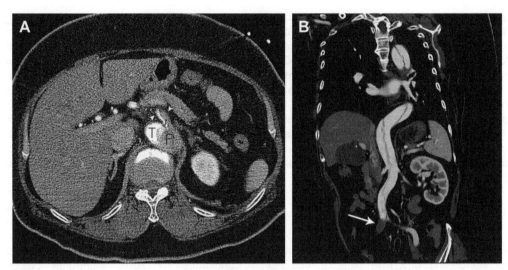

Fig. 8. Static obstruction in patients with Stanford type B dissection. (*A*) The proximal portion of celiac trunk (*arrowheads*) originating from true lumen (T) is severely narrowed by thrombosis of false lumen (F) on contrast-enhanced axial CT at the level of upper pole of left kidney in a patient with Stanford type B dissection. (*B*) Static obstruction of right common iliac artery (*arrow*) caused by thrombosis of false lumen is noted on coronal curved MPR image in a patient with Stanford type B dissection. Note the intimomedial flap in aorta.

occluded after stent-graft insertion, especially in cases without a reentry tear.[7]

There are two kinds of side branch involvement: static versus dynamic obstruction. Static obstruction can occur if the intimomedial flap directly extends into the affected side branch (**Fig. 8**). A possible solution for this complication is to insert a stent into the true lumen of the involved side branch. Conversely, dynamic obstruction indicates that the ostium of the affected side branch or aortic lumen before the side branch is occluded by an overlaying flap on the lumen (**Fig. 9**). This type of side branch involvement is caused by marked increase of false lumen pressure compared with that of the true lumen.[30] Stent-graft insertion into the severely compressed true lumen with or without fenestration of the intimomedial flap is the only good therapeutic option for dynamic obstruction of the branch vessel.

A simple way to discriminate true lumen from the false lumen is to demonstrate its communication with the uninvolved aortic segment. The larger

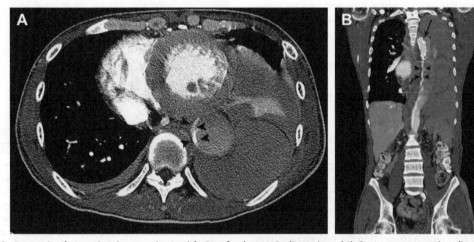

Fig. 9. Dynamic obstruction in a patient with Stanford type B dissection. (*A*) Severe compression (ie, dynamic obstruction) of true lumen (*arrowheads*) owing to high pressure of false lumen (F) is noted on contrast-enhanced axial CT image at the level of left ventricle in a patient with Stanford type B dissection. Note large amount of left hemothorax. (*B*) Dynamic obstruction (*arrowheads*) is also demonstrated on coronal MPR image. Note aortic stent-graft (*arrow*) inserted proximal to the site of dynamic obstruction.

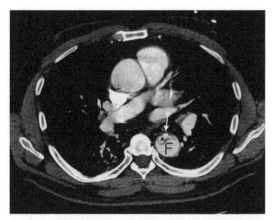

Fig. 10. Differentiation between true and false lumen in a patient with Stanford type B dissection. Beak sign (*arrowheads*) and larger lumen sign are noted in false lumen (F) on contrast-enhanced axial CT image at the level of mid-descending aorta. Intimal calcification (*arrow*) on the wall of true lumen is noted.

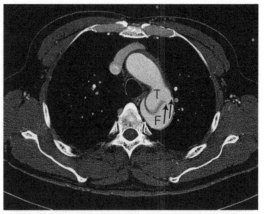

Fig. 12. A case of Stanford type B dissection showing intimomedial rupture sign. Both free ends (*arrows*) of intimomedial flap direct toward the false lumen (F) from true lumen (T) on contrast-enhanced axial CT image at the level of aortic arch.

lumen (**Fig. 10**) is typically the false lumen because the pressure in the false lumen is higher than that of true lumen.[7,18,21] In some cases, the velocity of blood flowing through the small true lumen is higher than that of large false lumen, resulting in lesser opacification of the false lumen (see **Fig. 1**).[7,18] The false lumen may show a beak sign manifested as an acute angle between the intimomedial flap and outer false lumen on axial CT images.[7,18,21] Intraluminal thrombus is more frequently encountered in the false lumen (46%) rather than true lumen (6%) owing to slow flow in the acute setting.[31] Although it has a low

sensitivity, the cobweb sign (**Fig. 11**) is typical of the false lumen, and corresponds to strands from incompletely torn connective tissue of the aortic media.[32] The intimomedial rupture sign (**Fig. 12**) is also helpful to distinguish the true lumen from false lumen. This sign refers to the discontinued ends of intimomedial flap at the site of entry tear

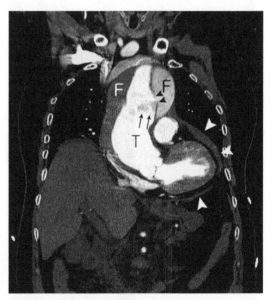

Fig. 13. Bidirectional blood flow through the entry tear in a patient with Stanford type A dissection. The presence of contrast material noted in false lumen (F) indicates flow direction from true lumen to false lumen through the entry tear (*black arrowheads*) on coronal MPR image. Conversely, low attenuation (*arrows*) noted in true lumen (T) suggests flow direction from false lumen to true lumen. Note hemopericardium (*white arrowheads*).

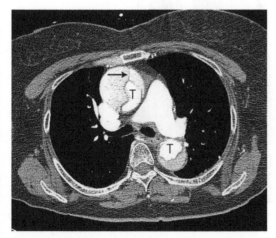

Fig. 11. Cobweb sign in a patient with Stanford type A dissection. Cobweb (*arrow*) is noted in false lumen of ascending aorta on contrast enhanced axial CT image at the level of main pulmonary artery. Attenuation of true lumen (T) is denser than that of false lumen due to slow flow of false lumen.

that point toward false lumen.[33] It is indicative of the direction of blood flow through entry tear from true to false lumen. However, the direction of blood flow through the entry tear can be bidirectional or reversed depending on the cardiac phase (**Fig. 13**).[15] Intimal calcification occurs along the wall of the true lumen or true lumen side of intimo-medial flap (see **Fig. 10**).

Consistent with Laplace's law, a large false lumen is more likely to be associated with aortic rupture than a small false lumen.

INTRAMURAL HEMATOMA

Similar to classic AD, the pathogenesis of IMH is not fully understood. Hypertension is a major predisposing factor of IMH as it is for classic AD. Although IMH can be caused by blunt trauma of the aortic wall or penetrating atherosclerotic ulcer (PAU),[6] two major pathophysiological mechanisms of IMH are bleeding of the vasa vasorum and intimal tear with complete thrombosis of false lumen. Spontaneous rupture of the vasa vasorum that supplies the aortic media is a primary event of first theory. Cases of IMH observed without an intimal tear at autopsy or during surgery support this theory. According to the second theory, IMH results from complete thrombosis of false lumen in an otherwise classic AD with an entry tear. Several recent reports suggest that most IMH results from an entry tear similar to classic AD[34–37] rather than bleeding of the vasa vasorum. Park

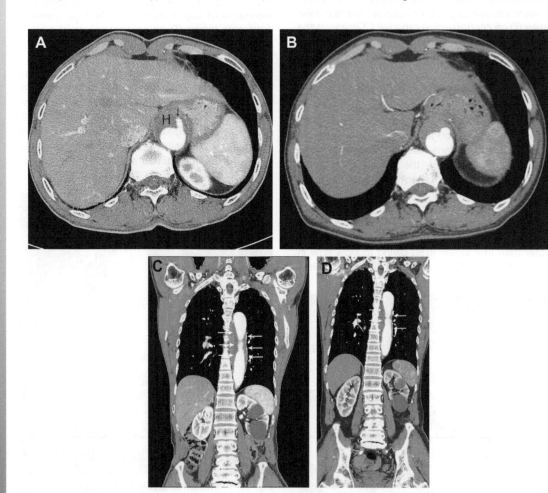

Fig. 14. Stanford type B intramural hematoma (IMH) with ulcer-like projection (ULP) in a 70-year-old man. (*A*) IMH (H; maximal thickness, 18 mm) with ULP (*arrow*; depth, 16 mm; width, 7 mm) is noted in descending thoracic aorta on contrast-enhanced axial CT image at the level of upper pole of left kidney. The lack of atherosclerotic change in the aortic lumen may suggest the diagnosis of IMH with intimal tear rather than IMH with PAU. However, definite differentiation between the two entities is difficult. (*B*) On follow-up CT performed on 15 months later, ULP (depth, 6.5 mm; width, 8 mm) is slightly decreased compared with A. (*C*) Coronal MPR image performed on same day with *A* shows extent of intramural hematoma (*arrows*) more intuitively. (*D*) On coronal MPR image performed on same day as *B*, thickness of IMH (*arrows*) is also decreased compared with C.

and colleagues[34] reported that intimal defects were identified during surgery in 27 patients (73.0%) among 37 patients with type A IMH, whereas preoperative CT detected intimal defects in only 13 patients (35.1%). Therefore, small intimal defects were identified in only 14 cases during surgery. As a result, they proposed that most IMH develops from intimal tear, not from bleeding of the vasa vasorum. They also suggested that it is unlikely that intimal defect is a secondary event followed by vasa vasorum bleeding. If intimal defect were a secondary event, the incidence of detection of intimal defects during surgery should have increased as the time interval between initial CT and surgery increases. However, no such increase was observed. They postulated that a small entry tear without a reentry

tear is likely to form IMH,[38] whereas a large entry tear with reentry tear would predispose to the formation of classic AD.

Several reports indicate that IMH associated with an ulcerlike projection (ULP) has less favorable outcome (ie, complications such as overt AD or rupture) compared with IMH without ULP, regardless of when the ULP is visualized.[39,40] ULP seems to be a more reasonable terminology to describe this entity than PAU or intimal tear, as it is often not confirmed pathologically. Because of the prognostic implications, radiologists should give special attention to detecting ULP when evaluating patients with IMH. ULP has been considered to represent the site of the entry tear or a PAU.[41–44] IMH can be preoperatively divided into IMH with ULP (**Fig. 14**) and IMH

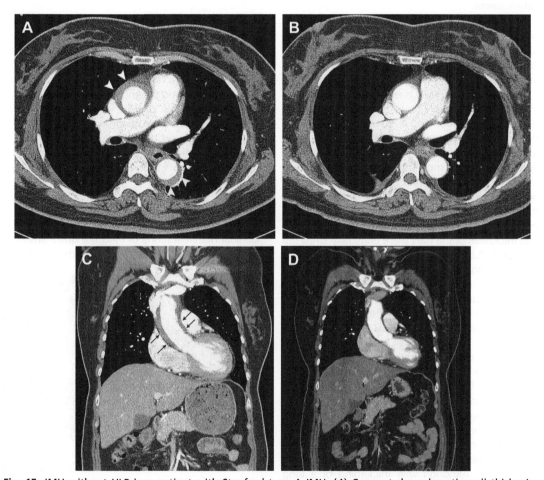

Fig. 15. IMH without ULP in a patient with Stanford type A IMH. (*A*) Crescent shaped aortic wall thickening (*arrowheads*) (diameter, 8 mm) is noted in ascending and descending aorta without the evidence of ULP or aortic rupture on contrast-enhanced axial CT image at level of right main pulmonary artery. Maximal aortic diameter including false lumen is within normal range (37 mm). The combination of these findings may suggest benign prognosis of this IMH. (*B*) IMH involving ascending and descending aorta is nearly disappeared on follow-up axial CT image performed 10 months later. (*C*) Coronal MPR image performed on same day as *A* shows intramural hematoma (*arrows*) involving ascending aorta. (*D*) Marked improvement of IMH is noted on coronal MPR image performed on same day with *B*.

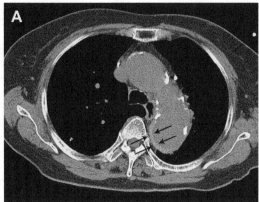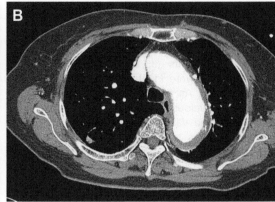

Fig. 16. Typical high attenuation of IMH on pre–contrast-enhanced CT in a patient with Stanford type B intramural hematoma. (*A*) High-density thickening of aortic wall (*arrows*) is noted on pre–contrast-enhanced axial CT image at the level of aortic arch. (*B*) After administration of contrast materials, IMH does not show contrast enhancement.

without ULP (**Fig. 15**) based on CT findings, although this may be changed at surgery. IMH with ULP can be further subdivided into IMH with intimal tear and IMH with PAU pathologically.

The treatment for IMH is essentially the same as classic AD. However, there is debate about the optimal treatment of type A IMH. Some studies reported that the prognosis of type A IMH is more favorable than that of Stanford type A dissection[45,46]; however, most of the studies that recommended conservative treatment of type A IMH did not disclose the size of the aorta or thickness of the IMH. In one study that recommended a conservative approach,[45] the mean diameter of the aorta and thickness of the IMH were unusually small (35 mm and 5.5 mm, respectively), making such a conclusion difficult to generalize.[34] Park and colleagues[34] suggested that type A IMH be treated by surgery unless all of the following criteria are satisfied: no aortic aneurysm (ie, aortic diameter <5 cm); small thickness of IMH (ie, <10 mm); no evidence of aortic rupture such as pericardial, mediastinal, or pleural hemorrhage; and no intimal defect in the proximal aorta on CT (see **Fig. 15**).

The major CT finding on pre–contrast-enhanced CT is crescentic or ring-shaped high attenuation of the aortic wall (**Fig. 16**).[6,7,18,21] Aortic wall thickening demonstrated on contrast-enhanced CT may be missed without special attention or alternatively may be confused with atheromatous mural thrombus.[6,7] Although wall thickening of a long segment in a nondilated aorta and a smooth internal border favor IMH rather than mural thrombus,[18,21] a pre–contrast-enhanced CT is highly recommended for definitive diagnosis of IMH.

Several CT findings are associated with an adverse outcome of IMH. Sueyoshi and colleagues[39] suggested that new ULP occurring

on follow-up CT is predictive of an adverse outcome. Thickness of IMH greater than 11 mm was associated with progression of IMH to frank aortic dissection.[46] Normal aortic diameter more likely led to a good prognosis for IMH.[47] However, the natural history of IMH varies from complete resolution to formation of aortic aneurysm or pseudoaneurysm, overt dissection, or aortic rupture.[48] Therefore, patients in whom IMH is not operated on should be followed closely to detect complications.

PENETRATING ATHEROSCLEROTIC ULCER

Clinical manifestations of PAU are quite similar to classic AD although the former tends to occur in

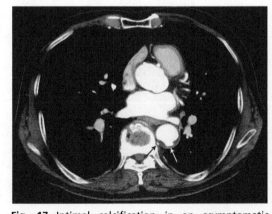

Fig. 17. Intimal calcification in an asymptomatic patient with atheromatous ulcer. Although atheromatous ulcer (*white arrow*) has a similar appearance with PAU, atheromatous ulcer does not extend over intimal calcification (*black arrow*) and expected aortic margin on contrast-enhanced axial CT image at the level of left atrium. This is an important differential point to distinguish atheromatous ulcer from PAU.

elderly patients with severe atherosclerosis and hypertension. By definition, PAU forms when ulcerated atherosclerotic plaque breaks down the internal elastic lamina and propagates into the media, often resulting in IMH. The most common site of PAU is the middle or lower thoracic descending aorta. Therefore, the typical CT finding of PAU is ULP in the middle or lower descending thoracic aorta often accompanied by IMH and severe atherosclerotic change of aortic wall.[49]

PAU should be differentiated from atheromatous ulcer in which ulceration is confined within intima. The location of intimal calcification can be helpful in this situation.[6] Atheromatous ulcer (**Fig. 17**) often overlies the expected aortic contour and calcified intima, whereas PAU extends outwardly beyond the expected aortic margin

and calcified intima.[6,7,18] However, if there is a calcified mural thrombus, differentiation between two entities can be challenging.

Park and colleagues[34] suggested that CT findings of IMH with an entry tear cannot be reliably differentiated from IMH with PAU. In most studies of the natural history of PAU, the diagnosis of PAU was not confirmed pathologically,[50–53] thus making inclusion of some cases of IMH with intimal tear highly probable.

In addition, a precise understanding of the natural history of PAU is further complicated because a variable proportion of asymptomatic cases of PAU were included in most previous studies. As a result, the natural history of PAU is reported to range from fairly benign[50,51] to extremely malignant.[52,54] Therefore, a well-designed

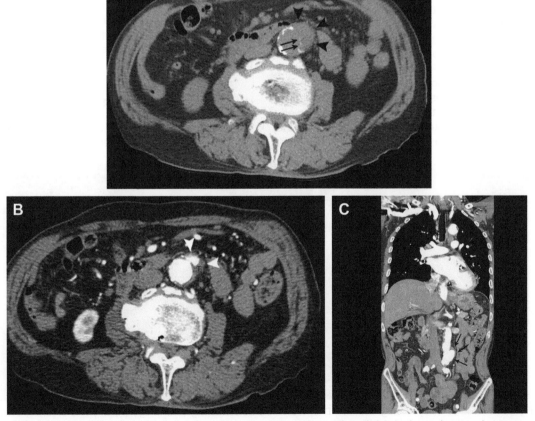

Fig. 18. Abdominal saccular pseudoaneurysm in an asymptomatic patient. Abdominal saccular pseudoaneurysm (*arrowheads*) is noted on pre–contrast (*A*) and contrast-enhanced (*B*) axial CT image at the level of distal abdominal aorta. Note the low attenuation of aortic wall thickening or mural thrombus (T) and intimal calcification (*arrows*) overlying saccular pseudoaneurysm. (*C*) Coronal MPR image also shows distal abdominal saccular pseudoaneurysm (*arrows*).

prospective study in which PAU is confirmed pathologically is needed to elucidate its natural history and prognosis as well as CT features that distinguish IMH with PAU from IMH with intimal tear.

CT features of asymptomatic PAU can be similar or identical to that of saccular pseudoaneurysm. It is often accompanied by aortic wall thickening of low attenuation on pre–contrast-enhanced CT (**Fig. 18**), which corresponds to chronic IMH or mural thrombus, whereas IMH of high attenuation on pre–contrast-enhanced CT is often demonstrated in PAU cases presented with AAS. Therefore, it is rational to classify asymptomatic PAU separately from PAU with acute IMH which is a subtype of AAS.

There is also debate about the relationship between the size of PAU and natural history.[55] One study suggested that a depth (>10 mm) and diameter of ulcer (>20 mm) are independent predictors of lesion progression such as further thickening of IMH, progression into overt AD, or aortic rupture on follow-up CT.[52] In contrast, Cho and colleagues[53] suggested that there are no predictors of adverse outcomes except for aortic rupture at presentation. Therefore, interval change on follow-up CT rather than size of the PAU on initial CT is likely to be more reliable in determining treatment options or prognosis.[49]

As IMH with PAU tends to occur in elderly patients with comorbidities, it is usually treated conservatively unless accompanied by impending or frank rupture. With recent advances in interventional technique, stent-graft insertion may be the best option in such patients.

THE ROLE OF TRIPLE RULE-OUT PROTOCOL IN PATIENTS WITH UNSPECIFIED ACUTE CHEST PAIN

Rapid and accurate diagnosis of AAS can be life saving, as the highest mortality occurs in the initial 48 hours. Unfortunately, studies reported that a delayed diagnosis of more than 24 hours after admission occurs in up to 39% of AD.[2,3] This is mainly caused by a significant overlap of clinical symptoms among AAS and ACS or PE, and relatively infrequent occurrence of AAS.[4,5] Accordingly, emergency department (ED) physicians and cardiologists risk misdiagnosing AAS as ACS or PE (**Fig. 19**). As the treatment of AAS is quite different from ACS or PE, catastrophic results may occur if patients with AAS mistakenly receive anticoagulant therapy such as heparin or a thrombolytic agent.

As AAS cannot always be reliably differentiated from ACS and PE on clinical grounds, an accurate, noninvasive imaging modality is desirable to make this distinction.[56,57] A triple rule-out protocol, essentially an ECG-gated study of the entire thorax aimed at these three diagnoses can be valuable. However, because of the fairly high radiation dose, the triple rule-out protocol should be performed only in patients with unspecified acute chest pain in whom the potential benefit justifies the radiation dose.[57,58]

UNSTABLE AORTIC ANEURYSM

Thoracic aortic aneurysm is diagnosed when the diameter of the aorta exceeds 5 cm.[18] The size

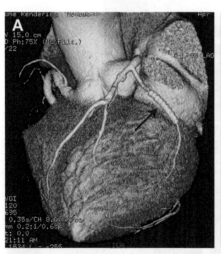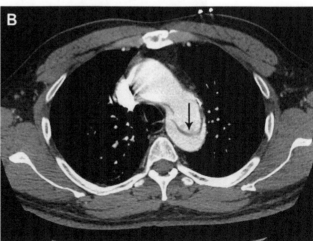

Fig. 19. A case of delayed diagnosis of AD as ACS. Volume rendering (VR) image (*A*) shows a coronary stent (*arrow*) inserted in proximal left circumflex artery on coronary CT angiography performed on 10 months before the onset of symptoms. Because of the history of coronary heart disease and nonspecific nature of chest pain in this patient, the ED physician considered non-ST elevated myocardial infarction (NSTEMI) or unstable angina (UA) as a first diagnostic concern. However, contrast-enhanced axial CT image (*B*) performed 48 hours after the onset of symptoms at the level of aortic arch demonstrates Stanford type B dissection (*arrow*).

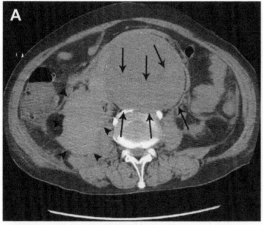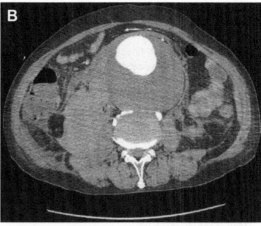

Fig. 20. Ruptured abdominal aortic aneurysm in a 69-year-old man. Abdominal aortic aneurysm about 10 cm in diameter is noted on pre–contrast (*A*) and post–contrast (*B*) enhanced axial CT image at the level of distal abdominal aorta. Faint high attenuation of aneurysmal wall (*arrows*) is consistent with crescent sign. Note hematoma (*arrowheads*) of high attenuation around right psoas muscle which indicates rupture of aortic aneurysm.

threshold for surgical repair of a thoracic aortic aneurysm in the ascending and descending aorta is 5.5 cm and 6.5 cm, respectively.[59] As the diameter of thoracic aortic aneurysm increases, the risk of aortic rupture increases according to Laplace's law. Rapid increase in the size of the thoracic aortic aneurysm (ie, aortic diameter increase more than 1 cm per year) also strongly correlates with aortic rupture.[60] Endovascular stent-graft repair is an alternative therapeutic option in patients with a large aortic aneurysm accompanied by multiple comorbidities. Thoracic aortic aneurysm often does not produce symptoms by itself, but may be associated with vague chest pain resulting from compression of adjacent structures.

In contrast, unstable aortic aneurysm is characterized by severe chest pain. High attenuation of the aneurysmal aortic wall on pre–contrast-enhanced CT (ie, crescent sign) indicates hemorrhage or hematoma into aortic wall (ie, impending aortic rupture) (**Fig. 20**).[61] Three-dimensional post-processing techniques help to measure accurately the size of aortic aneurysm and to discriminate which aneurysms have suitable anatomy for aortic stent-graft insertion.[27,62]

SUMMARY

MDCT plays an important role in the rapid and accurate diagnosis of AAS. Precise understanding of the current concepts and various CT features of subtypes of AAS is helpful in diagnosing AAS and improving patient outcome.

REFERENCES

1. Hirst AE Jr, Johns VJ Jr, Kime SW Jr. Dissecting aneurysms of the aorta: a review of 505 cases. Medicine 1958;37:217–79.
2. Viljanen T. Diagnostic difficulties in aortic dissection. Retrospective study of 89 surgically treated patients. Ann Chir Gynaecol 1986;75:328–32.
3. Klompas M. Does this patient have an acute thoracic aortic dissection? JAMA 2002;287:2262–72.
4. Hagan PG, Nienaber CA, Isselbacher EM, et al. The international registry of acute aortic dissection (IRAD): new insights into an old disease. JAMA 2000;283:897–903.
5. Abcarian PW, Sweet JD, Watabe JT, et al. Role of a quantitative D-dimer assay in determining the need for CT angiography of acute pulmonary embolism. AJR Am J Roentgenol 2004;182:1377–81.
6. Macura KJ, Corl FM, Fishman EK, et al. Pathogenesis in acute aortic syndromes: aortic dissection, intramural hematoma, and penetrating atherosclerotic aortic ulcer. AJR Am J Roentgenol 2003;181:309–16.
7. Chiles C, Carr JJ. Vascular diseases of the thorax: evaluation with multidetector CT. Radiol Clin North Am 2005;43:543–69.
8. Roberts WC. Aortic dissection: anatomy, consequences, and causes. Am Heart J 1981;101:195–214.
9. Larson EW, Edwards WD. Risk factors for aortic dissection: a necropsy study of 161 cases. Am J Cardiol 1984;53:849–55.
10. Murdoch JL, Walker BA, Halpern BL, et al. Life expectancy and causes of death in the Marfan syndrome. N Engl J Med 1972;286:804–8.

11. Matter SG, Kumar AG, Lumsden AB. Vascular complications in Ehlers-Danlos syndrome. Am Surg 1994;60:827–31.

12. Rogers FB, Osler TM, Shackford SR. Aortic dissection after trauma: case report and review of the literature. J Trauma 1996;41:906–8.

13. Rashid J, Eisenberg MJ, Topol EJ. Cocaine-induced aortic dissection. Am heart J 1996;132:1301–4.

14. Pumphrey CW, Fay T, Weir I. Aortic dissection during pregnancy. Br Heart J 1986;55:106–8.

15. Khan IA, Nair CK. Clinical, diagnostic, and management perspectives of aortic dissection. Chest 2002; 122:311–28.

16. von Kodolitsch Y, Schwartz AG, Nienaber CA. Clinical prediction of acute aortic dissection. Arch Intern Med 2000;160:2977–82.

17. Manghat NE, Morgan-Hughes GJ, Roobottom CA. Multi-detector row computed tomography: imaging in acute aortic syndrome. Clin Radiol 2005;60(12): 1256–67.

18. Bhalla S, West OC. CT of nontraumatic thoracic aortic emergencies. Semin Ultrasound CT MR 2005;26:281–304.

19. Salvolini L, Renda P, Fiore D, et al. Acute aortic syndromes: role of multi-detector row CT. Eur J Radiol 2008;65:350–8.

20. Batra P, Bigoni B, Manning J, et al. Pitfalls in the diagnosis of thoracic aortic dissection at CT angiography. Radiographics 2000;20:309–20.

21. Castaner E, Andreu M, Gallardo X, et al. CT in nontraumatic acute thoracic aortic disease: typical and atypical features and complications. Radiographics 2003;23:S93–110.

22. Johnson TR, Nikolaou K, Wintersperger BJ, et al. Optimization of contrast material administration for electrocardiogram-gated computed tomographic angiography of the chest. J Comput Assist Tomogr 2007;31:265–71.

23. Roos JE, Willmann JK, Weishaupt D, et al. Thoracic aorta: motion artifact reduction with retrospective and prospective electrocardiography-assisted multi-detector row CT. Radiology 2002;222: 271–7.

24. Morgan-Hughes GJ, Marshall AJ, Roobottom CA. Refined computed tomography of the thoracic aorta: the impact of electrocardiographic assistance. Clin Radiol 2003;58:581–8.

25. Yoshida S, Akiba H, Tamakawa M, et al. Thoracic involvement of type A aortic dissection and intramural hematoma: diagnostic accuracy-comparison of emergency helical CT and surgical findings. Radiology 2003;228:430–5.

26. Hayter RG, Rhea JT, Small A, et al. Suspected aortic dissection and other aortic disorders: multi-detector row CT in 373 cases in the emergency setting. Radiology 2006;238:841–52.

27. Fattori R, Napoli G, Lovato L, et al. Descending thoracic aortic diseases: stent-graft repair. Radiology 2003;229:176–83.

28. Therasse E, Soulez G, Giroux MF, et al. Stent-graft placement for the treatment of thoracic aortic diseases. Radiographics 2005;25:157–73.

29. Iezzi R, Cotroneo AR, Marano R, et al. Endovascular treatment of thoracic aortic diseases: follow-up and complications with multi-detector computed tomography angiography. Eur J Radiol 2008;65:365–76.

30. Williams DM, Lee DY, Hamilton BH, et al. The dissected aorta: part III. Anatomy and radiologic diagnosis of branch-vessel compromise. Radiology 1997;203:37–44.

31. Lepage MA, Quint LE, Sonnad SS, et al. Aortic dissection: CT features that distinguish true lumen from false lumen. AJR Am J Roentgenol 2001;177:207–11.

32. Williams DM, Joshi A, Dake MD, et al. Aortic cobwebs: an anatomic marker identifying the false lumen in aortic dissection-imaging and pathologic correlation. Radiology 1994;190:167–74.

33. Kapoor V, Ferris JV, Fuhrman CR, et al. Intimomedial rupture: a new CT finding to distinguish true from false lumen in aortic dissection. AJR Am J Roentgenol 2004;183:109–12.

34. Park KH, Lim C, Choi JH, et al. Prevalence of aortic intimal defect in surgically treated acute type A intramural hematoma. Ann Thorac Surg 2008;86: 1494–500.

35. Beauchesne LM, Veinot JP, Brais MP, et al. Acute aortic intimal tear without a mobile flap mimicking an intramural hematoma. J Am Soc Echocardiogr 2003;16:285–8.

36. Berdat PA, Carrel T. Aortic dissection limited to the ascending aorta mimicking intramural hematoma. Eur J Cardiothorac Surg 1999;15:108–9.

37. Neri E, Capannini G, Carone E, et al. Evolution toward dissection of an intramural hematoma of the ascending aorta. Ann Thorac Surg 1999;68: 1855–6.

38. Vilacosta I, Román JA. Acute aortic syndrome. Heart 2001;85:365–8.

39. Sueyoshi E, Matsuoka Y, Imada T, et al. New development of an ulcerlike projection in aortic intramural hematoma: CT evaluation. Radiology 2002;224:536–41.

40. Jang YM, Seo JB, Lee YK, et al. Newly developed ulcer-like projection (ULP) in aortic intramural haematoma on follow-up CT: is it different from the ULP seen on the initial CT? Clin Radiol 2008;63: 201–6.

41. Eyler WR, Clark MD. Dissecting aneurysms of the aorta: roentgen manifestations including a comparison with other types of aneurysms. Radiology 1965;85:1047–57.

42. Nienaber CA, von Kodolitsch Y, Petersen B, et al. Intramural hemorrhage of the thoracic aorta.

Diagnostic and therapeutic implications. Circulation 1995;92:1465–72.

43. Krinsky GA, Rofsky NM, DeCorato DR, et al. Thoracic aorta: comparison of gadolinium-enhanced three-dimensional MR angiography with conventional MR imaging. Radiology 1997;202:183–93.

44. Coady MA, Rizzo JA, Elefteriades JA. Pathologic variants of thoracic aortic dissections: penetrating atherosclerotic ulcers and intramural hematomas. Cardiol Clin 1999;17:637–57.

45. Shon DW, Jung JW, Oh BH, et al. Should ascending aortic intramural hematoma be treated surgically? Am J Cardiol 2001;87:1024–6.

46. Song JM, Kim HS, Song JK, et al. Usefulness of the initial noninvasive imaging study to predict the adverse outcomes in the medical treatment of acute type A aortic intramural hematoma. Circulation 2003; 108(Suppl 1):II324–8.

47. Evangelista A, Dominguez R, Sebastia C, et al. Long-term follow-up of aortic intramural hematoma: predictors of outcome. Circulation 2003;108:583–9.

48. Sueyoshi E, Matsuoka Y, Sakamoto I, et al. Fate of intramural hematoma of the aorta: CT evaluation. J Comput Assist Tomogr 1997;21:931–8.

49. Hayashi H, Matsuoka Y, Sakamoto I, et al. Penetrating atherosclerotic ulcer of the aorta: imaging features and disease concept. Radiographics 2000;20:995–1005.

50. Quint LE, William DM, Francis IR, et al. Ulcerlike lesions of the aorta: imaging features and natural history. Radiology 2001;218:719–23.

51. Hirris JA, Bis KG, Glover JL, et al. Penetrating atherosclerotic ulcers of the aorta. J Vasc Surg 1994;19:90–8.

52. Ganaha F, Miller DC, Sugimoto K, et al. Prognosis of aortic intramural hematoma with or without penetrating atherosclerotic ulcer: a clinical and radiological analysis. Circulation 2002;106:342–8.

53. Cho KR, Stanson AW, Potter DD, et al. Penetrating atherosclerotic ulcer of the descending thoracic aorta and arch. J Thorac Cardiovasc Surg 2004; 127:1393–401.

54. Coady MA, Rizzo JA, Hammond GL, et al. Penetrating ulcer of the thoracic aorta: what is it? How do we recognize it? How do we manage it? J Vasc Surg 1998;27:1006–15.

55. Jean J, Waite S, White CS. Nontraumatic thoracic emergencies. Radiol Clin North Am 2006;44:273–93.

56. Takakuwa KM, Halpern EJ. Evaluation of a "triple rule-out" coronary CT angiography protocol: use of 64-section CT in low-to-moderate risk emergency department patients suspected of having acute coronary syndrome. Radiology 2008;248:438–46.

57. Lee HY, Yoo SM, White CS. Coronary CT angiography in emergency department patients with acute chest pain: triple rule-out protocol versus dedicated coronary CT angiography. Int J Cardiovasc Imaging 2009;25:319–26.

58. Picano E. Sustainability of medical imaging. BMJ 2004;328:578–80.

59. Coady MA, Rizzo JA, Elefteriades JA. Developing surgical intervention criteria for thoracic aortic aneurysms. Cardiol Clin 1999;17:827–39.

60. Scott RA, Tisi PV, Ashton HA, et al. Abdominal aortic aneurysm rupture rates: a 7-year follow-up of the entire abdominal aortic aneurysm population detected by screening. J Vasc Surg 1998;28:124–8.

61. Gonsalves CF. The hyperattenuating crescent sign. Radiology 1999;211:37–8.

62. Thurnher SA, Grabenwoger M. Endovascular treatment of thoracic aortic aneurysms: a review. Eur Radiol 2002;12:1370–87.

Multidetector CT Scan in the Evaluation of Chest Pain of Nontraumatic Musculoskeletal Origin

Travis J. Hillen, MD, MS, Daniel E. Wessell, MD, PhD*

KEYWORDS

• Multidetector CT • Chest pain • Musculoskeletal

Chest pain is a very common symptom resulting in emergency department visits and admissions to the hospital.[1,2] There are many potential causes of acute nontraumatic chest pain ranging from relatively benign causes, such as gastroesophageal reflux, to life-threatening causes, such as myocardial infarction. While history and physical examination, along with targeted basic diagnostic testing, remain the mainstay in the evaluation of chest pain, advanced imaging with a thin-collimation multidetector computed tomography scan (MDCT) plays an increasing role. In the emergency setting, MDCT is obtained routinely to evaluate acute chest pain in suspected cases of pulmonary embolism (PE) and aortic dissection. Additionally, at many sites the MDCT triple rule-out is being used for suspected coronary artery disease.

The MDCT-imaging protocols for PE and aortic dissection studies use relatively high kilovolts peak and mAs with thin collimation. These parameters are typically set to values that are very similar to those used in dedicated musculoskeletal imaging protocols. These imaging techniques, along with dedicated reconstructions using high-resolution reconstruction kernels and multiplanar reformatting, allow for superb imaging of the

thoracic musculoskeletal structures. Thus, the images obtained with thin-collimation MDCT are excellent for evaluating PE and aortic dissection,[3] plus other causes of chest pain, including chest pain of musculoskeletal origin.

Musculoskeletal diseases are very common causes of chest pain in the general population (approximately 10%–15% adults and 24% children).[4–6] One of the most common causes of musculoskeletal chest pain, costochondritis, is routinely diagnosed by physical examination and not by chest CT scan.[7,8] However, many other causes of musculoskeletal chest pain can be visualized on thin-collimation MDCT examinations. These include (1) infectious causes, such as discitis/osteomyelitis and sternoclavicular septic arthritis; (2) rheumatic causes, such as ankylosing spondylitis (AS), with and without fracture; and synovitis, acne, palmoplantar pustulosis, hyperostosis, and osteitis (SAPHO); and (3) systemic diseases resulting in bone findings, such as osteoporosis with insufficiency fractures, neoplasm (with or without pathologic fracture), and sickle cell disease with bone infarcts or avascular necrosis. These entities are not the most common causes of acute nontraumatic chest pain and may

This article originally appeared in *Radiologic Clinics of North America*, Volume 48, Issue 1, January 2010.
Division of Diagnostic Radiology, Section of Musculoskeletal Radiology, Mallinckrodt Institute of Radiology, Washington University School of Medicine, 660 South Euclid Avenue, Campus Box 8131, St Louis, MO 63110, USA
* Corresponding author.
E-mail address: wesselld@mir.wustl.edu (D.E. Wessell).

Thorac Surg Clin 20 (2010) 167–173
doi:10.1016/j.thorsurg.2009.12.012
1547-4127/10/$ – see front matter © 2010 Elsevier Inc. All rights reserved.

not even be in the initial differential diagnosis when a thin-collimation MDCT chest CT scan is ordered. However, in total they do account for a significant minority of the causes of acute chest pain. Given the excellent capability of thin-section MDCT with coronal and sagittal reformatting to depict these musculoskeletal disease entities, the cardiothoracic imager must have a basic familiarity with their imaging appearances.

INFECTIOUS CAUSES OF CHEST PAIN
Discitis/Osteomyelitis

Discitis/osteomyelitis is an uncommon cause of chest pain but is important to diagnose given the consequences of recognition failure. In adults, discitis can have a slow insidious onset and the classic signs of infection, fever and chills, may not be present. A common presentation is back pain. In adults, the infection is thought to most often arise via hematogenous spread of infection at another site (eg, upper respiratory tract infection, urinary tract infection). The most common infectious organism is *Staphylococcus aureus*, which accounts for greater than 50% of infections. Infection begins in the disk with loss of disk space and subsequent invasion or destruction of the adjacent vertebral body. The CT scan findings of early discitis/osteomyelitis are subtle and difficult to visualize in the axial plane.[9] MDCT with sagittal and coronal reformatations improves identification of early disk-height loss and endplate destruction.[10] On the sagittal and coronal reformatted images, all of the disk spaces can be viewed simultaneously and thus even subtle changes at

a single level are readily seen as being different from the adjacent levels. As the disease progresses the vertebral body involvement may become more advanced and potentially result in vertebral body collapse.

In some cases, there may be concomitant development of adjacent soft tissue infection or epidural abscess. While the disk and vertebral body involvement is often best seen on sagittal or coronal reformatted images with bone windowing, the adjacent soft tissue involvement is often best seen on the transverse (axial) images with soft tissue windowing. The exact extent and character of the soft tissue component may be better evaluated with magnetic resonance imaging.

Discitis/osteomyelitis may present with acute chest pain (**Fig. 1**). Sagittally reformatted images clearly demonstrate the disk-centered process with adjacent vertebral body destruction and provide a useful adjunct to transverse images. Windowing for bone and soft tissue allows for evaluation of both the involvement of the vertebral bodies and the adjacent soft tissues.

Disk space narrowing is very common owing to degenerative disk disease. The main diagnostic dilemma with dicsitis/osteomyelitis is differentiating it from degenerative disk disease. Degenerative disk disease results in disk-space narrowing, but is differentiated from discitis/osteomyelitis by the absence of endplate destruction at the adjacent vertebral bodies. In degenerative disk disease, the endplates can appear quite irregular because of remodeling, but are usually between normal and increased in density, without any destruction of the endplates. Additionally, discitis

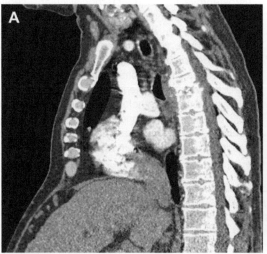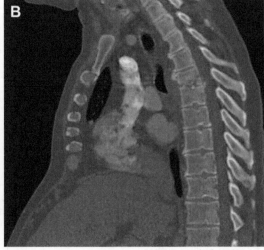

Fig. 1. Mid-sagittal image from a PE protocol MDCT examination for acute chest pain with soft-tissue (*A*) and bone (*B*) windowing demonstrating disk-centered destruction of midthoracicvertebral bodies with associated phlegmon consistent with discitis/osteomyelitis.

usually involves a single disk space while degenerative disk disease often, but not always, involves multiple levels. One important exception is discitis/osteomyelitis due to atypical organisms such as mycobacteria and fungi, which can involve multiple contiguous levels. Additionally, the indolent nature of these atypical infections can result in increased density of the vertebral bodies. The presence of an adjacent soft tissue mass or paraspinal fluid collection favors a diagnosis of discitis/osteomyelitis, be it of pyogenic or atypical origin.

Sternoclavicular Septic Arthritis

Sternoclavicular joint septic arthritis accounts for less than 1% of septic arthritis in the general population.[11] The most common organism is *Staphylococcus aureus*. The risk factors include intravenous drug abuse, diabetes mellitus, central line infection, immunosuppression, and distant infection. As with any suspected septic arthritis, in the vast majority of cases synovial fluid analysis is crucial and joint aspiration is often the best initial diagnostic and potentially therapeutic procedure. Therefore, it should not be delayed by advanced imaging. However, as in the case of discitis/osteomyelitis, septic arthritis may not be in the initial differential diagnosis and, thus, advanced imaging of this entity with CT scan may be obtained. CT scan findings include erosions of the manubrium and clavicle at the sternoclavicular joint with fluid and adjacent soft tissue swelling (**Fig. 2**) that, depending on the severity of the infection, can extend into the mediastinum.[12] The sternoclavicular joints can be evaluated on either the straight transverse images or on oblique coronal reformatted images set up off a midline sagittal image along the body of the sternum.

RHEUMATIC CAUSES OF CHEST PAIN
AS

AS is an inflammatory disorder that typically begins as inflammation at the tendinous and ligamentous insertions on the bones. The disorder typically waxes and wanes with new reactive bone formation occurring with each flare of the disease. AS classically affects the axial joints with findings of sacroiliitis and progressive ossification of the spinal ligaments, disks, and facet joints. Approximately one-half million people in the United States have AS, with a 3 to 1 ratio of men to women. A common early presenting feature of the disease includes the presence of chest pain,[13] which often worsens with expansion of the thoracic cavity. Because of this, the chest pain in AS can easily be mistaken for pleuritic chest pain. Thus, it is common for patients with

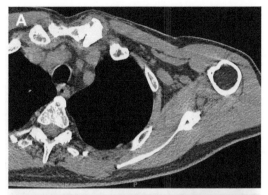

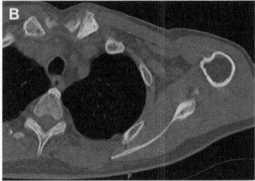

Fig. 2. Transverse (axial) image with soft tissue (*A*) and bone (*B*) windowing from a MDCT examination of the chest in a patient with suspected sternoclavicular osteomyelitis. There is joint-centered destruction of the left sternoclavicular joint with associated abscess. As should be the case with any case of suspected septic arthritis, the left sternoclavicular joint was aspirated and the patient underwent subsequent irrigation and debridement of the left sternoclavicular joint.

AS to undergo thin-section MDCT of the chest as part of the evaluation of their chest pain.

While they are easily recognizable on conventional lateral radiographs of the thoracic spine, the gracile syndesmophytes, which are characteristic of AS, are not as easily recognizable on direct transverse (axial) CT scan images. Sagittal reformats readily depict the syndesmophytes and coronal reformats satisfactorily demonstrate the ossification that can be seen within the costal cartilages. In suspected cases, correlation with any available pelvic imaging may be helpful to evaluate for the classic changes of sacroiliitis or ankylosis of the sacroiliac joints.

With increasing ossification of the spine, there is less mobility and increasing risk for fracture. Patients with AS may develop spinal fractures with even minor trauma (**Fig. 3**). Spinal fracture in a patient with AS can have serious consequences, including spinal instability with neurologic defects

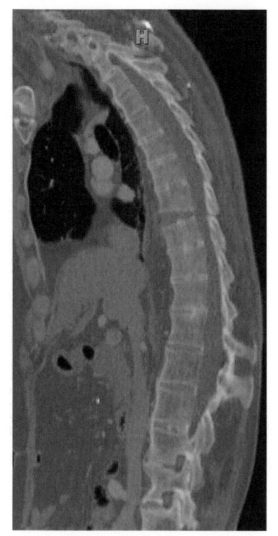

Fig. 3. Sagittal reformatted image obtained from a thin-section MDCT examination performed for aortic dissection. This patient's acute upper back pain was thought to be due to aortic dissection given his relatively minor trauma. Note the findings of AS, including ossification of the spinal ligaments and disks. There is a fracture of the ossified anterior and posterior longitudinal ligaments with associated widening of the disk space between T9 and T10. Fractures through the syndesmophytes at the T9-T10 level with widening of the disk space at this level suggest disruption of the anterior and posterior longitudinal ligaments. Although not seen on this midline sagittal image, the fracture extended to involve the posterior elements. The patient also underwent MR imaging, which confirmed disruption of the anterior and posterior longitudinal ligaments without signal abnormality in the cord. The patient subsequently underwent surgical stabilization via an instrumented posterior spinal fusion from T7 to T12.

secondary to central canal stenosis or hematoma.[14,15]

SAPHO Syndrome

SAPHO syndrome is a rare disease of unknown cause with findings including synovitis, acne, palmoplantar pustulosis, hyperostosis, and osteitis. Approximately 28% of patients with palmoplantar pustulosis have anterior chest wall pain and 18% of these patients have radiographic anterior chest wall changes.[16] Usually, SAPHO involves the anterior chest wall followed by the spine.[17,18] MDCT evaluation of the anterior chest wall demonstrates hyperostotic and erosive changes (**Fig. 4**) with joint space narrowing most commonly at the sternocostoclavicular joint and hyperostosis and ankylosis at the costochondral junctions.[17] The use of reformatted images in the coronal oblique plane oriented parallel to the sternum effectively demonstrates these findings. Patients with SAPHO also commonly have findings in the spine, including erosions of the vertebral body corners, osteosclerosis, paravertebral ossifications, and discovertebral junction lesions.[17–19] The differential diagnosis for the lesions of the anterior chest wall and spine includes inflammatory and crystalline arthropathies. However, the physical examination findings described above should help lead to the diagnosis.

SYSTEMIC DISEASES WITH MUSCULOSKELETAL FINDINGS
Osteoporosis with Insufficiency Fracture

Osteoporosis is a common disorder associated with aging, characterized by decreased bone mineral density affecting more women than men. With decreasing bone mineral density, there is resultant increased risk for fracture. Common locations for osteoporotic fractures include the femur, spine, pelvis, and sacrum. In 1995 alone, the estimated expense for the treatment of osteoporotic fractures was $13.8 billion.[20] Osteoporotic compression fractures in the thoracic spine commonly result in both back and chest pain.[21] Another cause of chest pain related to osteoporotic fractures includes sternal insufficiency fractures, which are often, but not always, associated with increasing thoracic kyphosis (**Fig. 5**).[22,23] Sternal insufficiency fractures have been shown to cause chest pain similar to the chest pain of myocardial infarction and PE.[24–26] MDCT evaluation of both vertebral compression fractures and sternal insufficiency fractures is best performed in the sagittal plane. Compression fractures of the spine are characterized by anterior loss of vertebral body height. If severe enough,

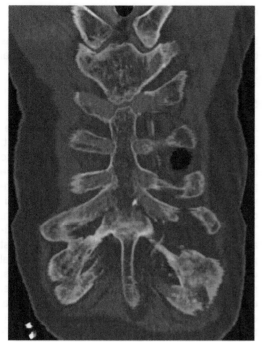

Fig. 4. Oblique coronal reformatted image along the plane of the sternal body from a MDCT examination originally ordered as a PE protocol to evaluate the patient's chest pain and shortness of breath. Examination demonstrates hyperostosis of the costochondral junctions with associated sternoclavicular erosions or inflammatory arthritis in a patient with SAPHO. While this can be an age-related change, the extensive ossification along with ankylosis, and the erosions at the right sternoclavicular joint, suggest SAPHO syndrome. Given the imaging findings, the clinical examination can be directed to evaluate for typical skin changes.

they can extend into the posterior aspect of the vertebral body and be associated with retropulsion of bone fragments resulting in central canal narrowing. Sternal insufficiency fractures are characterized as either buckling (displaced) or nondisplaced.[22,23]

Neoplasm with or Without Pathologic Fracture

Metastatic disease to the skeleton is the third most common location of metastases and is much more common than primary malignancy of the skeleton.[27] Metastases or primary skeletal neoplasms of the bones in the chest can involve the spine, ribs, sternum, scapulae, and clavicles. Metastases are often painful with or without associated pathologic fracture.[28] Fractures of metastases to bones in the chest often occur with no trauma or only minimal trauma and may result in chest pain.[29] MDCT is more sensitive than conventional

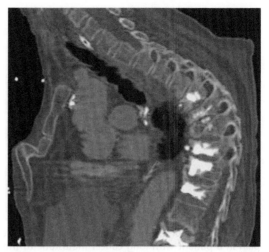

Fig. 5. PE protocol MDCT examination for acute chest pain in a patient with osteoporosis from chronic steroid treatment post-lung transplantation shows a marked thoracic kyphosis secondary to multiple vertebral insufficiency fractures and associated sternal insufficiency fractures.

radiographs at detecting metastases and is able to detect metastases in bone marrow before cortical destruction has occurred.[28,30] Imaging features are varied depending on the primary malignancy and the extent of involvement of the bones. Typically, the lesions are lytic, blastic (sclerotic), or a combination of both (**Fig. 6**). In addition to the detection of metastases, MDCT is often used as imaging guidance for skeletal biopsy if the primary cancer is not known.

Sickle Cell Disease with Bone Infarcts

Sickle cell anemia is the most common single gene disorder affecting black Americans. Acute chest pain in sickle cell disease is most often the result of either pain crisis or acute chest syndrome. Pain crisis is the most common cause of hospitalization in patients with sickle cell disease and is the result of acute bone ischemia or infarct.[31] Acute chest syndrome is defined as an acute illness associated with an infiltrate on chest radiography.[32] It is thought to represent a common clinical manifestation of several different pathologic processes, including fat embolism secondary to bone infarct, infection, or vascular occlusion.[33] MDCT is sometimes used in the evaluation of sickle cell disease associated acute chest pain to evaluate for causes of the chest pain including PE. The bone infarcts associated with acute chest pain are not readily identified by MDCT in the acute setting. However, manifestations of chronic bone infarction (**Fig. 7**) and avascular necrosis

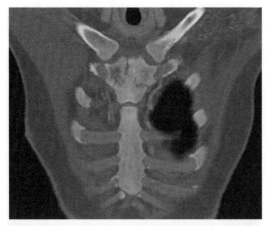

Fig. 6. PE protocol MDCT examination for acute chest pain in a patient with lung cancer metastatic to the manubrium with a pathologic fracture. The patient had a known history of lung cancer and the MDCT examination was obtained to evaluate for suspected PE. While the presence of the lesion was evident on the straight transverse (axial) images, the extent of the lesion and the associated pathologic fracture is better elucidated on the coronal reformats.

are often seen on MDCT examinations in patients with sickle cell disease as H-shaped vertebral bodies, humeral head avascular necrosis, and as chronic infarcts in ribs, scapula, or vertebral bodies.[34]

SUMMARY

Acute nontraumatic chest pain is a common presenting symptom to the emergency department. Often, it is evaluated by MDCT with PE, aortic dissection, or coronary artery protocols. The parameters used for these MDCT protocols are very similar to those used in protocols for dedicated imaging of the musculoskeletal system. Thus, these studies are not only effective in evaluating for these traditional vascular causes of chest pain, but also in evaluating musculoskeletal causes of chest pain, including those of infectious, rheumatologic, and systemic causes. In essence, every MDCT of the chest is also a musculoskeletal examination of the chest and anyone interpreting these images must be familiar with the MDCT-imaging appearance of common musculoskeletal causes of acute nontraumatic chest pain.

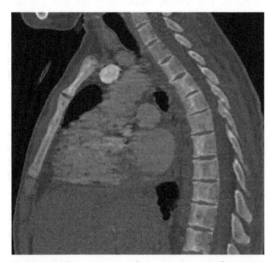

Fig. 7. Mid-line sagittal reformatted image from a PE protocol MDCT examination of the chest. Bone findings of sickle cell disease, including sternal and vertebral body bone infarcts and multiple H-shaped vertebral bodies. The extensive areas of patchy increased bone density seen in the vertebral bodies and sternum are classic for old bone infarcts. In the acute setting, these infarcts can be extremely painful. While infarcts are typically not visible on MDCT in the acute setting, the presence of old bone infarcts on an otherwise normal MDCT examination of the chest should raise suspicion that an acute bone infarct may be the cause of the patient's pain.

REFERENCES

1. Clinical policy for the initial approach to adults presenting with a chief complaint of chest pain, with no history of trauma. American College of Emergency Physicians. Ann Emerg Med 1995;25:274.
2. Graff LG, Dallara J, Ross MA, et al. Impact on the care of the emergency department chest pain patient from the Chest Pain Evaluation Registry (CHEPER) study. Am J Cardiol 1997;80:563.
3. Johnson TRC, Nikolaou K, Wintersperger BJ, et al. ECG-gated 64-MDCT angiography in the differential diagnosis of acute chest pain. AJR Am J Roentgenol 2007;188:76.
4. Karlson BW, Herlitz J, Pettersson P, et al. Patients admitted to the emergency room with symptoms indicative of acute myocardial infarction. J Intern Med 1991;230:251.
5. Selbst SM, Ruddy RM, Clark BJ, et al. Pediatric chest pain: a prospective study. Pediatrics 1988; 82:319.
6. Kocis KC. Chest pain in pediatrics. Pediatr Clin North Am 1999;46:189.
7. Disla E, Rhim HR, Reddy A, et al. Costochondritis. A prospective analysis in an emergency department setting. Arch Intern Med 1994;154:2466.
8. Habib PA, Huang GS, Mendiola JA, et al. Anterior chest pain: musculoskeletal considerations. Emerg Radiol 2004;11:37.
9. Stabler A, Reiser MF. Imaging of spinal infection. Radiol Clin North Am 2001;39:115.

10. Tali ET. Spinal infections. Eur J Radiol 2004;50:120.

11. Ross JJ, Shamsuddin H. Sternoclavicular septic arthritis: review of 180 cases. Medicine (Baltimore) 2004;83:139.

12. Pollack MS. Staphylococcal mediastinitis due to sternoclavicular pyoarthrosis: CT appearance. J Comput Assist Tomogr 1990;14:924.

13. Dawes PT, Sheeran TP, Hothersall TE. Chest pain—a common feature of ankylosing spondylitis. Postgrad Med J 1998;64:27.

14. Wang YF, Teng MMH, Chang CY, et al. Imaging manifestations of spinal fractures in ankylosing spondylitis. AJNR Am J Neuroradiol 2005;26:2067.

15. Hitchon PW, From AM, Brenton MD, et al. Fractures of the thoracolumbar spine complicating ankylosing spondylitis. J Neurosurg 2002;97(2 Suppl):218.

16. Jurik AG. Anterior chest wall involvement in patients with pustulosis palmoplantaris. Skeletal Radiol 1990;19:271.

17. Cotton A, Flipo RM, Mentre A, et al. SAPHO syndrome. Radiographics 1995;15:1147.

18. Boutin RD, Resnick D. The SAPHO syndrome: an evolving concept for unifying several idiopathic disorders of bone and skin. AJR Am J Roentgenol 1998;170:585.

19. Laredo JD, Vuillemin-Bodaghi V, Boutry N, et al. SAPHO syndrome: MR appearance of vertebral involvement. Radiology 2007;242:825.

20. Ray NF, Chan JK, Thamer M, et al. Medical expenditures for the treatment of osteoporotic fractures in the United States in 1995: report from the National Osteoporosis Foundation. J Bone Miner Res 1997;12:24.

21. Patel U, Skingle S, Campbell GA, et al. Clinical profile of acute vertebral compression fractures in osteoporosis. Rheumatology 1991;30:418.

22. Cooper K. Insufficiency fractures of the sternum: a consequence of thoracic kyphosis? Radiology 1988;167:471.

23. Chen C, Chandnani V, Kang HS, et al. Insufficiency fracture of the sternum caused by osteopenia: plain film findings in seven patients. AJR Am J Roentgenol 1990;154:1025.

24. Rutledge DI. Spontaneous fracture of the sternum simulating myocardial infarction. Postgrad Med 1962;32:502.

25. Vassalo L. Spontaneous fracture of the sternum simulating pulmonary embolism. Br J Clin Pract 1969;23:288.

26. Schapira D, Nachtigal A, Scharf Y. Spontaneous fracture of the sternum simulating myocardial infarction. Clin Rheumatol 1995;14:478.

27. Berretoni BA, Carter JR. Current concepts: review mechanisms of cancer metastasis to bone. J Bone Joint Surg 1986;68:308.

28. Rosenthal DI. Radiologic diagnosis of bone metastases. Cancer 1997;80:1595.

29. Rubens RD. Bone metastases—the clinical problem. Eur J Cancer 1998;34:210.

30. Helms CA, Cann CE, Brunelle FO, et al. Detection of bone-marrow metastases using quantitative computed tomography. Radiology 1981;140:745.

31. Kumar DS, Yadavali RP, Concepcion LA, et al. Acute chest pain in a young woman with a chronic illness. Br J Radiol 2008;81:261.

32. Lane P. Sickle cell disease. Pediatr Clin North Am 1996;43:639.

33. Lonergan GF, Cline DB, Abbondanzo SL. From the archives of the AFIP: sickle cell anemia. Radiographics 2001;21:971.

34. Keeley K, Buchanan GR. Acute infarction of long bones in children with sickle cell anemia. J Pediatr 1982;101:170.

Cross-Sectional Evaluation of Thoracic Lymphoma

Young A Bae, MD[a,b], Kyung Soo Lee, MD[a,*]

KEYWORDS

- Lymphoma • CT • Hodgkin lymphoma
- Thoracic neoplasms

Lymphomas are a diverse group of neoplastic disorders. They are divided into Hodgkin lymphoma (HL) and non-Hodgkin lymphoma (NHL) and further subdivisions depend on the histologic types.[1]

The presence and distribution of thoracic involvement are important in both tumor staging and treatment, especially when radiation therapy is planned.[2] Intrathoracic involvement is commoner in HL than NHL.[3,4] Although HL represents only 10% to 15% of all cases of lymphomas, approximately 85% of patients with HL have intrathoracic disease at presentation.[5] NHL represents about 85% to 90% of all cases of lymphoma and approximately 40% to 45% of patients with NHL have intrathoracic disease at the initial presentation.[4]

Although HL and NHL may have overlapping imaging findings, there are some significant differences in their radiologic features. In this article, we demonstrate the diverse radiologic features of thoracic lymphomas.

MEDIASTINAL INVOLVEMENT OF LYMPHOMAS

HL is the most common lymphoma presenting with mediastinal lymphadenopathy and most frequently involves lymph nodes in anterior mediastinal and paratracheal areas in a contiguous manner, and thus involves in decreasing order of frequency the nodes in the hilar, subcarinal, peridiaphragmatic, paraesophageal, and internal mammary areas (**Fig. 1**).[1] Nodular sclerosing HL, the commonest subtype, has a unique predilection for the nodes in the anterior mediastinum.

On CT, HL is characterized by the presence of a discrete anterior mediastinal mass with a lobulated contour. The tumor most commonly demonstrates homogeneous soft-tissue attenuation, although large lymph node masses may demonstrate heterogeneity with complex low attenuation representing necrosis, hemorrhage, or cystic degeneration (**Fig. 2**).[6] In the series by Hopper and colleagues,[7] necrotic and cystic-appearing mediastinal lymph nodes were noticed at presentation in 21% of cases of HL. Necrosis is observed most commonly in the nodular sclerosing and mixed cellularity cell types of HL and was not seen in the lymphocyte predominant variety.

In NHL, thoracic involvement is present in up to 45% of cases[8] and, most often, mediastinal lymphomatous involvement occurs as a disseminated or recurrent form of extrathoracic lymphoma. Generally, involved lymph nodes tend to be larger as compared with those in HL and have a predilection for noncontiguous or hematogenous spread to thoracic and distant nodal and extranodal sites.[9,10] Unlike HL, in which anatomic sites of involvement are important, the histologic subtype and tumor bulk are more important prognostic factors in NHL.

This article originally appeared in *Radiologic Clinics of North America*, Volume 46, Issue 2, March 2008.
This study was supported by the SRC/ERC Program of MOST/KOSEF (R11-2002-103).
[a] Department of Radiology, Center for Imaging Science, Samsung Medical Center, Sungkyunkwan University School of Medicine, 50, Ilwon-Dong, Kangnam-Ku, Seoul 135-710, Republic of Korea
[b] Department of Radiology, Hallym University College of Medicine, Pyongchon, Kyungki-do 431-070, Republic of Korea
* Corresponding author.
E-mail address: kyungs.lee@samsung.com (K.S. Lee).

Thorac Surg Clin 20 (2010) 175–186
doi:10.1016/j.thorsurg.2009.12.013

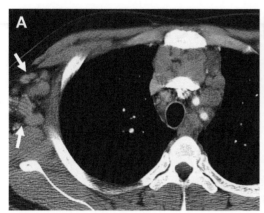
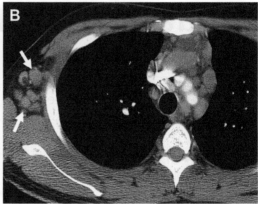

Fig. 1. Hodgkin lymphoma (nodular sclerosing type) in a 26-year-old man. (*A, B*) Transverse mediastinal-window CT (5.0-mm section thickness) scans obtained at levels of left innominate vein show conglomerated lymph node enlargement showing contiguous growth in prevascular (anterior mediastinal) and bilateral paratracheal areas. Also note enlarged lymph nodes (*arrows*) in the right axillary area.

Nodes in the paratracheal and anterior mediastinal areas are still the most common sites for NHL involvement followed by those in the subcarinal, hilar, posterior mediastinal (para-aortic, paravertebral, and retrocrural), and pericardial areas.[8] It is difficult to differentiate HL from NHL on the basis of nodal distribution alone.[1] Although lymphoma is one of the commonest mediastinal tumors, it is uncommon for either NHL or HL to be limited to the mediastinum at the time of diagnosis. The sole mediastinum involvement occurs in only about 5% of lymphoma cases.[11] On CT, the majority of tumors have a relatively homogeneous soft tissue density; large tumors commonly contain areas of low attenuation due to hemorrhage or necrosis (**Fig. 3**). Enlarged nodes in contiguous lymph node groups are frequently present.

Although there are many subtypes of NHL, large B-cell lymphoma and lymphoblastic lymphoma are the most common subtypes, primarily involving the anterior mediastinum (**Table 1**). Primary mediastinal large B-cell lymphomas usually present with large and lobulated anterior mediastinal masses and occur predominantly in young adults with a median age of 26 years (see **Fig. 3**).[12] Low attenuation areas of necrosis (see **Fig. 3**) within the mass were seen in 50% and calcification in 5%.[13] Also they often directly invade adjacent structures. Lymphoblastic lymphomas are highly aggressive and high-grade lymphomas, arising from thymic lymphocytes.[14] They usually occur in patients in the first to second decades of life. The involvement of extrathoracic structures and bone marrow is

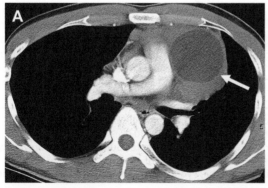
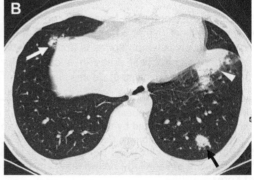

Fig. 2. Hodgkin lymphoma (nodular sclerosing type) in a 23-year-old man. (*A*) Transverse mediastinal-window CT (7.0-mm section thickness) scan shows left anterior mediastinal mass containing necrotic low-attenuation area (*arrow*) within mass. (*B*) Lung-window CT scan shows multiple poorly defined nodules (*arrows*) in both lower lobes and area of consolidation (*arrowhead*) in left lower lobe.

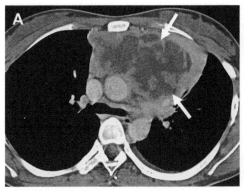
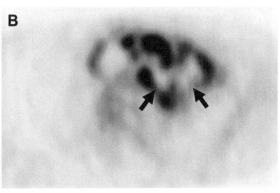

Fig. 3. Non-Hodgkin lymphoma (diffuse large B-cell type) in a 23-year-old woman. (*A*) Transverse mediastinal-window CT (3.0-mm section thickness) scan at the level of carina demonstrates large heterogeneous mass in anterior mediastinum containing large necrotic low attenuation areas (*arrows*). Also note small amount of left pleural effusion. (*B*) Transverse PET scan obtained at similar level to *A* demonstrates avid FDG uptake in peripheral portion of mass (maximum standardized uptake value = 16.9). Central portions of tumor are necrotic and show no significant FDG uptake (*arrows*).

commoner at presentation than in large B-cell lymphoma.[15]

Lymphoma is the third most common (12%, range; 1%–25%) malignant cause of superior vena cava syndrome following non–small cell lung cancer (50%, range; 43%–59%) and small cell lung cancer (22%, range; 7%–39%) (**Fig. 4**). Complete relief of symptoms is achieved with chemotherapy in approximately 80% of patients with NHL.[16]

Recurrent disease is common in the pericardial and internal mammary lymph nodes, since these nodes are usually not included in the radiation field.[1]

Dystrophic calcification may develop in involved lymph nodes following mediastinal radiation (**Fig. 5**).[17,18] The time interval between radiation and the appearance of calcification may be 1 to 9 years. Lymph node calcification before treatment is unusual, but has been associated with aggressive HL or NHL.[19]

When interpreting lymphomatous involvement of each nodal station based on CT images (**Table 2**), professional judgment should be used. A normal-sized lymph node may be involved with lymphoma and be PET (positron emission tomography) avid. Conversely, a lymph

Table 1
Frequent thoracic-primary lymphomas and their manifestations

Sites	Cell Types (WHO Classification)	Age/M:F Ratio	Common Imaging Findings
Mediastinum			
	Mediastinal (thymic) large B-cell lymphoma	Young adults/slightly F > M	Large lobulated anterior mediastinal mass ± low attenuation areas
	Lymphoblastic lymphoma	Young adults/M > F	
	Angioimmunoblastic lymphoma	Patients > 50 y/slightly M > F	Extensive hilar or mediastinal lymphadenopathy with enlargement of multiple nodal groups
Lung			
	Marginal zone lymphoma of BALT	Usually 6th and 7th decades/slightly F > M	Single or multiple nodule(s) and area(s) of consolidation
	Diffuse large B-cell lymphoma	Middle aged or elderly/slightly M > F	

Abbreviations: BALT, bronchus-associated lymphoid tissue; F, female; M, male; WHO, World Health Organization.

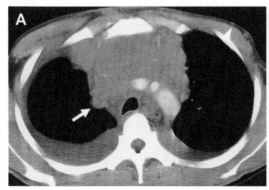
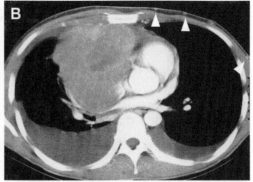

Fig. 4. Hodgkin lymphoma (nodular sclerosing type) in a 36-year-old man. Transverse mediastinal-window CT (5.0-mm section thickness) scans obtained at levels of aortic arch (*A*) and inferior pulmonary vein (*B*), respectively, show large anterior mediastinal mass. Also note total occlusion of superior vena cava (*arrow*) by mediastinal mass and collateral vessels (*arrowheads*) in left anterior chest wall. Bilateral pleural effusions are associated.

node could remain enlarged after successful treatment of lymphoma due to post-treatment changes.

[18]F-fluorodeoxyglucose (^{18}F-FDG) PET or PET-CT provides whole body images that allow a comprehensive assessment of disease extent during staging workup and follow-up evaluation. PET or PET-CT helps detect more disease sites and involved organs than conventional staging procedures including CT, and has a major impact on staging.[20] PET mostly upstaged disease when compared with CT.[21–23] Upstaging includes the detection of increased FDG uptake in normal-sized lymph nodes (usually <10 mm in diameter) as well as in extranodal sites. In addition, PET or PET-CT is of value for monitoring the response to various therapeutic protocols, for prognostic stratification, and for detection for relapse during follow-up.[24]

PET or PET-CT is superior to CT in differentiation of viable tumor, necrosis, and fibrosis.[25] With anatomic imaging modalities only, it is difficult to differentiate viable tumor from post-therapy changes such as scarring or fibrosis. Residual abnormalities after therapy in lymphomas are often encountered. However, only a maximum of 10% to 20% of residual masses is reported to be positive for lymphoma at the end of treatment.[26] In these situations of treatment completion or of partial cycle(s) of chemotherapy, ^{18}F-FDG PET has a high prognostic value as a valid imaging tool for post-treatment evaluation of malignant NHL and HL, as compared to conventional anatomic imaging techniques.[27]

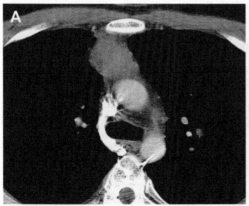
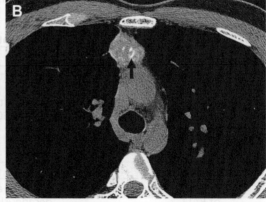

Fig. 5. Non-Hodgkin lymphoma (diffuse large B-cell type) in a 29-year-old man. (*A*) Transverse mediastinal-window CT (7.0-mm section thickness) scan obtained at level of azygos arch shows homogeneous soft tissue mass in anterior mediastinum. (*B*) CT scan obtained at same level as *A* 13 months after completion of radiation therapy demonstrates that tumor has decreased in size and contains dystrophic calcifications (*arrow*) within remaining tumor.

Table 2 Recommendations for upper limits of normal lymph node size in a short-axis diameter at CT		
Site	Location	Short-axis Nodal Diameter, mm
Axilla		10
Mediastinum	Subcarinal	12
	Paracardiac	8
	Retrocrural	6
	All other sites	10

Data from Hricak H, Husband J, Panicek DM. Oncologic imaging: essentials of reporting common cancers. Philadelphia: Saunders Elsevier; 2007.

LUNG

Pulmonary involvement is identified more often in HL than in NHL. The lung is more frequently involved in disseminated or recurrent disease than in primary disease.[3,28,29] Pulmonary parenchymal involvement may present with variable patterns. The commonest feature of pulmonary involvement is a direct extension from hilar or mediastinal nodes toward the lungs (**Fig. 6**); however, recurrences in the lung may be seen without associated lymphadenopathy. Other appearances include pulmonary nodules (with or without cavitation) (**Fig. 7**), lobar or segmental consolidation with air bronchograms representing peribronchial tumor infiltration without destruction of bronchial

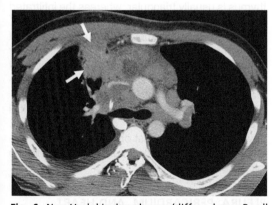

Fig. 6. Non-Hodgkin lymphoma (diffuse large B-cell type) showing direct lung involvement from adjacent mediastinal lymphadenopathy in a 17-year-old man. Transverse mediastinal-window CT (5.0-mm section thickness) scan obtained at level of main bronchi shows lymph node enlargement in anterior and middle mediastinal and left hilar areas. Note direct lung involvement from adjacent lymphadenopathy (*arrows*).

wall (**Fig. 8**), reticular pattern with bronchovascular bundle and interlobular septal thickening (**Fig. 9**), disseminated small nodules, cavitating masses, endobronchial lesion per se, and atelectasis or obstructive pneumonia secondary to endobronchial or nodal obstruction (**Fig. 10**).[4,25,30–32] When these findings are seen in a patient with newly diagnosed lymphoma, pulmonary involvement of lymphoma should be considered. In treated patients, however, it is often difficult to differentiate between pulmonary involvement and other benign conditions such as infection, radiation pneumonia, or drug-induced lung disease.[33,34] It is important to determine whether the tumor originated from lung parenchyma (primary pulmonary lymphoma), whether it originated in nodal tissue and direct spread to the adjacent lung, or whether it originated in nodal tissue and hematogenously spread to extranodal sites.[35]

Primary pulmonary lymphoma is rare and is encountered usually in NHL. The frequency of lymphoma arising from the lung is estimated to be less than 1% of all lymphomas.[36] The disease usually takes the form of bronchus-associated lymphoid tissue (BALT) lymphoma. In the BALT lymphoma, tumor infiltration develops in multiple extranodal mucosal sites through the lungs.[37] According to a report,[38] BALT lymphoma may manifest diverse patterns of lung abnormality on CT, but single or multiple nodule (or nodules) and area (or areas) of consolidation are the main patterns that occur in a majority (**Fig. 11**). Other patterns include the findings of bronchiectasis and cellular bronchiolitis and diffuse interstitial lung disease. Pleural involvement is rare. Another important finding is the indolent nature of the lesions. On PET-CT, most tumors showed subtle FDG uptake (see **Fig. 11**). It should be noted that some cases of BALT lymphoma would show increased uptake of ^{18}F-FDG, whereas others would not.

Most cases of primary high-grade pulmonary lymphoma are of B-cell type (**Fig. 12**); occasional cases of anaplastic lymphoma or peripheral T-cell lymphoma have also been reported.[39–41] Some tumors appear to be derived from the low-grade B-cell lymphoma.[42] Others occur in patients who have organ transplants (post-transplant lymphoproliferative disorder [PTLD]) or occur in association with AIDS (AIDS-related lymphoma [ARL]). The most common type of lymphoma in PTLD and ARL is B-cell NHL. PTLD represents an abnormal proliferation of lymphoid cells that is induced by the Epstein-Barr virus and progresses because of a compromised immune system. Nearly all patients (approximately 90%) with PTLD are positive for Epstein-Barr virus.[36] ARL is the major cause of parenchymal nodule (or nodules) in AIDS

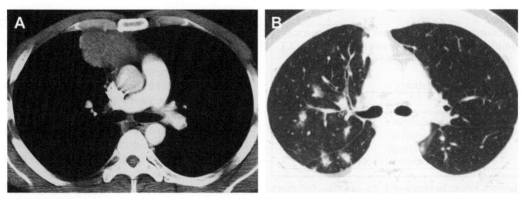

Fig. 7. Hodgkin lymphoma (nodular sclerosing type) in a 35-year-old man. (*A*) Transverse mediastinal-window CT (7.0-mm section thickness) scan obtained at level of right upper lobar bronchus shows homogeneous right anterior mediastinal mass. (*B*) Transverse lung-window CT scan shows multiple pulmonary nodules in both lungs with ill-defined margin.

patients, which often coexisted with a pleural effusion or axillary lymphadenopathy.[43]

On CT, lymphomas in patients with PTLD and ARL commonly manifest as multiple bilateral nodules (**Fig. 13**) or occasionally as a single nodule or mass. The nodules tend to have well-defined margins and do not show evidence of cavitation. Rarely, the lymphomas appear as a diffuse disease with numerous small nodules and thickening of interstitium.

High-grade lymphomas show avid FDG uptake; therefore PET imaging is useful for staging high-grade lymphoma[35,44] and to monitor response to therapy.

THYMUS

Current staging and treatment methods consider the thymus as a nodal site, and thymic involvement

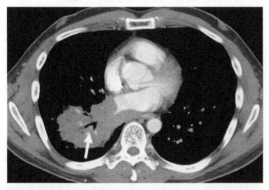

Fig. 8. Hodgkin lymphoma (nodular sclerosing type) in a 42-year-old man. Transverse mediastinal-window CT (5.0-mm section thickness) scan shows homogeneous soft-tissue mass in right lower lobe. Note air bronchograms (*arrow*) within tumor.

does not change the stage of the disease.[45] In adults, the thymus is regarded enlarged if it is greater than 15 mm in the largest diameter. The two morphologic criteria that suggest the presence of an enlarged thymus are a triangular configuration of the thymus or the presence of cyst(s) within it.[2,45,46] Although thymic enlargement is seen in 30% to 56% of patients with intrathoracic involvement at presentation in HL,[3,5] it is often impossible to differentiate the thymic enlargement from thymus infiltrated with tumor on the basis of CT appearance alone.

Post-therapeutic enlargement of the thymus may represent recurrent disease, thymic rebound (hyperplastic thymus), or development or persistence of thymic cysts.[3,45,46] The hyperplastic thymus is usually triangular, whereas the infiltrated thymus is quadrilateral with a lobulated border.[47] When thymic enlargement is present in adults, if the thymus was not the original site of disease or if there is no other evidence of disease relapse, it should be considered that this is due to hyperplasia rather than to tumor infiltration.[48,49]

Thymic cysts may occur in HL either at the initial presentation (21%–50%) or after treatment. Thymic cysts may persist or enlarge and this indicates neither residual or recurrent disease nor an increased risk of relapse.[45]

PLEURA, PERICARDIUM, AND HEART INVOLVEMENT

Pleural effusions are observed at presentation in approximately 10% of patients in HL[4,5] and eventually develop in approximately 30%, most often in association with other intrathoracic manifestations of the disease.[30] They are not of prognostic significance unless associated with

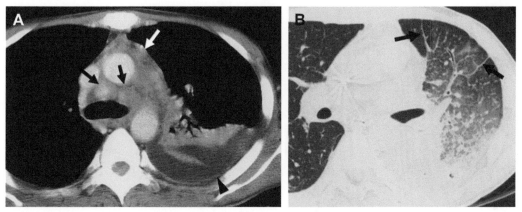

Fig. 9. Non-Hodgkin lymphoma (angioimmunoblastic type) in a 33-year-old man. (*A*) Transverse mediastinal-window CT (10-mm section thickness) scan obtained at level of azygos arch shows lymph node enlargement in anterior mediastinal and paratracheal areas (*arrows*). Also note left pleural effusion with pleural thickening (*arrowhead*). (*B*) Transverse lung-window CT scan demonstrates smooth interlobular septal thickening (*arrows*) with diffuse ground-glass opacity in left lung that represents lymphomatous infiltration with or without edema.

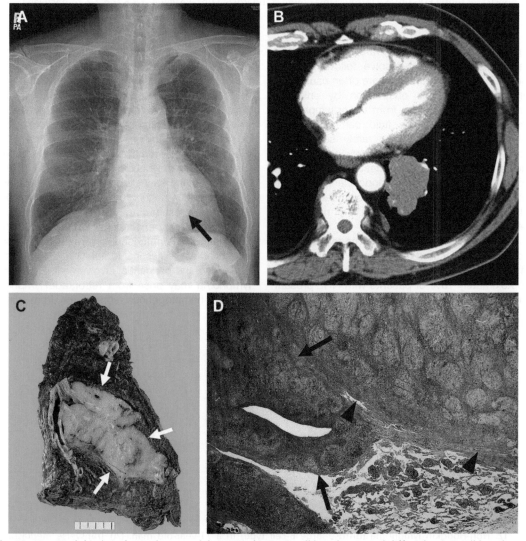

Fig. 10. Non-Hodgkin lymphoma (extranodal marginal zone B-cell lymphoma and diffuse large B-cell lymphoma) in a 72-year-old man. (*A*) Chest radiograph shows vertically oriented masslike lesion in left retrocardiac area (*arrow*). (*B*) Transverse mediastinal-window CT (1.0-mm section thickness) scan obtained at ventricular level shows a mass with homogeneous attenuation and lobulated contour in left lower lobe. (*C*) Gross pathologic specimen shows a gray tan and firm mass on left basal trunk and posterolateral basal segmental bronchus (*arrows*). (*D*) Low-magnification (hematoxylin-eosin stain, original magnification ×40) photomicrograph discloses monocytoid B-cell lymphocytic infiltration involving airways (*arrows*) and lung parenchyma (*arrowheads*).

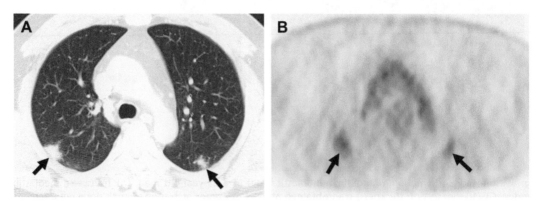

Fig. 11. Marginal zone B-cell lymphoma of bronchus-associated lymphoid tissue in a 47-year-old man. (*A*) Transverse lung-window CT (5.0-mm section thickness) scan shows two subpleural nodules (*arrows*) with poorly defined margin in right upper lobe and superior segment of left lower lobe. (*B*) Transverse PET scan obtained at similar level to *A* demonstrates subtle FDG uptake (*arrows*) (maximum standardized uptake value = 2.6 and 2.2, respectively).

a pleural mass, because they rarely contain malignant cells and usually resolve following treatment.[2,3,5,33] Pleural effusions are often caused by lymphatic or venous obstruction by enlarged lymph nodes rather than from direct lymphomatous involvement.[50] The fluid can be serous, chylous, pseudochylous, or rarely serosanguinous.[51] However, NHL may rarely present with pleural effusion as a sole manifestation, most often occurs in the setting of immunodeficiency (primary effusion lymphoma, [PEL]; approximately 3% of AIDS-related lymphomas and <1% of non–AIDS-related lymphomas).[52]

Pleural involvement by lymphoma may occur in both HL and NHL and represents a manifestation of systemic disease.[2,53–56] According to a report, approximately 16% of patients with NHL present with, or subsequently develop, pleural involvement

during the course of the disease.[57] They may manifest as a solitary nodule or multiple, broad-based pleural mass, or a combination of the two, and usually are associated with pleural effusion (**Fig. 14**). It is important to recognize the pleural involvement (which is frequently overlooked on conventional imaging), because that finding of pleural involvement may significantly affect patient management and because unrecognized pleural involvement increases the risk of treatment failure.

Pericardial effusion, by contrast with pleural effusion, is presumed to represent lymphomatous invasion of the pericardium. It may arise from lymphatic or hematogenous spread or by direct extension of mediastinal tumor.[49]

Cardiac and pericardial involvement (**Fig. 15**) of lymphoma may arise from retrograde lymphatic spread, hematogenous spread, or from direct

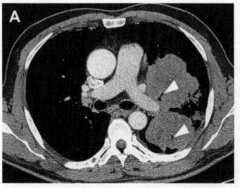
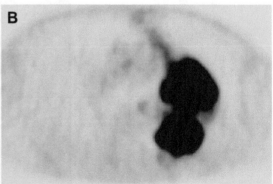

Fig. 12. Non-Hodgkin lymphoma (diffuse large B-cell type) in a 71-year-old man. (*A*) Transverse mediastinal-window CT (2.5-mm section thickness) scan obtained at subcarinal level shows large masslike consolidative lesions in left upper lobe and left lower lobe. Note these masses have internal air bronchograms (*arrowheads*). (*B*) Transverse PET scan obtained at similar level to *A* demonstrates high FDG uptake (maximum standardized uptake values = 20.5 in both lesions) within masses.

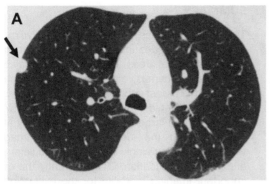
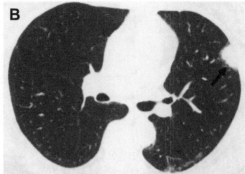

Fig. 13. AIDS-related (large B-cell type) lymphoma in a 56-year-old woman. Transverse lung-window CT (5.0-mm section thickness) scans obtained at levels of azygos arch (*A*) and bronchus intermedius (*B*), respectively, show two subpleural nodules (*arrows*), one each in right upper lobe and left upper lobe, with well-defined margins.

extension of mediastinal lymphadenopathy. According to a report,[58] the prevalence of cardiac and pericardial involvement by malignant lymphoma (both HL and NHL) at autopsy is estimated at 8.7%.

The incidence of pneumothorax is increased in patients who have HL. In one study of 1977 patients who had the lymphoma, the complication was 10 times higher than expected, most patients being younger than 30 years of age.[59] Treatment with radiotherapy, lung involvement, radiation fibrosis, and infection appear to be risk factors.

CHEST WALL AND THORACIC SKELETAL INVOLVEMENT

Chest wall involvement occurs in about 6.4% of cases in HL[5] and may represent an initial

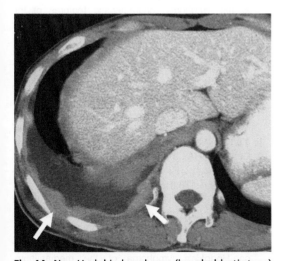

Fig. 14. Non-Hodgkin lymphoma (lymphoblastic type) in a 24-year-old man. Transverse mediastinal-window CT (10.0-mm section thickness) scan obtained at level of liver dome shows pleural effusion and enhancing uneven pleural thickening in right hemithorax (*arrows*).

manifestation of the disease or a site of recurrence in HL (**Fig. 16**). Detection of chest wall invasion is of clinical relevance, because it is associated with higher relapse rates and requires more aggressive therapy.[2] Most patients with chest wall involvement have associated intrathoracic disease.[3,60] Parasternal and thoracic spine involvements are often secondary to extension of anterior (especially internal mammary chain) and posterior mediastinal lymphadenopathy, respectively.[2,3,61] Isolated chest wall masses are uncommon and are usually a manifestation of NHL, especially large B-cell lymphoma.

Approximately 5% to 20% of patients with HL manifest bone involvement during the course. But, the bone involvement is seen in only 1% to 4% at presentation.[33,62–64] The thoracic skeleton usually, but not invariably, is affected by direct extension of tumor from the mediastinum or lungs.

BREAST

Breast lymphoma accounts for approximately 0.15% of all malignant breast tumors.[65] Primary breast lymphoma accounts for only 0.1% to 0.5% of all breast tumors;[66] approximately 2.0% of extranodal lymphomas involve the breasts. Most breast lymphomas are B-cell lymphomas and rarely, T-cell or histiocytic lymphomas.[67,68] The diagnosis of primary breast lymphoma depends on the absence of systemic lymphoma (with the exception of ipsilateral axillary nodes) and no previous diagnosis of extramammary lymphoma. Regardless of histologic subtype, breast lymphomas manifest most frequently as a single, lobular or irregular mass with indistinct margin at mammography and a solid, hypervascular irregular mass with indistinct margin or an echogenic boundary at ultrasound.[69,70]

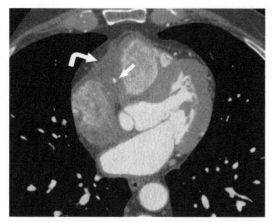

Fig. 15. Non-Hodgkin lymphoma (diffuse large B-cell type) in a 63-year-old woman. Transverse mediastinal window image of ECG-gated CT (2.5-mm section thickness) scan shows low-attenuation infiltrative mass lesion at right atrium/right heart border (*curved arrow*). Mass is indistinguishable from muscle and replaces epicardiac fat. There is encasement of right coronary artery (*arrow*) within lesion.

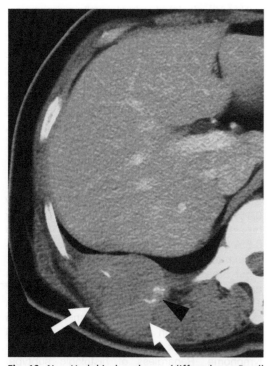

Fig. 16. Non-Hodgkin lymphoma (diffuse large B-cell type) in a 46-year-old woman. Transverse medias-tinal-window CT (7.0-mm section thickness) scan shows well-defined solid mass in right posterior chest wall (*arrows*). Also note rib destruction (*arrowhead*).

SUMMARY

Thoracic lymphomas most frequently involve medi-astinal lymph nodes in the anterior mediastinum and paratracheal areas. The lymphomas may also involve lung, thymus, pleura, pericardium, chest wall, and the breast and their radiologic manifesta-tions are diverse. Lymphomas (mostly BALT lymphoma and large B-cell lymphoma) may arise primarily from the lung with various imaging features including single or multiple nodule(s) and area(s) of consolidation. CT is currently the most important imaging modality for the evaluation of thoracic lymphoma but FDG PET also plays a crucial role in the clinical management of these cases.

REFERENCES

1. Sharma A, Fidias P, Hayman LA, et al. Patterns of lymphadenopathy in thoracic malignancies. Radio-graphics 2004;24:419–34.
2. Guermazi A, Brice P, de Kerviler EE, et al. Extrano-dal Hodgkin disease: spectrum of disease. Radio-graphics 2001;21:161–79.
3. North LB, Libshitz HI, Lorigan JG. Thoracic lymphoma. Radiol Clin North Am 1990;28:745–62.
4. Filly R, Bland N, Castellino RA. Radiographic distribu-tion of intrathoracic disease in previously untreated patients with Hodgkin's disease and non-Hodgkin's lymphoma. Radiology 1976;120:277–81.
5. Castellino RA, Blank N, Hoppe RT, et al. Hodgkin disease: contributions of chest CT in the initial staging evaluation. Radiology 1986;160:603–5.
6. Tateishi U, Müller NL, Johkoh T, et al. Primary medi-astinal lymphoma: characteristic features of the various histological subtypes on CT. J Comput Assist Tomogr 2004;28:782–9.
7. Hopper KD, Diehl LF, Cole BA, et al. The signifi-cance of necrotic mediastinal lymph nodes on CT in patients with newly diagnosed Hodgkin disease. AJR Am J Roentgenol 1990;155:267–70.
8. Castellino RA, Hilton S, O'Brien JP, et al. Non-Hodg-kin lymphoma: contribution of chest CT in the initial staging evaluation. Radiology 1996;199:129–32.
9. Castellino RA. The non-Hodgkin lymphomas: prac-tical concepts for the diagnostic radiologist. Radi-ology 1991;178:315–21.
10. Keller AR, Kaplan HS, Lukes RJ, et al. Correlation of histopathology with other prognostic indicators in Hodgkin's disease. Cancer 1968;22:487–99.
11. Levitt LJ, Aisenberg AC, Harris NL, et al. Primary non-Hodgkin's lymphoma of the mediastinum. Cancer 1982;50:2486–92.
12. Lazzarino M, Orlandi E, Paulli M, et al. Primary medi-astinal B-cell lymphoma with sclerosis: an aggres-sive tumor with distinctive clinical and pathologic features. J Clin Oncol 1993;11:2306–13.

13. Shaffer K, Smith D, Kirn D, et al. Primary mediastinal large-B-cell lymphoma: radiologic findings at presentation. AJR Am J Roentgenol 1996;167:425–30.

14. Thomas DA, Kantarjian HM. Lymphoblastic lymphoma. Hematol Oncol Clin North Am 2001;15:51–95.

15. Duwe BV, Sterman DH, Musani AI. Tumors of the mediastinum. Chest 2005;128:2893–909.

16. Wilson LD, Detterbeck FC, Yahalom J. Superior vena cava syndrome with malignant causes. N Engl J Med 2007;356:1862–9.

17. Fishman EK, Kuhlman JE, Jones RJ. CT of lymphoma: spectrum of disease. Radiographics 1991;11:647–69.

18. Brereton HD, Johnson RE. Calcification in mediastinal lymph nodes after radiation therapy of Hodgkin's disease. Radiology 1974;112:705–7.

19. Apter S, Avigdor A, Gayer G, et al. Calcification in lymphoma occurring before therapy: CT features and clinical correlation. AJR Am J Roentgenol 2002;178:935–8.

20. Podoloff DA, Macapinlac HA. PET and PET/CT in management of the lymphomas. Radiol Clin North Am 2007;45:689–96.

21. Bangerter M, Moog F, Buchmann I, et al. Whole-body 2-[18F]-fluoro-2-deoxy-D-glucose positron emission tomography (FDG-PET) for accurate staging of Hodgkin's disease. Ann Oncol 1998;9:1117–22.

22. Young CS, Young BL, Smith SM. Staging Hodgkin's disease with 18-FDG PET. Clin Positron Imaging 1998;1:161–4.

23. Foo SS, Mitchell PL, Berlangieri SU, et al. Positron emission tomography scanning in the assessment of patients with lymphoma. Intern Med J 2004;34:388–97.

24. Bar-Shalom R. Normal and abnormal patterns of 18F-fluorodeoxyglucose PET/CT in lymphoma. PET Clinics 2006;1:231–42.

25. Rademaker J. Hodgkin's and non-Hodgkin's lymphomas. Radiol Clin North Am 2007;45:69–83.

26. Surbone A, Longo DL, DeVita VT, et al. Residual abdominal masses in aggressive non-Hodgkin's lymphoma after combination chemotherapy: significance and management. J Clin Oncol 1998;6:1832–7.

27. Kostakoglu L, Coleman M, Leonard JP, et al. PET predicts prognosis after 1cycle of chemotherapy in aggressive lymphoma and Hodgkin's disease. J Nucl Med 2002;43:1018–27.

28. Brennan DD, Gleeson T, Coate LE, et al. A comparison of whole-body MRI and CT for the staging of lymphoma. AJR Am J Roentgenol 2005;185:711–6.

29. Radin AI. Primary pulmonary Hodgkin's disease. Cancer 1990;65:550–63.

30. Fisher AM, Kendall B, Van Leuven BD. Hodgkin's disease: a radiological survey. Clin Radiol 1962;13:115–27.

31. Diehl LF, Hopper KD, Giguere J, et al. The pattern of intrathoracic Hodgkin's disease assessed by computed tomography. J Clin Oncol 1991;9:438–43.

32. Mentzer SJ, Reilly JJ, Skarin AT, et al. Patterns of lung involvement by malignant lymphoma. Surgery 1993;113:507–14.

33. Sandrasegaran K, Robinson PJ, Selby P. Staging of lymphoma in adults. Clin Radiol 1994;49:149–61.

34. Lewis ER, Caskey CI, Fishman EK. Lymphoma of the lung: CT findings in 31 patients. AJR Am J Roentgenol 1991;156:711–4.

35. Even-Sapir E, Lievshitz G, Perry C, et al. Fluorine-18 fluorodeoxyglucose PET/CT patterns of extranodal involvement in patients with Non-Hodgkin lymphoma and Hodgkin's disease. Radiol Clin North Am 2007;45:697–709.

36. Lee KS, Kim Y, Primack SL. Imaging of pulmonary lymphomas. AJR Am J Roentgenol 1997;168:339–45.

37. Cordier JF, Chailleux E, Lauque D, et al. Primary pulmonary lymphomas. A clinical study of 70 cases in nonimmunocompromised patients. Chest 1993;103:201–8.

38. Bae YA, Lee KS, Han J, et al. Marginal zone B-cell lymphoma of bronchus-associated lymphoid tissue (BALT): imaging findings in 21 patients. Chest 2008;133:433–40.

39. Close PM, Macrae MB, Hammond JM, et al. Anaplastic large-cell Ki-1 lymphoma: pulmonary presentation mimicking military tuberculosis. Am J Clin Pathol 1993;99:631–6.

40. Cheng AL, Su IJ, Chen YC, et al. Characteristic clinicopathologic features of Epstein-Barr virus-associated peripheral T-cell lymphoma. Cancer 1993;72:909–16.

41. Harrison NK, Twelves C, Addis JB, et al. Peripheral T-cell lymphoma presenting with angioedema and diffuse pulmonary infiltrates. Am Rev Respir Dis 1988;138:976–80.

42. Koss MN. Pulmonary lymphoid disorders. Semin Diagn Pathol 1995;12:158–71.

43. Sider L, Gabriel H, Curry DR, et al. Pattern recognition of the pulmonary manifestations of AIDS on CT scans. Radiographics 1993;13:771–84.

44. Marom EM, McAdams HP, Butnor KJ, et al. Positron emission tomography with fluoro-2-deoxy-D-glucose (FDG-PET) in the staging of posttransplant lymphoproliferative disorder in lung transplant recipients. J Comput Assist Tomogr 2004;19:74–8.

45. Wernecke K, Vassallo P, Rutsch F, et al. Thymic involvement in Hodgkin disease: CT and sonographic findings. Radiology 1991;181:375–83.

46. Heron CW, Husband JE, Williams MP. Hodgkin disease: CT of the thymus. Radiology 1988;167:647–51.

47. Luker GD, Siegel MJ. Mediastinal Hodgkin disease in children: response to therapy. Radiology 1993;189:737–40.

48. Kissin CM, Husband JE, Nicholas D, et al. Benign thymic enlargement in adults after chemotherapy: CT demonstration. Radiology 1987;163:67–70.

49. Fletcher BD, Xiong X, Kauffman WM, et al. Hodgkin disease: use of Tl-201 to monitor mediastinal involvement after treatment. Radiology 1998;209:471–5.

50. Rademaker J. Diagnostic imaging modalities for assessment of lymphoma with special emphasis on CT, MRI, and ultrasound. PET Clinics 2006;1:219–30.

51. Strickland B. Intra-thoracic Hodgkin's disease. Part II. Peripheral manifestations of Hodgkin's disease in the chest. Br J Radiol 1967;40:930–8.

52. Pileri SA, Leoncini L, Falini B. Revised European-American lymphoma classification. Curr Opin Oncol 1995;7:401–7.

53. Schmutz GR, Fisch-Ponsot C, Regent D, et al. Computed tomography (CT) and magnetic resonance imaging (MRI) of pleural masses. Crit Rev Diagn Imaging 1993;34:309–83.

54. Manoharan A, Pitney WR, Schonell ME, et al. Intra-thoracic manifestations in non-Hodgkin's lymphoma. Thorax 1979;34:29–32.

55. Berkman N, Breuer R, Kramer MR, et al. Pulmonary involvement in lymphoma. Leuk Lymphoma 1996; 20:229–37.

56. Vega F, Padula A, Valbuena JR, et al. Lymphomas involving the pleura: a clinicopathologic study of 34 cases diagnosed by pleural biopsy. Arch Pathol Lab Med 2006;130:1497–502.

57. Das DK, Gupta SK, Ayyagari S, et al. Pleural effusions in non-Hodgkin's lymphoma. A cytomorphologic, cytochemical and immunologic study. Acta Cytol 1987;31:119–24.

58. McDonnell PJ, Mann RB, Bulkley BH. Involvement of the heart by malignant lymphoma: a clinicopathologic study. Cancer 1982;49:944–51.

59. Yellin A, Benfield JR. Pneumothorax associated with lymphoma. Am Rev Respir Dis 1986;134:590–2.

60. Carlsen SE, Bergin CJ, Hoppe RT. MR imaging to detect chest wall and pleural involvement in patients with lymphoma: effect on radiation therapy planning. AJR Am J Roentgenol 1993;160:1191–5.

61. Cho CS, Blank N, Castellino RA. Computerized tomography evaluation of chest wall involvement in lymphoma. Cancer 1985;55:1892–4.

62. Gaudin P, Juvin R, Rozand Y, et al. Skeletal involvement as the initial disease manifestation in Hodgkin's disease: a review of 6 cases. J Rheumatol 1992;19: 146–52.

63. Edeiken-Monroe B, Edeiken J, Kim EE. Radiologic concepts of lymphoma of bone. Radiol Clin North Am 1990;28:841–64.

64. Sullivan WT, Solonick DM. Case report 414: nodular sclerosing Hodgkin disease involving sternum and chest wall. Skeletal Radiol 1987;16:166–9.

65. Rosen PP. Lymphoid and hematopoietic tumors. In: Rosen PP, editor. Rosen's breast pathology. Philadelphia: Lippincott-Raven; 1997. p. 757–78.

66. Giardini R, Piccolo C, Rilke F. Primary non-Hodgkin's lymphomas of the female breast. Cancer 1992;69: 725–35.

67. Arber DA, Simpson JF, Weiss LM, et al. Non-Hodgkin's lymphoma involving the breast. Am J Surg Pathol 1994;18:288–95.

68. Jeon HJ, Akagi T, Hoshida Y, et al. Primary non-Hodgkin malignant lymphoma of the breast. An immunohistochemical study of seven patients and literature review of 152 patients with breast lymphoma in Japan. Cancer 1992;70:2451–9.

69. Liberman L, Giess CS, Dershaw DD, et al. Non-Hodgkin lymphoma of the breast: imaging characteristics and correlation with histopathologic findings. Radiology 1994;192:157–60.

70. Yang WT, Lane DL, Le-Petross HT, et al. Breast lymphoma: imaging findings of 32 tumors in 27 patients. Radiology 2007;245:692–702.

Index

Moving?

Make sure your subscription moves with you!

To notify us of your new address, find your **Clinics Account Number** (located on your mailing label above your name), and contact customer service at:

Email: journalscustomerservice-usa@elsevier.com

800-654-2452 (subscribers in the U.S. & Canada)
314-447-8871 (subscribers outside of the U.S. & Canada)

Fax number: 314-447-8029

Elsevier Health Sciences Division
Subscription Customer Service
3251 Riverport Lane
Maryland Heights, MO 63043

*To ensure uninterrupted delivery of your subscription, please notify us at least 4 weeks in advance of move.

Printed and bound by CPI Group (UK) Ltd, Croydon, CR0 4YY

12/10/2024

01773394-0002